£35.

The Public–Private Mix for Health

Plus ça change, plus c'est la même chose?

Edite

Alan

Forev

John

Secretai

The Nu

D1421605

The N

FOR RESE

STUDIES I

Radcliffe Publishing

Oxford • Seattle

Radcliffe Publishing Ltd
18 Marcham Road
Abingdon
Oxon OX14 1AA
United Kingdom

www.radcliffe-oxford.com
Electronic catalogue and worldwide online ordering facility.

British Library Cataloguing in Publication Data

A catalogue record for this book is available from the British Library.

ISBN 1 85775 701 7

Typeset by Anne Joshua & Associates, Oxford
Printed and bound by TJ International Ltd, Padstow, Cornwall

Contents

Foreword   v

Preface   vi

List of contributors   vii

The Nuffield Trust   x

1 International healthcare reform: what goes around, comes around
Alan Maynard   1

2 The pervasive role of ideology in the optimisation of the public–private mix in public healthcare systems
Alan Williams   7

3 Efficient purchasing in public and private healthcare systems: mission impossible?
Cam Donaldson, Karen Gerard and Craig Mitton   21

4 The public–private mix in the UK
Rudolf Klein   43

5 UK healthcare reform: continuity and change
Alan Maynard   63

6 The mix of public and private payers in the US health system
Uwe Reinhardt   83

7 Political wolves and economic sheep: the sustainability of public health insurance in Canada
Bob Evans with Marko Vujicic   117

8 Public–private mix for health in France
Lise Rochaix and L Hartmann   141

9 The public–private mix in Scandinavia
Kjeld Møller Pedersen   161

10 Public–private mix for healthcare in Germany
Martin Pfaff and Axel Olaf Kern   191

11 The public–private mix in health services in New Zealand
Nicholas Mays and Nancy Devlin   219

12 The role of the private sector in the Australian healthcare
system
Jane Hall and Elizabeth Savage 247

13 Common challenges in healthcare markets
Alan Maynard 279

14 Enduring problems in healthcare delivery
Alan Maynard 293

Index 311

Foreword

In 1982 my predecessors Gordon McLachlan and Alan Maynard edited a mile-stone book – *The Public–Private Mix for Health: the relevance and effects of change* – on the mixed health economy at a time when the concept in the UK was a challenge to the accepted structure and financing of healthcare. Attitudes and practices have no doubt changed in the last 23 years and will continue to do so. In 2001 and 2003, the Trust, with the Australian government, organised two bilateral conferences on sustainable financing and quality in healthcare, and these forums reinforced the view of the change at the macro-economic level, of the importance of strong overall government stewardship and of the acceptance of the limits to public expenditure.

The contributors to this second, equally important, volume describe the public–private mix in health in the US, Canada, France, Scandinavia, Germany, New Zealand and Australia. They show both the universality of the problems facing healthcare provision in the UK and abroad and some of the different routes to the best and most equitable service. Alan Maynard brings out the historical, inter-national and practical lessons that can be learnt for UK policy.

This book is an important contribution to the debate and sits alongside the Policy Futures programme of work of The Nuffield Trust, which this year will publish its second report on future trends in healthcare, highlighting the challenges of 'Who Cares?', 'The Shape of the System' and 'Who Pays?'. The Trust warmly welcomes the publication of this book and the discussions that it will undoubtedly provoke.

John Wyn Owen CB
Secretary
The Nuffield Trust
January 2005

Preface

Over the 30 years I have worked in York, I have benefited enormously from the friendship and intellectual stimulation of numerous colleagues, including Alan Williams, Karen Bloor, Tony Culyer, Mike Drummond, Diane Dawson, Hugh Gravelle, Trevor Sheldon, Peter Smith and Andrew Jones. Outside York, colleagues in Aberdeen, the London School of Economics, the Centre for Health Economics Research and Evaluation at the University of Technology in Sydney and many others have knowingly, and sometimes unwittingly, educated and stimulated me! Particular mention is made of Elias Mossialos (LSE), Jane Hall and colleagues (Sydney), Steve Birch (McMaster, Canada), John Hutton (Medtap) and Nick Freemantle (Birmingham). To all these able and kind people, my sincere thanks for their support in times good and not so good.

I have been involved in NHS management for 20 years and since 1997, have been Chair of York Hospitals Trust. In these roles, I have learnt much about the difficult choices faced by practitioners and the challenges of NHS management. This has tempered (slightly!) my zeal to get them to 'be reasonable and do it my way'. Thanks to them all for tolerance of my emphasis on evidence and management by measurement. I hope these experiences have been salutary for us all!

I would like to acknowledge the Trojan efforts of Anne Burton and Karen Bloor, who have revised drafts, pursued references and brought this enterprise to a conclusion.

Finally, I would like to acknowledge the stimulus and support offered to me by Gordon McLachlan. It was with him that I edited the first Nuffield volume on *The Public–Private Mix for Health* in 1982. His combination of insight, rigour and mischief inspired me to believe that health policy might yet be 'confused' by facts rather than non-evidence based opinion and unsubstantiated beliefs.

Alan Maynard
University of York
January 2005

List of contributors

Nancy Devlin
Professor of Economics
City Health Economics Centre
Department of Economics
City University, London, UK
formerly
Associate Professor in Economics
Department of Economics
University of Otago, New Zealand

Cam Donaldson
Health Foundation Chair in Health Economics and Public Service Fellow in the
    ESRC/EPSRC Advanced Institute of Management Research (AIM)
Centre for Health Services Research
School of Population and Health Sciences and Business School (Economics)
University of Newcastle upon Tyne, UK

Bob Evans
Professor of Economics
Centre for Health Services and Policy Research
University of British Columbia, Canada

Karen Gerard
Senior Lecturer
Health Care Research Unit
Faculty of Medicine, Health and Life Sciences
University of Southampton, UK
and
Senior Visiting Fellow
Health Economics Research Centre
Institute of Health Sciences
University of Oxford, UK

Jane Hall
Professor of Health Economics
Centre for Health Economics Research and Evaluation
University of Technology, Sydney, Australia

L Hartmann
Service d'épidemiologie et santé publique
CHRU
Lille, France

Axel Olaf Kern
Research Associate
Institute for Economics
University of Augsburg, Germany

Rudolf Klein
Visiting Professor
London School of Economics, UK
and
Emeritus Professor
University of Bath, UK

Alan Maynard
Professor of Health Economics
York Health Policy Group
Department of Health Sciences
University of York, UK

Nicholas Mays
Professor of Health Policy
London School of Hygiene and Tropical Medicine
University of London, UK
and
Principal Advisor
Social Policy Branch
The Treasury, New Zealand

Craig Mitton
Research Scientist
Centre for Healthcare Innovation and Improvement
British Columbia Research Institute for Children's and Women's Health
and
Assistant Professor
Department of Health Care and Epidemiology
University of British Columbia, Canada

Kjeld Møller Pedersen
Professor of Economics
University of Southern Denmark

Martin Pfaff
Professor of Economics
Institute for Economics
University of Augsburg, Germany

Uwe Reinhardt
Professor of Political Economy
Princeton University, USA

Lise Rochaix
Professor
Groupe de Récherches en Economie Quantitative d'Aix-Marseille et Institut d'Economie Publique
Marseille, France

Elizabeth Savage
Senior Lecturer
Centre for Health Economics Research and Evaluation
University of Technology, Sydney, Australia

Marko Vujicic
World Health Organization and World Bank

Alan Williams
Professor of Economics
Centre for Health Economics
University of York, UK

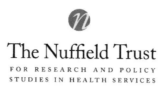

The Nuffield Trust

FOR RESEARCH AND POLICY
STUDIES IN HEALTH SERVICES

The Nuffield Trust is one of the leading independent health policy charitable trusts in the UK. It was established as the Nuffield Provincial Hospitals Trust in 1940 by Viscount Nuffield (William Morris), the founder of Morris Motors. In 1998 the Trustees agreed that the official name of the trust should more fully reflect the Trust's purposes and, in consultation with the Charity Commission, adopted the name The Nuffield Trust for Research and Policy Studies in Health Services, retaining 'The Nuffield Trust' as its working name.

The Nuffield Trust's mission is to promote independent analysis and informed debate on UK healthcare policy. The Nuffield Trust's purpose is to communicate evidence and encourage an exchange around developed or developing knowledge in order to illuminate recognised and emerging issues.

It achieves this through its principal activities:

- Bringing together a wide national and international network of people involved in UK healthcare through a series of meetings, workshops and seminars.
- Commissioning research through its publications and grants programme to inform policy debate.
- Encouraging interdisciplinary exchange between clinicians, leglislators, academics, healthcare professionals and management, policy makers, industrialists and consumer groups.
- Supporting evidence-based health policy and practice.
- Sharing its knowledge in the home countries and internationally through partnerships and alliances.

To find out more please refer to our website or contact:

The Nuffield Trust
59 New Cavendish St
London
W1G 7LP
Website: www.nuffieldtrust.org.uk
Email: mail@nuffieldtrust.org.uk
Tel: +44 (0)20 7631 8458
Fax: +44 (0)20 7631 8451

Charity number: 209201

Chapter 1

International healthcare reform: what goes around, comes around

Alan Maynard

Introduction

This book, written over 20 years after the publication of a similar collection of essays,[1] examines again the complexities, frustrations and progress of healthcare systems in a leading group of rich countries. Like its predecessor, it offers few panaceas, but the insights of its authors show that the political and economic challenges of healthcare reform are now better articulated, if still often largely unmet. The resilience of some of the obstacles to efficient reform articulated over 20 years ago and examined again here demonstrates the power of public and private interest groups in resisting changes that will benefit the patient. The ongoing battle between funders, providers and consumers is the business of healthcare, like many other markets. The characteristic of healthcare, however, is its resistance to change and the preservation of inefficient practices by management techniques appropriate for Dickensian times.

Despite differences in culture, history and resourcing, the nature and performance of healthcare systems worldwide are very similar. Political debates about healthcare reform are dominated by covert ideological arguments, and the policies these debates produce are generally ill-focused in terms of resolving well-evidenced common performance and incentive problems. As a consequence, the political necessity is created for the next often-irrelevant 'redisorganisation' of structures, epitomised nicely in the behaviour of successive Dutch and British governments, both having adopted, abandoned and readopted reforms in the past 15 years. Such changes usually fail to define the causes of inefficiencies in performance and pay scant attention to how better systems of incentives can be implemented to remedy performance problems. A common international belief is that performance deficiencies can be remedied by spending more and changing delivery structures. The evidence base demonstrates the futility of such a belief.

Healthcare continues to be characterised by sometimes well-evidenced deficiencies that are not the primary focus of reformers. There are well-chronicled deficiencies in healthcare delivery, in particular well-evidenced, unexplained and unmanaged variations in clinical practice,[2,3] the failure to deliver evidence-based and appropriate healthcare to manage major killers such as hypertension, diabetes and asthma,[4] the prevalence of medical errors[5] which kill thousands of patients and create avoidable morbidity for many more, and the absence of health-related quality-of-life measures of the success of healthcare in improving the functioning of patients.[6]

Often these manifestations of inefficiency in the delivery of healthcare are either ignored or not central to the practices of policy makers. When they are explicitly discussed, they are often submerged in medical capture, e.g. Thatcher's attempts to create a medical audit system in 1989 failed, and those of Blair risk the same fate. As Starr remarked 20 years ago, 'The dream of reason did not take power into account'.[7]

As it was then, so it is now. Apparent and real inefficiencies are regularly 'rediscovered' in healthcare funding and provision, and ambitious programmes of reform or social experimentation are engineered by well-meaning bureaucrats in the public and private sectors. Often these reformers readopt the policies of the past in the hope that the changes they create will, at worst, create diversion from criticism, and at best marginally improve the performance of the healthcare system. Often the diversion effects are short-lived and performance improvements transitory as powerful provider groups subvert reform and game the new system to their own advantage.

The international experience

The inclination of policy makers worldwide to 'make smoke' with ill-designed reforms that divert attention from the fundamental failures in the delivery of public and private healthcare can be seen in the experiences of all countries in the chapters that follow. However, the three initial chapters address issues of common interest.

The ideological nature of the policy discourse in health and healthcare is shrewdly examined by Alan Williams. This discourse, both ubiquitous and covert, succeeds in diverting much intellectual and research effort into unproductive cul-de-sacs, but its dominance should not be ignored. Policy making in healthcare is not a value-free activity!

Cam Donaldson, Karen Gerard and Craig Mitton evaluate the lessons that can be learnt from the policy emphasis on purchasing, evident in the UK reform and managed care in the US. They provide a clear illustration of the poor quantity and quality of the evidence, often drowned by opinion, and argue that the task of developing efficient purchasing is certainly a longer-term enterprise – indeed, it may be 'mission impossible'.

Rudolf Klein studies the politics of the public–private mix for health in the UK, arguing for the uncertainty of the future nature of this mix. This uncertainty is, in part, a product of the Blair Government's rush for change, particularly in reducing waiting times. In order to meet their goal, they have provided public funding for marginal increases in private provision to create additional capacity and catalyse a hoped-for change in NHS efficiency. The owners of this capacity have an equity stake in future NHS funding, which may be of significant political importance.

The past 15 years of the UK NHS are examined in Chapter 5. The Thatcher reforms were bold in design and modest in effect, as politicians belatedly recognised that an efficient national market might lose them votes and destabilise the system. Initially, the reform was palliated by increased growth in expenditure and then by declining political interest in competition as an engine of creating dissonance and change. Initially, the Blair Government maintained relative funding stability and parsimony, and adopted an anti-market rhetoric. Subsequently, it has increased NHS funding at unparalleled rates and gradually shifted its stance on competition, adopting measures that are potentially more radical than those of Thatcher. Spending has been accompanied by a plethora of structural reforms and target setting, which consumed much of the limited managerial capacity of the system. Consequently, many fundamental deficiencies in the NHS remain unresolved and, because of capacity restraints in the short term, much of the new funding has been absorbed by price increases (e.g. doctors' pay) with modest impact on the levels of NHS activity and the quality of care. Frustration with the pace of change has led to policies that have challenged NHS provision monopolies by enhancing the role of private providers.

Uwe Reinhardt provides a comprehensive and insightful analysis of the healthcare system, public and private, in the US. In 2003, over 15% of the US GDP was spent on healthcare and prices continue to rise at 8%. The US system is capable of providing some of the best healthcare in the world, but continues to exhibit profound inefficiency and inequity. While the Democrats continue to contemplate national health insurance, the Bush Administration has adopted 'patch-up' policies, such as an expensive system of pharmaceutical benefits for the elderly under Medicare, appearing more focused on vote acquisition than the efficient and equitable improvement of access and quality of care.

The affordability of public healthcare in the Canadian context is the issue addressed by Bob Evans – an issue pertinent to all healthcare systems with a large public sector. Evans demonstrates that although the wolves are at the door of the Canadian public system, it is remarkably robust, but in danger of fundamental damage by flirtation with private options. He concludes that the sustainability of Canadian Medicare is a moral issue, 'defining the mutual obligations of the members of the community'.

France's healthcare system is in severe crisis, as illustrated by Lise Rochaix and L Hartmann in Chapter 8. Although the hospital system is constrained by budget limits, the primary or ambulatory sector is replete with perverse incentives, e.g. free choice of doctors and open-ended pharmaceutical budgets. The previous socialist government introduced substantial tax finance on the UK NHS model and the current conservative regime is seeking to reduce demand with co-payments and restriction of benefits.

In Scandinavia (Denmark, Sweden, Norway and Finland), healthcare is publicly financed and generally publicly provided. Kjeld Pedersen's analysis shows that private insurance and provision are making only minor inroads in these fundamentally unchanging systems. He notes that in three of the four Scandinavian countries, the share of the GDP spent on health has been reduced, and that public dissatisfaction with the service has increased. One of the causes for complaint is the length of waiting times, which Scandinavia, in common with others, has managed with marginal increases in private provision while maintaining public systems.

Like the French system, German healthcare faces considerable cost pressures. The Dutch may lament having to wait four weeks for treatment and the British and the Danes have a target of six months, while the Germans have practically immediate access to treatment because of overprovision of hospital capacity and ambulatory care. The Schroeder Government, faced with costs of reunification, the need to reflate the economy and the cost of the public sector, finds itself in breach of European Union budget deficit limits. 2004 has seen the introduction of patient co-payments and the Government is seeking to use incentives to improve efficiency, e.g. the progressive introduction of diagnostic related group tariffs to reduce the length of hospital stays. Such policies inevitably have an effect on employment and the voting intentions of a healthcare labour force in excess of three million are a powerful constraint on efficient adjustment.

In the Antipodes, Australia and New Zealand are reforming in opposite ways. The creation of a market mechanism and the purchaser–provider split in New Zealand produced both little evaluation and few observable benefits, despite the competing polemics of the National and Labour Parties. In 1999, the new Labour Government abandoned the purchaser–provider split and returned to a structure very similar to the one in place before the National Government market reforms. The principal policy challenges for government remain the existence of waiting times for elective hospital care and price barriers to utilisation in primary care, which the present Government plans to remove over time.

In contrast to New Zealand, the Australian government is determined to reduce the size of its public system – Medicare. Jane Hall and Elizabeth Savage show how a combination of subsidies and taxes has induced more Australians to acquire some level of private health insurance. They note that the opportunity cost of this policy ($A 2.5 billion) could have produced more healthcare if used in the public sector. These subsidies have affected the balance of public–private hospital funding and have been accompanied by price controls for general practitioners, which has led them to increase patient payments. Such radical attempts to privatise the universal Medicare system need careful evaluation. However, they have also shifted attention from the problems of the public sector and this will be a nice challenge for the Australian government after the 2004 election.

The final chapters seek to bring together the lessons from these diverse but often similar experiences. The nature of healthcare markets worldwide is very similar. These market characteristics require sophisticated and careful regulation. The problems of the monopoly power of professions and commercial entities such as the pharmaceutical industry, the uneven or asymmetrical distribution of knowledge and power between consumers and providers, the absence of price barriers to consumption and equity goals make the pursuit of social goals such as efficiency and equity difficult and complex.

Despite the worldwide efforts of healthcare reformers, common problems remain, of which perhaps the most significant are variations in clinical practice and the absence of measures of success (i.e. improvements in the health of the population). Lack of reform in these areas is the product of a failure to define and rank policy goals and incentivise change based on scientific evidence rather than the opinion of 'experts'. While there may be some progress in addressing problems of efficiency common to public and private healthcare systems, there will continue to be disagreement over the distribution of the burden of funding healthcare and the rules determining patient access to care.

Choices in the financing and provision of healthcare are determined by ethics and ideology. Thankfully, the dominant ethic in most countries continues to be that of mutual obligation to ensure universal access to medical care for our fellow citizens. This basic ethic of a civilised society continues to be challenged but, in healthcare as in other matters, united we stand, divided we fall!

References

1   McLachlan G, Maynard A (eds) (1982) *The Public–Private Mix for Health: the relevance and effects of change*. London: Nuffield Provincial Hospitals Trust.

2   Fisher ES, Wennberg DE, Stukel TA, Gottlieb DJ, Lucas FL, Pinder EL (2003) The implications of regional variations in medicare spending. Part 1: The content, quality, and accessibility of care. *Ann Intern Med.* 138: 273–87.

3   Fisher ES, Wennberg DE, Stukel TA, Gottlieb DJ, Lucas FL, Pinder EL (2003) The implications of regional variations in medicare spending. Part 2: Health outcomes and satisfaction with care. *Ann Intern Med.* 138: 288–98.

4   Rand Corporation. The First National Report Card on Quality of Health Care in America. [Online] [access 2004 May]. Available from URL www.rand.org/publications

5   Kohn L, Corrigan J, Donaldson M (eds) (1999) *To Err Is Human: building a safer health system*. Washington, DC: National Academy Press.

6   Kind P, Williams A. Measuring success in healthcare – the time has come to do it properly. *Health Policy Matters* (9). Department of Health Sciences, University of York. [Online] [access 2004 May]. Available from URL www.york.ac.uk/healthsciences/pubs/hpmindex.htm

7   Starr P (1984) *Social Transformation of American Medicine*. New York: Basic Books.

Chapter 2

The pervasive role of ideology in the optimisation of the public–private mix in public healthcare systems

Alan Williams

Introduction

Ideology affects not only what we seek to achieve, but also how we judge reality. While the former influence is obvious, the latter is not. It comes about through the questions we ask, the way we formulate problems, the analytical methods we adopt and the evidence we seek. By deciding to tackle an issue in a particular way, even those who believe themselves to be ideologically neutral may find themselves unwittingly working within an implicit ideological stance. The problem of optimising the public–private mix in healthcare is particularly vulnerable to this danger, as I shall argue here.

Optimising the public–private mix can be addressed at two levels. At the macro level it concerns the relative sizes and roles of the public healthcare sector and the private healthcare sector when acting as alternative routes by which an individual can gain access to healthcare. In the simplest possible terms, this is typically a clash between individual access being determined by somebody else's judgements about 'need', and access being determined by an individual's own willingness and ability to pay (frequently mediated by private insurance arrangements). But in the present context, it is a lower (micro) level that is the main focus of attention. Again in the simplest terms, this focuses on whether it would be more efficient for the public sector to subcontract some of its activities to the private sector, while still setting its own broad priorities by individual need assessment rather than by individual willingness and ability to pay. The idea is that an 'internal market' is created in which the public sector becomes the purchaser on behalf of the individual, with the public purchaser simply choosing the most efficient provider (whether public or private) and offering that source of provision to the individual on the same terms as purely public provision would have been offered. The individual should, therefore, be indifferent between the two.

I would argue that this perception of the internal market as a value-neutral way of pursuing public sector objectives is an illusion, because the conventional way in which 'efficiency' is measured is not value-free. We do need to confront our own ideological positions openly and honestly, and seek to make explicit the ideological position upon which current healthcare policy is based, and adopt analytical methods appropriate to that ideological position. So instead of seeking to make economic analysis as value-neutral as possible, we should be seeking to make it as value-compatible as possible.

Ideology and analytical method

The first danger we need to recognise is the failure to realise that optimisation requires evaluation, and that *evaluation requires values*. Policy recommendations cannot emerge directly from a positive analysis – only from a normative analysis. The closest a positive analysis can get to being directly policy-relevant is a statement such as 'if you wish to maximise X, the most cost-effective way of doing so, in the circumstances assumed within this analysis, would be to do Y'. This does not imply that policy makers should actually *do* Y, even if their objective is to maximise X and even if the circumstances are those assumed in the analysis, because the costs of doing so may be too high. More fundamentally still, the circumstances assumed within the analysis may not be close enough to the real-world context in which policy is being formulated for the conclusion (that Y would be the best thing to do) to hold. Evaluation inevitably requires abstraction and simplification. A well-conducted, formal evaluation will make these abstractions and simplifications explicit. If they do not seem to be appropriate, a formal evaluation based on different assumptions should be sought. But rejecting a systematic formal evaluation and then replacing it with a more comfortable informal evaluation is extremely dangerous, because the absence of explicit simplifications and abstractions does not mean there aren't any, but simply that they are hidden. They may have been hidden deliberately, but it is also possible that the analysts themselves are not aware of them. So even a conditional statement of the type 'if . . . then . . .', supposedly based on a purely factual analysis, carries the danger that it is ideologically biased. In this case the ideological bias flows from the analyst's decisions about the assumptions that need to be made in order to make the analysis acceptable to policy makers. The assumed nature of the healthcare market is a classic example of such a quasi-factual (but also perhaps ideological) judgement concerning how a system works and therefore how it is to be modelled in a 'positive' analysis.[1 i]

The second danger surrounds the *choice of the appropriate statistical techniques* to be employed, which is frequently seen as a technical matter to be left to the experts. Policy decisions are always about populations, although they are then applied to individuals. So the key judgement that has to be made is whether we should treat a particular individual 'i' as a typical member of population 'x'. Two aspects of the conventional statistical wisdom are particularly noteworthy here. The first is the choice of 'significance' level by which we should judge whether an inevitably uncertain finding about population x is secure enough to act upon in the case of individual i. Conventionally, these significance levels are set at the 1% or 5% levels, meaning that a finding should only be acted on if there is a 99% or 95% chance (respectively) of it being correct. Given the uncertainties surrounding most policy decisions these tests are far too stringent, and in any case it is not for the analyst to determine what risks of error are worth taking in a particular policy context. It would be better if the risks were simply stated and the policy maker left to decide whether the resulting conclusions are robust enough to act upon. The second 'technical' judgement which has strong political implications is the choice of measure of central tendency when summarising data from a heterogeneous population. The conventional wisdom is that if the distribution of the data is 'normal' (i.e. bell-shaped when plotted on a graph) the arithmetic mean should be used, but when the distribution is skewed (i.e. is not symmetrical, but instead, when plotted on a graph, has a long tail on one side or the other) it is better to use the median. Some analysts prefer always to use the mean, because it enables more of the information about individuals to remain in play, and the relationship of the mean to various measures of dispersion is well known and handy to work with. But in a policy context, this choice between mean and median is a decision about how the data from different individuals shall count. The median gives no special weight to the individuals with extreme values, but the arithmetic mean does, so what is really at stake here is 'whose values count for what', which in a policy context is hardly a value-neutral decision.

This brings me to economic principles, and the third danger, which is *the belief that mainstream economics is value-free*. We owe the conventional analytical framework employed by economists in determining the 'efficiency' of any set of social arrangements to Pareto and the 'New' Welfare Economics. It was developed in order to circumvent two major restrictions on what was held to be acceptable in a proper scientific enterprise. The first was that there is no scientific way of measuring individual utility in a cardinal manner, and the second was that there is no scientific way in which interpersonal comparisons of welfare can be made. To overcome the first problem, only ordinal measurement is acceptable (i.e. statements can be made about which alternative is better or worse, but not about *how much* better or *how much* worse). To overcome the second problem, any judgements about better or worse are only acceptable from an individual who is referring solely to his or her own well-being. Within that restricted realm the rule to be adopted for one social situation to be judged to be better than another (i.e. 'Pareto-preferred'), is that at least one person must be better off and no one must be worse off (the 'no-loser constraint'). Both of these strict positions about acceptability have been diluted in practice, because there are hardly any real-life alternatives to the status quo that could be declared 'Pareto-preferred'. The main dilution has been to replace the 'no-loser constraint' with a compensation principle, namely, to calculate whether the money value of the gains to the gainers exceeds the money value of the losses to the losers. This would be a good way round the second restriction if such compensation were actually paid, but it isn't. And, because it is only hypothetical, we are left with the implicit judgement that whatever the resulting distribution of gains and losses is, it is socially acceptable and can be ignored. This excludes any policy interest there may be in trading off the maximisation of some good Y against improving the interpersonal distribution of Y. By declaring as 'efficient' (or cost-effective) a situation in which total gains exceed total losses (but in which the gainers do not actually compensate the losers), the analyst has accepted an ideological position which, even in its strict form, many people would not accept. The ideological position in question is that if one person is better off and no one is worse off, society is a better place, *irrespective of who the solitary gainer is*. If the solitary gainer is already the best-off person in that society, and everyone else is on the breadline, this may indeed not be a view shared by many. But this is only an extreme example of a more general concern that may be felt about the degree of inequality in a society. Such a concern may be a dominant one in a particular public policy setting. And it is certainly a major concern in a public healthcare system. Indeed it may be the very *raison d'être* for having such a system.

Rival ideologies

It is one thing to point out that no analysis can be entirely value-free, and another to argue that analysts are the unwitting agents of some particular ideological position. I do, however, think that many analysts are in that trap, so I now want to examine that danger in a little more detail, again with the optimising of the public–private mix in healthcare firmly in mind.

The two main ideological positions in this field are the libertarian and the egalitarian.[2,3 ii] In their polarised forms, the contrasts between them are set out in Table 2.1.

Table 2.1 Libertarian and egalitarian ideologies compared In their polarised forms

	Libertarians believe that	Egalitarians believe that
Basics	Freedom of choice is a good in itself	All members of society have equal rights to basic goods
	Individuals are the best judges of their own welfare	It is for the society to determine what these basic goods are
	Social welfare is no more than the sum of individuals' welfare	Social welfare depends on how these goods are distributed within the society
Achievement	Achievement must be rewarded	Lack of achievement must not be punished
Misfortune	Private charity is the proper way to show social concern	Collective mechanisms are needed if people are to be dealt with equitably
Freedom	Freedom is a supreme good in itself and should not be sacrificed lightly	Freedom is about real opportunities for choice, and these may need to be curtailed for some in order that they can be enlarged for others
Equality	Equality before the law is the key concept, with freedom dominating equality if ever they conflict	Equality of opportunity is the key concept. In its absence, compensation of the deprived becomes a moral obligation

It will be seen that the libertarian position is well-served by conventional economic analysis, which assumes that the consumer is sovereign, that individuals are the best judges of their own welfare, that social welfare is no more than the aggregate welfare of the individuals who comprise that society and that concerns about distributive justice can be neglected (to be taken up elsewhere, if at all). By contrast, the conventional economic analysis does not serve the egalitarian position at all well, and egalitarian concerns have somehow or other to be grafted onto this framework, where they appear as awkward accretions on an otherwise elegant and familiar intellectual structure. The ultimate insult is then to argue that any position other than the pure 'welfarist' position lacks a firm theoretical basis and is not proper economics. Attempts to measure well-being in cardinal terms are held to be unacceptable, the making of interpersonal comparisons of welfare is unacceptable, the inclusion of any items in a social welfare function other than the utilities of the individuals in that society is unacceptable, and venturing outside the realm of 'efficiency' is unacceptable, because only by working within the concept of 'efficiency' (it is said) are economists able to avoid ideological commitment!

Ideology and objectives

When it comes to specifying the objectives of a public healthcare system, non-welfarists may not have much in common with each other ideologically, apart from their rejection of the strict welfarist position.[3][iii] Similarly, within the non-welfarist fold, egalitarians may have little in common with each other apart from their desire to equalise *something*. It is well established that many different answers can and are given to the question 'Equality of what?' by those who claim to hold an egalitarian stance in matters of health and healthcare.[4–7][iv] My own personal egalitarian stance in the healthcare field targets people's lifetime experience of health, because I believe that this is fundamental to the opportunities people have to 'flourish' in any society. The adverse effects of a life that in health terms is nasty, brutish and short are so pervasive that any broad notion of social justice must give quality-adjusted life-expectancy a major role. All other targets for equalisation seem to me to be merely instrumental. But this is not a view shared by all. Indeed at the other extreme from my particular consequentialist stance are those who believe that if we have ensured equal opportunity for access to healthcare for those in like circumstances, we shall have discharged our ethical duty as far as social justice is concerned, and, whatever is the outcome of such a process in terms of the distribution of health in that community, it should be considered a just one.[6][v]

This difference of perspective is clearly of the utmost importance for the role of the public sector in health and healthcare. If you are a procedural or access-focused egalitarian, it is not necessary to discover the effects of publicly provided healthcare on people's lifetime experience of health. From that standpoint, if opportunities are equal, outcomes are unimportant. But if you are a consequentialist, the situation is reversed. From that standpoint, if in order to equalise lifetime experience of health some people would have to be denied access to publicly provided healthcare altogether, so be it!

Both these extreme positions need to be moderated by seeing the desire for greater equality (of something or other) not as the sole objective of publicly provided healthcare, but as one of its two principal objectives, the other being the maximisation of population health. In general, the desire to reduce inequality will entail some sacrifice in overall population health. If this were not so, the egalitarian objective would be redundant, and a single-minded policy of maximisation would deal with distributive justice coincidentally and costlessly. This will not normally be the case, so whatever kind of egalitarian you are, you will have to think about trade-offs between maximisation and inequality reduction.

Note, however, that within the non-welfarist world in which this discussion is being conducted, it is not individual utility (or patient satisfaction or even *public* satisfaction) that is being maximised or equalised, but health (or accessibility to healthcare) measured according to some standard set of socially determined values. One source of tension in the optimisation of public and private healthcare turns on this distinction, and it is focused on consumer 'choice'. The basic issue is whether consumer choice in healthcare is a good thing in itself (even if exercised unwisely) or whether it needs to be severely circumscribed at the individual level in the interests of other individuals. For instance, if the public healthcare system offers only such healthcare as meets some cost-effectiveness test, I think that although an individual has the right to refuse whatever treatment is on offer (provided that by so doing he or she does not constitute a danger to others), that individual does not have the right to demand something different from what is on offer. There may be occasions when there are appropriate alternatives that are both cost-effective, in which case choice should be offered. Where choice is costless, and where people want it, it should be offered. But choice will rarely be costless, so if it is held to be a good thing in its own right we have a third trade-off candidate to enter into the competition for resources.

One way of avoiding this would be to argue that the private healthcare system is the vehicle through which consumer choice operates, and that anyone who wants something different from what the public sector offers should go there instead. This is already what happens in the UK with respect to elective surgery, where people can 'choose' not to wait for the treatment which the public system will eventually offer free of charge, and instead pay directly or through private insurance for earlier treatment in the private sector. But this 'choice' is only available to those with the right kind of private health insurance or to those willing and able to pay directly. Even those who avail themselves of this facility would not necessarily argue that this recourse to the private sector is socially just from an egalitarian standpoint. They would be more likely to argue from a libertarian position that it is unduly oppressive to deny people the right to spend their legitimately earned money on healthcare if that is what they wish to do (and, by so doing, to free up public sector resources for use by those poorer than themselves). There is clearly a trade-off at societal level here between tolerating unequal access to health and healthcare, and offering people more choice.

Ideology and trade-offs

It is possible to see ideological conflicts in rather stark terms. Those who are not with us are against us! Are you a libertarian or an egalitarian? Indeed there are some theories of distributive justice which are cast in such terms. In economists' terms, they specify constraints, which have to be satisfied before a social situation can be declared morally acceptable.[7][vi] No compromise is permissible; it is an on-or-off, black-or-white matter. But even among philosophers such extremism is rare, and it is widely recognised that principles of distributive justice are inevitably contestable, and a relativistic position is the only one that is ultimately tenable.[8][vii] As I have noted elsewhere,[9][viii] this leads us into the following situation:

> *Ethical discourse is typically inconclusive. There are good reasons why this should be so. The premises on which it is based are usually contestable. There is usually more than one principle in play. No single principle 'trumps' all others. The situations that are selected for analysis are complex ones where the appropriate resolution of the ethical difficulties is not self-evident . . .*
>
> *Helping people to be clear in their own minds about the ethical implications of their actions is not a trivial pursuit, and in the context of publicly accountable decision-making it is especially important, since the principal actors are expected to be able to provide justification for their actions, and not to behave arbitrarily or capriciously. But it is not sufficient for them merely to list the various things they claim to have taken into account. The citizenry are entitled to know what weight they gave to each, so that they can see what it was that proved decisive. Otherwise, the same bland listing of relevant principles could provide justification for almost any decision.*

This is the main reason why economists prefer the 'trade-off' concept to be used in such a context. It requires the elicitation of some quantified rate at which people would sacrifice one thing that they want in order to get more of something else that they want. It is a more complicated notion than it seems at first sight, because it not only depends on your general strength of preference for the one good over the other, but also on how much of each you currently have. Generally speaking, the more scarce something is, the greater the value attached to it relatively to other things. This is just as true of distributive justice as a 'good' as it is to food and shelter as 'goods'.

Seen in this light, it will be evident that the world is not populated by single-minded people who are pure libertarians or pure egalitarians. There may be a few 'pure' fanatics of this kind, but most of us seem to be 'impure' pluralists, who simultaneously embrace several ideological principles knowing full well that they will sometimes clash with each other and place us in a moral quandary. Looking within myself, I can identify completely with the twin objectives of maximising population health and reducing inequalities in its distribution between individuals over their lifetime, but I am also willing to go along to a very small extent with the notion that a public healthcare system should offer people choices wherever it costs little to do so, and I feel most strongly that individuals have the right to make lots of decisions about themselves which the paternalistic attitudes of the majority of health professionals think they are incapable of making wisely. But the professionals are right in arguing that making people better informed, so that they are less likely to regret their own decisions later, is not a costless activity, and we need to think hard about whether 'patient empowerment' is being pursued because it is likely to help with the pursuit of the two main objectives of a public healthcare system, or whether it is being pursued because it is regarded as a good in itself.[10] In the latter case it enters the field as a third trade-off candidate.

Ideology and 'World Health 2000'

The problems involved in appraising alternative social situations using explicit quantitative weights (because many different objectives are in play simultaneously) was well illustrated by the World Health Organization's report on *World Health 2000* (henceforth WHR2000). In their case, the alternative social situations were the healthcare systems of different countries, but they could equally well have been one country's healthcare system before and after some reform (e.g. in which an internal market had been introduced into a public healthcare system). It is not my purpose here to comment on the league tables of national health system performance which emerged from their method, but to use their broad approach as a vehicle for illustrating the difficulties encountered in this sort of enterprise.

The authors of WHR2000 identify four broad objectives (and several sub-objectives) that are being pursued by healthcare systems, to each of which they attach a numerical weight, these weights summing to 100. These are set out in Table 2.2.

The weights were derived by asking people to divide a pie containing 100 segments between rival objectives, according to their assessment of each objective's importance.[11][ix] This was done in four stages. The first cut was between health, responsiveness and fairness in financing (yielding 50:25:25 in Table 2.2), the second was between health level and health distribution (yielding 50:50), the third was between responsiveness level and responsiveness inequality (yielding 50:50) and the final one was between respect for persons and client orientation within responsiveness level (also yielding 50:50). People were also asked to rank alternatives, and eventually, after a bit of smoothing, this neat final scheme emerged. Whether or not the right people were asked is for discussion elsewhere,[12][x] but what I want to question here is whether the people whose data generated these weights realised the implications of their judgements (and even whether the authors of WHR2000 did so). It would be especially important to explore the influence of people's ideological positions on these weights, because one of the advantages claimed for the approach adopted in WHR2000 was that 'recommendations should be based on evidence rather than ideology'.[13][xi] My argument here is that the evidence you collect and the way you interpret it is heavily influenced by ideology, and that this is inevitable. It is not a matter of replacing ideology with evidence, but a matter of being explicit about the ideological underpinnings of your analysis. The great advantage of the WHR2000 approach is not its ideological neutrality, but its explicitness, which makes it possible for an outside observer to tease out its implied ideological position. That is what I now propose to do.

Dividing a nominal budget of points between rival claimants should imply that if performance improved by some given proportion on one dimension but declined by a similar proportion in an equally weighted dimension, then overall performance should be unchanged. If the scores within the two dimensions were normalised, then a one-unit change on either dimension has the same policy weight. But if a dimension carries only one tenth of the weight of the two just mentioned, then it requires a tenfold change in its normalised score to carry equal weight to the one-unit change just mentioned. When performance scores on dimensions change from one situation to another, it is the weighting of these *marginal* differences that matters.

Table 2.2 The scoring system used in the *World Health Report 2000* for measuring overall attainment

Concept	Weight (%)	Definition
Health level	25	Disability-adjusted life expectancy (adjusted to a 0–1 scale for the range 20–80 DALYs)
Health distribution	25	Equality of child survival* (an index of expected child survival up to the age of 5)
Responsiveness level	12.5	A composite index of the items listed below
of which		
Respect for persons	(6.25)	
of which		
Dignity	2.08	Observation of basic human rights
Confidentiality	2.08	Privacy of consultation and records
Autonomy	2.08	Choice of treatment options
Client orientation	(6.25)	
of which		
Promptness	2.5	Accessibility and waiting times
Amenities	1.875	Cleanliness, food quality, etc
Support	1.25	From community and care agencies
Choice	0.625	Between providers at each level
Responsiveness distribution	12.5	Extent of differences in responsiveness by those population subgroups selected for each country individually by its own 'key informants'
Fair financing	25	'The way health is financed is perfectly fair if the ratio of total health contribution to total non-food spending is identical for all households, independently of their income, their health status or their use of the healthcare system'
Composite index	100	

*To be replaced by an index of the equality of disability-adjusted life expectancy across individuals when these data are available.

Let me offer a numerical example to drive home this important point. I will focus on the ideologically highly charged issue of freedom of choice, which, as we saw from Table 2.1, is a key difference between the Libertarian and Egalitarian positions. In Table 2.2 this is represented as 'autonomy' under 'respect for persons' (which in turn is classified under 'responsiveness'), and is a sub-objective to which a weight of approximately 2.08 out of 100 is assigned. So if some reform had been introduced, which brought about a ten-point improvement (out of 100) in the range of choice that people had when hospital inpatient treatment was under consideration, the attainment score for that system would rise by 0.208

(out of 100) as a consequence. But suppose that a certain degree of sacrifice were required to achieve that, and suppose that this sacrifice would be in the level of overall population health (both because explaining the options fully to people took time and other health system resources, and because some people would choose the less cost-effective of the options presented). The question which then has to be considered is 'what price (in terms of population health) would it be worth paying to improve patient choice in this way?'

Suppose we are considering a country with a population of 50 million people who enjoy an average disability-adjusted life expectancy at birth (DALE) of 50 disability adjusted life years (DALYs) (which can be thought of as 50 years of healthy life). This would have contributed 12.5 (out of 100) to the overall attainment score, but we now need to reduce that by 0.208 if the scores before and after the postulated reform are to remain constant. This would happen if the DALE of that community fell from 50 to about 49.75, i.e. if everybody sacrificed three months of healthy life expectancy. Would this be too high a price to pay? If you are a Libertarian you might well argue that since freedom of choice is very highly valued, the loss of three months' life expectancy is a small price to pay for the benefits it brings to the freedom of the individual. But an Egalitarian might take a contrary view, and argue that the loss of 12.5 million healthy life-years by the whole community is a very high price to pay for a small improvement in the amount of choice offered for the small minority of the population who will be affected by such a change (since only a small fraction of the population is offered hospital inpatient treatment in any one year). The trouble is that the issue was not put in these *marginal trade-off* terms, so the opportunity cost of improving choice was not made explicit and the discussion between the Libertarians and the Egalitarians as sketched out above would not take place. Instead, it would have had to be conducted in the much more abstract form of deciding whether 25% and 2.08% were the right weights to attach to health level and choice of treatment respectively. What is needed is a question of the form 'How much of X do you think it is worth sacrificing in order to get some specified extra quantity of Y?', and I think that health level is the best 'numeraire' to use as the common point of reference ('X') whenever such questions are posed.

Ideology and value-compatibility

At one time there was a series of jokes in circulation which followed the pattern 'I am . . . You are . . . They are . . .', which were designed to show the way in which the same phenomenon is characterised from different standpoints. If used to illustrate my present argument it might run: 'I have principles, you have an ideology, they are bigoted'. *The Concise Oxford Dictionary* offers the following definition of ideology:

> *manner of thinking characteristic of a class or individual*

which seems to work as a definition equally well when applied both to my principles and to the attitudes of that bigot over there. That same dictionary suggests that a bigot is someone who, irrespective of reason, 'attaches dispropor-tionate weight to some creed or view'. It is well known that all reasonable people think and act as I would, so in this context 'disproportionate' means 'not in the same proportion as I think appropriate'. After all, I have principles, etc.

It is futile to attempt to exclude ideology from any evaluative process. What will surely ensue from such a misguided enterprise is not the exclusion of ideology but its concealment. This obfuscation may of course be deliberate, and that is why, when scrutinising any evaluative work, it is important to look carefully at the motives of the analysts, the interests of their sponsors and the use to which the results of the analysis are being put, and by whom. But that is not the only context in which eternal vigilance is called for. Much more difficult to detect are the unconscious ideological positions embedded in the conventional assumptions of 'mainstream' analytical methods. In economics this is epitomised by the tension between mainstream 'welfarism' and the various departures from it which are lumped together as 'non-welfarist' approaches, and which are regarded as rather eccentric, even idiosyncratic, and lacking a firm theoretical foundation. According to my tripartite classification, this means that the (principled) welfarists see the non-welfarists as 'bigoted' because they attach disproportionate weight to something welfarists are happy to neglect altogether, such as a concern for distributive justice.

But in the context of the public–private mix for health at a subcontracting level within an internal market, a more important issue to concentrate on is 'what are we maximising?'. For instance, is it patient satisfaction, or public satisfaction, or population health (to name but three possibilities)? Each requires a different optimisation framework, each will be perceived to have different importance according to the standpoint of the observer and each may lead to different conclusions about whether some proposed reform is good or bad. Maximising patient satisfaction is important for those in the healthcare system itself, since patients are the ones they see and deal with on a daily basis, and whose complaints and gratitude they experience. Public satisfaction is a much broader notion, probably more important to elected politicians seeking votes, for whom the image of the healthcare system as reported in the media is more relevant than the day-to-day reality of how the system actually operates. One only has to think about how waiting list data are reported in the media to see this. The boring news that the average waiting time for elective surgery has fallen from (say) seven weeks to six weeks is brushed aside, and what is highlighted is that some people had to wait 12 months, from which it is implied that 12 months is the wait you may expect. But neither improving patient satisfaction (e.g. by offering more choice) nor improving public satisfaction (by shortening maximum waiting times but at the cost of lowering the priority given to patients whose health is more susceptible to delay) will necessarily improve population health, so we must return once more to the trade-off problem. This can only be addressed within a framework that makes explicit all the rival objectives that are in play in the optimisation process, and this takes us back to the WHR2000 example, and the analytical lessons to be learned from it.

Ideology and polemics

My final observation concerns the respective roles of ideology and evidence in broader policy discussions about the public–private mix in healthcare. There are three basic formats in which this may occur. It could operate in a purely ideological realm, in which an idealised conception of System X is compared with an idealised version of System Y, with the criteria for the comparison of relative merits being drawn from the observer's own ideology. Thus if System X is a private system and System Y is a public system, then *in principle*, X will look better than Y from a Libertarian viewpoint, but Y will look better than X from an Egalitarian viewpoint, and there the matter ends. But since neither system is likely to live up to its ideals, a much stronger case can be made by each protagonist if they compare the actual performance of their opponent's favoured system with the idealised version of their own. This is likely to lead to a final format in which actual is compared with actual, which means that evidence has come to dominate the discussion. But the rivals are still appraising things from their own respective ideological standpoints, so even if each accepted the evidence as factually accurate, they would have quite different views about its relevance and importance.

Ideology affects not only what we seek to achieve, but also how we judge reality. While the former influence is obvious, the latter is not. It comes about through the questions we ask, the way we formulate problems, the analytical methods we adopt and the evidence we seek. By deciding to tackle an issue in a particular way, even those who believe themselves to be ideologically neutral may find themselves unwittingly working within an implicit ideological stance. The problem of optimising the public–private mix in healthcare is particularly vulnerable to this danger, as I hope I have convinced you in this chapter.

References

1 Rice T (1998) *The Economics of Health Reconsidered*. Chicago: Health Administration Press, especially Chapter 2.
2 Williams A (1997) Priority setting in public and private health care: A guide through the ideological jungle. In: Culyer AJ, Maynard AK (eds) *Being Reasonable about the Economics of Health: selected essays by Alan Williams*. Cheltenham: Edward Elgar, Chapter 5.
3 Tsuchiya A, Williams A (2001) Welfare economics and economic evaluation. In: Drummond M, McGuire A (eds) *Economic Evaluation in Health Care: merging theory with practice*. London: OHE & Oxford University Press, Chapter 2.
4 Sen AK (1980) Equality of what? In: McMurrin S (ed.) *The Tanner Lectures on Human Values*. Cambridge: Cambridge University Press.
5 Culyer AJ and Wagstaff A (1993) Equity and equality in health and health care. *Journal of Health Economics*. 12: 431–57.
6 Daniels N (1985) *Just Health Care*. Cambridge: Cambridge University Press.
7 Williams A, Cookson R (2000) Equity in health. In: Culyer AJ, Newhouse JP (eds) *Handbook of Health Economics*, vol. 1. North Holland: Elsevier Science BV, Chapter 35.
8 Chadwick R (1993) Justice in priority-setting. In: Smith R (ed.) *Rationing in Action*. London: BMJ Publishing Group, pp. 85–95.
9 Williams A (2001) How economics could extend the scope of ethical discourse. *Journal of Medical Ethics*. 27: 251–5.
10 Coulter A (2002) *The Autonomous Patient: ending paternalism in medical care*. London: Nuffield Trust.
11 Gakidou E, Murray CJL, Frenk J (2000) Measuring preferences on health system performance measurement. *GPE Discussion Paper Series No. 20*. Geneva: World Health Organization.

12 Williams A (2001) Science or marketing at WHO? *Health Economics.* **10**: 93–100.

13 WHO (2000) *World Health Report 2000 – Health Systems: improving performance.* Geneva: World Health Organization, p. 7.

Endnotes

i See, for instance, Rice T (1998) *The Economics of Health Reconsidered.* Health Administration Press, Chicago, and especially Chapter 2.

ii For a fuller discussion see Williams A (1997) Priority setting in public and private health care: A guide through the ideological jungle. Chapter 5 of Culyer AJ, Maynard AK (eds) *Being Reasonable about the Economics of Health: selected essays by Alan Williams.* Edward Elgar, Cheltenham.

iii See Tsuchiya A, Williams A (2001) Welfare economics and economic evaluation. Chapter 2 of Drummond M, McGuire A (eds) *Economic Evaluation in Health Care: merging theory with practice.* London: OHE & Oxford University Press.

iv Classic works posing this question and exploring different answers to it are Sen AK (1980) Equality of what? In: McMurrin S (ed.) *The Tanner Lectures on Human Values.* Cambridge University Press, and Culyer AJ, Wagstaff A (1993) Equity and equality in health and health care. *Journal of Health Economics.* **12**: 431–57.

v See Daniels N (1985) *Just Health Care.* Cambridge: Cambridge University Press.

vi See Williams A, Cookson R (2000) Equity in health. Chapter 35 of Culyer AJ, Newhouse JP (eds) *Handbook of Health Economics,* vol. 1. Elsevier Science BV.

vii Chadwick R (1993) Justice in priority-setting. In: Smith R (ed.) *Rationing in Action.* London: BMJ Publishing Group, pp. 85–95.

viii Williams A (2001) How economics could extend the scope of ethical discourse. *Journal of Medical Ethics.* **27**: 251–5.

ix See Gakidou E, Murray CJL, Frenk J (2000) Measuring preferences on health system performance measurement. *GPE Discussion Paper Series No. 20.* Geneva: World Health Organization.

x Williams A (2001) Science or marketing at WHO? *Health Economics.* **10**: 93–100.

xi WHO (2000) *World Health Report 2000 – Health Systems: improving performance.* Geneva: World Health Organization, p. 7.

Chapter 3

Efficient purchasing in public and private healthcare systems: mission impossible?

Cam Donaldson, Karen Gerard and Craig Mitton

Introduction

The perception of policy makers in most healthcare systems, public or private, is that the power rests on the provider side and that is where regulators need to act with respect to directing incentives. This would seem to rule out placing much reliance on the individual consumer, from the demand side of the market, as a driver of efficiency in resource allocation. However, there may still be a role for collective purchasing in some form, resulting in powerful provider units, such as hospitals, being faced with purchasing entities which can negotiate more effectively on behalf of groups of individuals.[1] These entities could be organised:

- on a population basis, as in many (usually taxation-based) publicly funded healthcare systems
- through consumers registering with an intermediary who receives a payment from the individual plus a subsidised payment from government to reflect the individual's risk status, as in other (usually social insurance) systems
- through consumers (or, more likely, their employers) paying the premium in full to register with an entity, such as a health maintenance organisation (HMO), as in private systems.[2][i]

Indeed, through the growth of 'internal markets' and 'managed care', this is the way that the purchasing function in many healthcare systems has developed over the past 20 years. But, what form has collective purchasing taken? Have attempts to introduce and strengthen the purchasing function actually led to any improvements in health services efficiency? These are the questions addressed in this chapter. The perspective is mainly a UK one; however, reference will be made to evidence from elsewhere when relevant.

In the following section, a brief theoretical perspective on the healthcare market is offered, focusing in particular on the inadequacy of relying on individual consumers as healthcare purchasers and the notions of efficiency against which alternative purchasing entities can be assessed. This is followed by a brief description of the main developments in purchasing in publicly funded healthcare systems over the past 15 years, focusing on the development of internal markets, including general practitioner (GP) fundholding, and reviewing the research evidence on these. The next section addresses the question of whether public systems have anything to learn from private healthcare systems by drawing on research evidence and recent experience with managed care from the US. In conclusion, the lessons from the experiences with public and private purchasing entities are drawn. It will be seen that, although private purchasers may *appear* more effective at the micro level, the reality is quite different, with the result that challenges for policy makers at the global level remain greater in private systems than in their public counterparts.[3][ii]

Theoretical perspectives

Problems of traditional economic models of healthcare markets have been reviewed by Evans,[4] McGuire *et al.*[5] and Donaldson and Gerard.[3,6] Among other things, market failure in healthcare results because the consumer cannot be relied on to be the arbiter of 'good' and 'bad' so is not a driving force for efficiency in resource allocation. The main reason for this, of course, is that the task of understanding issues of quality and price are too great (just imagine how problems of variations in healthcare vex the minds of governments, policy analysts and clinicians, never mind consumers). Furthermore, a 'consumerist' model fits well with more educated and prosperous people, but not with many others, and risk pooling between the healthy and the ill is challenged by the actuarial methods required for cross-subsidisation and whether the healthy (and, more likely, wealthy) would want such subsidisation to occur anyway.

The first of these reasons means that providers of care (especially physicians) are put in a strong position, as they not only act as 'agents' providing advice for consumers, but also, in order to maintain quality, they control entry into the market. Physicians, then, can recommend use of their own services, for which there will be little or no competition. This is likely to lead to a lack of both allocative efficiency (i.e. provision of a mix of services which does not maximise consumer well-being) and technical efficiency (i.e. services not being provided at minimum cost). In order to combat such inefficiencies and problems of risk pooling, public systems with universal coverage have arisen, as well as the more fragmented system, largely in the US, of employer-operated schemes. Within each of these, collective purchasers such as health authorities or managed care organisations have developed to negotiate with service providers on issues of the amounts and types of services to be delivered.[7]

One could characterise some kind of insurer or health authority as a principal and a provider (e.g. hospital) as an agent. Given asymmetry of information, the aim of the principal is to devise a contract inducing more effort from the agent and which minimises costs. Of course, for this to work, both the principal has to be satisfied that aims are achieved at acceptable cost and the agent has to be satisfied with the returns.[8] In many respects, the public and private purchasing schemes reviewed later in the chapter are examples of crude attempts to induce greater efficiency in the healthcare system through such a principal-agent model.

Despite the diminished role of the consumer in such systems, the principles for their evaluation remain rooted in traditional economic theory. Thus, notions of allocative efficiency (i.e. what types of healthcare to provide) and technical efficiency (i.e. how best to provide each type of healthcare) remain important. It is mainly the question of technical efficiency which is to be addressed in presenting evidence on different purchasing models. For the most part, alternative mechanisms will be compared in terms of cost per day, cost per case (mainly as reflected in length of stay) and effects on total costs (mainly as reflected in throughput), and less often (because of lack of data) in terms of effects on outcome, equity of outcome and equity of access. Once these later pieces of data are introduced, questions relating to allocative efficiency can be asked (but not necessarily answered).

Purchasing in publicly funded healthcare systems: developments and evidence

Traditionally, owing to the absence of market mechanisms in healthcare systems which are, for the most part, provided and/or financed by government, such as the UK National Health Service (NHS), there exists no natural pricing mechanism through which the supply of healthcare resources can be efficiently matched to demands. In theory, this may be overcome by introducing 'quasi-markets' or 'internal markets' which may be created through rules and regulations. According to the nature of these rules and regulations, incentive structures may be set up to reward providers and/or consumers for efficient behaviour. The 1990s saw wide experimentation with such systems.

For example, the basic contents of the reforms of the UK NHS were published in the White Paper on *Working for Patients*.[9] Then, district health authorities (DHAs) in England were responsible for purchasing secondary care on behalf of their catchment populations. Major acute hospitals became self-governing, offering services to DHAs in return for block funding or funding for a specified number of cases, with additional cases funded on a cost-per-case basis. The boards of directors of such hospitals were ultimately responsible to the Secretary of State and, subject to some restrictions, could acquire and dispose of assets, raise funds, retain operating surpluses and build up reserves, employ whatever staff they consider necessary, and determine pay and conditions of staff.

In this way, responsibility for finance and provision of services was separated, a DHA being faced with its own hospitals, self-governing hospitals and the private sector competing for contracts and cases. The DHA, it is claimed, would choose between providers on the basis of cost, outcome, availability, convenience, etc. It was responsible for ensuring purchasing of core services (such as accident and emergency departments) which must be provided locally and for monitoring quality of services (e.g. through patient surveys). Funding for training, research and specialised services were provided centrally for hospitals which happened to provide those services.

Similar proposals were implemented in New Zealand (from July 1993),[10] while in Sweden, the 26 county councils were already responsible for healthcare, and some of them (numbering 12 by 1995) implemented such reforms throughout the 1990s.[11][iii]

Unique to the UK was an additional proposal that general practices of a certain minimum size, if they so wished, be given more responsibility for the purchase of hospital services. They were given a budget to purchase elective inpatient services, outpatient services and diagnostic tests on behalf of their patients, similar to HMO arrangements in the US.[iv] Later, some practices evolved with 'community' or 'total' fundholding, extending the range of services which were purchased by the fundholder, and consortia of fundholders were created or more formal pooling of multi-fundholders took place.[16] The aim was that GPs too would choose care for patients on the basis of both cost and quality. Patients remained free to change practice, budget allocations being suitably adjusted. In DHAs where general practices opted for budgets, the DHA had its budget reduced by the amount allocated to these general practices for 'buying in' hospital services.

Further reforms have taken place in the UK since, but it is the ones described which have been evaluated and the more recent reforms, introduced since a change of government in 1997, do contain important remnants of the internal market (see below).

In addition to New Zealand and Sweden, other European countries are now attempting to undertake quasi-market reforms.[17] The same is true of countries which have a different model of a publicly funded system, encouraging competition among intermediaries, with whom individuals and families enrol; such intermediaries subsequently attempt to gain efficiencies from competing providers. However, many of these latter reforms remain at the proposal stage. The most notable are the 'Dekker' reforms for the Dutch healthcare system, whereby insurers (or sickness funds) purchase services from suppliers of health and social services on the basis of cost and quality.[18] The consumer pays the sickness fund a flat rate, which is risk-adjusted via a government subsidy.[19,20] However, this reform has struggled to introduce competition among the sickness funds. Despite this, other European countries, such as Switzerland and Germany,[17,21] many South American countries (e.g. Argentina, Chile and Columbia),[22] and the Russian Federation[23] have also tried to introduce such reforms. Of course, the main challenge has been to guarantee that the risk-adjustment component can compensate for most of the variation in health expenditures among enrolees, thus ensuring a fair distribution of funds and prevention of risk selection.

The basic aims of these reforms were to better integrate considerations of cost and quality in healthcare resource allocation decisions and, to some extent, achieve greater vertical integration (and thereby efficiency) in the financing of primary, secondary and tertiary care, whereby costs incurred in secondary or tertiary parts of the sector may be reimbursed by a primary care organisation (like a GP fundholder). This is similar to the idea behind managed care in the US but, ironically, may have actually led to increased fragmentation, as those working in purchasing and provider organisations might see less scope for collaboration and, thus, communication. The schemes have proved difficult to evaluate, with most of the evidence coming from the UK, New Zealand and Sweden.

Evidence on the purchasing function in publicly financed systems

In short, there has been little rigorous evaluation of the role of health authorities as purchasers of care, the main reason for this being that all health authorities in the UK became purchasers at the beginning of the reforms, so there was little scope for comparative analysis.[24] The same is true in New Zealand,[12,25] but in

Sweden, with some county councils implementing such reforms at different times, more scope existed for comparative analysis.[11]

What is now known is that the reformed system of health authority purchasing in the UK, at least initially, mirrored the old style of system. This contrasted with the more immediate impacts of GP fundholding, i.e. GPs 'shopping around' for services in attempts, for example, to reduce their patients' waiting times. Health authorities, perhaps inevitably, were more influenced by policy directives from the centre (i.e. the Department of Health).[26] Initially, in the main, 'block' contracts were established between health authorities and providers.[27] These were open-ended with respect to levels of activity and expected outcomes, which, again, basically mirrored the old-style NHS. Only later, did cost and volume contracts, which specified, among other things, actual numbers to be treated by a provider, become more established (though not on a widespread basis). Central policy directives also hampered progress in New Zealand. Indeed, the failure of health authorities to generate competition, in part, led to their replacement with a central agency, the Health Funding Authority.[13] At this point, a purchaser–provider split was still maintained, but one based more on cooperation than competition. The 'split' has now been abolished. Scotland, too, has dismantled its internal market, with providers operating under their local health board as in the NHS pre-1990.

Ability to make providers compete did exist, to some extent, in the UK. For example, Appleby et al.[28] showed that only 8% of acute hospitals in a major region of England (West Midlands) had a monopoly of their main surgical specialties within a 30-mile radius. As well as being constrained by policy directives from the centre, there are two other main reasons why the potential to induce competition was not taken up more extensively by UK health authorities. First, the sheer enormity of the task may have prevented them from taking action. Unlike GPs, health authorities had to purchase the full range of health services. It is also unlikely that they would have staff specialised enough to challenge the plans of providers.[29] Second, the potential to de-stabilise providers by making potentially large resource shifts is likely to have inhibited many purchasers from making such shifts.[24] This is not surprising in the politically charged atmosphere of healthcare provision.

Swedish county councils were less hampered by central directives because they had previously held responsibility for healthcare funding and provision, a factor likely to have led to more positive results there. Gerdtham et al.[30] estimated that those county councils in which reforms were implemented reduced costs (by about 13%) relative to county councils which remained with the status quo. Tambour and Rehnberg[31] found that, during the period 1991 to 1994, productivity (measured only in terms of activity) for both internal market and 'control' county councils improved, with the rate of productivity being higher in internal market councils. But they found that market mechanisms were only one factor in productivity gains, with the resource allocation system (e.g. performance-based review) and other healthcare reforms also having an impact. Further work from Sweden suggests that internal market reforms did aim to reduce costs but failed to generate much competition between hospitals.[32] This study also presents evidence that quality of healthcare was not adversely affected by the reforms.

Neither should one be too pessimistic about the impact of the reforms in the UK. Ham[33] describes what happened to healthcare in London in 1991. Given the population and number of hospitals, particularly relatively expensive teaching hospitals, in London, this is precisely the place where one would have expected the UK reforms to have an impact. Indeed, this is what happened. Almost immediately after the reforms were introduced, purchasers shifted resources out of central London hospitals to those in less costly and more accessible surrounding areas. These resource movements were sufficient to create problems with respect to the sustainability of some central London hospitals and led to the suspension of the internal market in London and a review of health services in the UK capital, led by Sir Bernard Tomlinson. The review gave greater priority to community and primary care services, while London's hospitals were given more resources to enable them to cope with the changes. Eventually, hospitals were closed or rationalised. It might be argued that such rationalisation led to little real change, while others might say that a combination of market signals and government management led to a more orderly process of change than would otherwise have been the case. Yet, the internal market still had an impact. Ham[33] claims that other major cities experienced similar changes, but at a slower pace than in London.

Among the UK's 1991 'internal market' reforms, GP fundholding was one of the most studied. By 1997, half the population was covered by fundholding practices, which controlled over 10% of hospital and community health service spending, but like the other reforms, evaluation of this aspect suffered from the lack of a planned and rigorous overall evaluation. In addition to challenges in evaluating internal markets already pointed out, there were a series of changes in the NHS which were all introduced around the same time, hampering the ability to attribute any observed changes to fundholding alone. The feature that practices voluntarily self-selected into the fundholding scheme is a further confounder: fundholders tended to be better resourced and located in more affluent areas than non-fundholders, so they were not a random sample.[34] There is also documented evidence showing that practices entering in the first wave were measurably different from those entering later.[35–37] The differences between fundholders and non-fundholders may not be attributable to fundholding status *per se*, but to other (unmeasured) differences in these practices.

The body of literature on fundholding has been comprehensively reviewed by Goodwin *et al.*[16] including evidence related to efficiency and equity. Despite comparator problems, there is some consensus in the literature that, at least initially, fundholders were able to curb the rise in prescription costs compared with non-fundholders.[38] This reduction was achieved largely via a lower cost per item of prescribing, through measures like increased use of generic alternatives, although there is also some evidence of reduced volumes.[38] After the first few years of entry into fundholding, continued cost reductions, as one would expect, were observed to level off as savings were more difficult to achieve.

More specifically related to purchasing was the impact of fundholding on rate of referrals to specialists and emergency care. It was hoped that by having GPs bear the financial responsibility for their referral decisions to specialists, inappropriate referrals would be reduced, thus freeing resources for more appropriate use. On the other hand, there was also a concern that fundholders might have an incentive to shift costs to health authorities, i.e. by referring patients to emergency care which came out of health authority budgets rather than those of the fundholders. The small body of literature on these issues is inconclusive; it appears that, in England, referral rates did not alter after the introduction of fundholding, while in Scotland, the introduction of the scheme did lead to reduced rates of referral for certain groups.[39,40]

Other results on fundholding relate to impacts on prices charged to fund-holders, the location of care, administrative costs and the investment of any surpluses. Propper et al.[41] have shown, through rigorous regression analyses, that market forces, measured by variables such as numbers of NHS providers in a given area and market share counted for by a provider, have had an impact in reducing prices charged to fundholders across eight common procedures. There also appear to be more services provided by fundholding practices after they became fundholders, such as more outreach clinics by hospital clinicians, resulting in a shift in the location of secondary care, although, again, it is not clear that this is attributable to fundholding per se. The administrative costs of fundholding were high, with some estimates suggesting that they were not outweighed by the cost savings.[29] A further issue is whether the savings achieved by fundholders, and the practice-based investments made by the fundholders with these savings, repres-ented an efficiency improvement. There is much debate but little evidence on this question.

Despite great difficulties in measuring changes in quality in a comprehensive manner, there is now some limited evidence on the overall impact of internal markets. After controlling for important characteristics (such as hospital size and teaching status) and exploiting the policy changes of the 1990s (whereby there was no competition until 1991, actively encouraged competition until 1995, less encouragement in 1996 and active discouragement post 1997), Propper et al.[42] show that there was a negative relationship between mortality post-treatment for heart attack and competition. Of course, a fall in quality may be expected to accompany a fall in costs and such a relationship, between competition and outcomes, may not exist for other services.

With respect to equity, there were two specific issues which arose regarding the impact of fundholding. First of all, the potential for 'cream skimming' was a concern, whereby fundholders would have the incentive to select only healthy patients since ill patients would jeopardise the fundholders' ability to make savings on their budget, though there is no evidence that this was an issue. In all probability, the provision limiting the per patient liability of the fundholder to £5000 per annum is responsible for this. The second issue was that patients of fundholders would receive preferential access to care, because of their improved ability to negotiate favourable terms with hospitals. There is some evidence that this did in fact occur and that it represented 'two-tierism' in access to care, which arose because fundholding did not cover all practices.

Overall, with respect to equity impacts of the UK internal market reforms, British Household Panel Survey data, analysed by Propper[43] showed that the pattern of use of GP and inpatient services remained stable over the period 1990/1 (before the UK reforms) to 1993/4 (two years after). Use was still slightly in favour of the poor, after adjusting for indicators of need, so equity (or inequity) in healthcare delivery remained largely unaffected by healthcare purchasing.

In 1997, the new English Labour Government replaced health authority and fundholding purchasing with primary care groups (PCGs) (now trusts, PCTs) which are responsible for the purchase of most hospital, community and primary care for their populations. These PCTs cover all practices, and cooperation rather than competition is encouraged between purchasers and providers.[44] They are typically much smaller than health authority purchasers. The encouragement of cooperation does, to some extent, dilute the incentive effects on the PCTs, especially when combined with central government initiatives, such as National Service Frameworks and national treatment guidelines to which trusts are expected to adhere. Although difficult to interpret in terms of attribution to these reforms, increases in hospital activity have not been as great as during the 1989–90 to 1996–97 period, with the total number of GP consultations falling between 1996–7 and 1998–9.[44] A more sophisticated, but still limited, case-weighted activity index, measuring units of resources used per unit of activity, showed improvements in 'efficiency' during the period of the internal market and has fallen since.[44] Waiting lists did, however, decline, from 1.16 million in 1997 to 1.039 million in 2001,[44] but it is unclear whether this is due to greater cooperation, 'throwing money at it' or some other reason. For example, it has been suggested that success on waiting lists has resulted merely because, among the plethora of performance criteria introduced since the 'abolition' of the UK internal market post 1997, those related to waiting times are more easily measured.[45,46]

Despite the apparent success on waiting lists, Le Grand[44] attributes the lack of success on other indicators at least in part to a lack of the incentives that would be induced by competitive pressures. It could be argued, then, that the purchasing function has been made weaker, with consequent (possible and slight) adverse effects. The recent proposals for (re?-) introduction of Foundation Hospitals in the UK may, in part, be a response to this problem; hospitals are ranked according to how well they perform and, if ranked in the lowest category, they are given a period of time to reach certain targets. Failure to meet these, means that private management teams and those from other (say, neighbouring) hospitals can compete to take over the management of the 'failing' hospitals. Those in the top category are given more freedom to raise capital to further develop services. This 'franchise' scheme remains unevaluated, although where it seems to differ from the earlier version of the UK internal market is in the increased emphasis put on providers rather than purchasers, further weakening the purchasing function. Reflecting a point raised by McGuire and Hughes[7] in the context of internal markets more generally, it is unclear the extent to which (now smaller) purchasing units will be able to exert their authority against (still) large 'three-star' Foundation Hospitals. This could be characterised as leading to less of a focus on population health as more resources are 'sucked' into acute services, which may or may not be efficient. Prime issues should be the objectives of such reforms and evaluation of whether these objectives are met, and in this sense, such reforms are the means to an end, not the end in themselves.

In summary, the evidence is not clear cut, but it does seem that efficiency improvements, however small, arose from internal markets, and some of them must be attributable to purchasing. It could also be argued that GP fundholding displayed the greatest potential within the UK set of reforms to improve efficiency in healthcare provision. Even were this potential not fully exploited, it seems to have even less chance of success now. To make up for any losses, fundholding may have to reappear, although for political reasons, this would likely be in a rebadged form.

Purchasing in privately funded healthcare systems: are there lessons for an NHS?

The managed care 'revolution'

Traditionally, hospital care in the US was dominated by large institutions, principally of three types:

- privately owned for-profit
- voluntary not-for-profit
- publicly owned.

Third-party payers such as insurance companies would reimburse all 'reasonable' medical expenses incurred in such institutions. With third-party payment, neither consumers nor providers had incentives to control costs, especially as most consumers would have their premiums paid by their employers (fourth-party payment?!).

The cost escalation induced by rapidly developing technology and incentives embodied within the above structure led to the managed care 'revolution' in the US, over the past 20–30 years, which was partially an attempt to introduce stronger purchasing to gain a degree of cost control within the system.

The main innovations in this regard were the introduction of HMOs and, subsequently, preferred provider organisations (PPOs). These innovations had a strong influence on the reforms in publicly financed systems discussed in the previous section.

HMOs arrange and pay for comprehensive healthcare for a fixed periodic per capita payment (or 'premium') which is paid by the consumer (usually with a subsidy from employers or social security). The premium is set in advance and is independent of the volume of services provided to the individual during the period. A range of remuneration schemes are used, such as salaries, fee-for-service (FFS),[v] capitation and 'bonus' schemes related to activity rates.

An important difference between HMOs and purchasers in publicly funded healthcare systems is that HMOs still operate in a competitive system, within which there will still be incentives to tailor premiums to individuals' risk status (experience rating). In all likelihood, this will give rise to the poorest risks, usually the least well off members of society, facing the highest premiums, and thus opting out of health insurance.[vi] The main issue here, in assessing the efficiency of HMOs, is whether cost reductions are real or apparent, arising simply from HMOs attracting a lower-risk, and thus lower-cost, clientele. Doctor-demand inducement is not likely to be very prevalent, as not only must doctors compete for custom, usually on an annual basis, but also the annual HMO budget is fixed in advance. Doctors will be cost-conscious, since the residual between the budget and expenditure accrues to the HMO and, thereby, to them, causing high-spending doctors to be financially penalised.

Consumers select the healthcare plan of their choice on an annual basis, so greater choice is thought to exist. Because consumers usually receive only a fixed subsidy towards payment (or a fixed percentage of the premium) the argument is that they too have an incentive to be cost-conscious. HMOs have always had user charges, particularly for drugs,[47] but their use is becoming more widespread.

PPOs have arisen in the US as a result of attempts by insurance companies to enter into competition with HMOs. Premiums are paid by employers or are shared between employer and employee. Price at the point of use of services is zero. Insurers contract selectively with providers (e.g. primary care doctors and hospitals who provide care below a certain cost per case), contracting on the basis of both a negotiated fee schedule, which the preferred providers accept as payment in full, and acceptance of utilisation review. User charges and deductibles tend to be lower in PPOs than under previous private insurance arrangements.[48]

Once more, experience rating will almost inevitably develop within a care system based on PPOs, leaving the more costly groups without cover for healthcare unless they are subsidised. There is also more financial risk to primary care providers with respect to the volume of services provided. With FFS as the basis for payment the doctor can, to some extent, still manipulate utilisation, though this is limited, as if cost per case rises above a certain level the doctor may not be selected as a preferred provider at the next review. The incentive for hospitals to keep costs down arises because a set of prices has been agreed in advance.

Patients can choose between a limited set of providers or elect another provider on less favourable terms, so incentives also exist on the demand side. One specific advantage of PPOs is that they have enabled employers in the US to move quickly to control healthcare costs for employees who are already under FFS schemes. Companies either organise schemes themselves or persuade insurance companies to do it. The latter cooperate, as this provides a means of competing with HMOs.

Again, highlighting similarities across public and private systems and noting that managed care is not so new, one system which has parallels to the UK internal market and the Dutch governments' reforms is the selective contracting scheme in California. Introduced in July 1982, and a forerunner to PPOs, this scheme permits Medicaid and private insurers to contract selectively with hospitals and other providers of care, the aim being to stimulate price competition among these providers. Both Medicaid and private insurers can negotiate terms and conditions with each specific provider, whom they will reimburse for services to their subscribers. Previously, this could not be done because of the threat of antitrust prosecution of funders by providers. The California State Medicaid programme has used the system to negotiate discounts with hospitals, as have private payers.[49]

Evidence on managed care: has the revolution been sustained?

In the US, a comprehensive review of work up to the mid-1990s found that, on average, HMO patients consume fewer hospital resources due to shorter lengths of stay, fewer ancillary resources used and a lower rate of admission.[50] More recent work has confirmed these findings and furthered the issue by examining not just the effect on hospitals of HMO versus non-HMO plans, but also investigating the impact of the level of HMO penetration and the degree of competition between HMOs. For example, Robinson[51] examined the impact of HMOs in California from 1983 to 1993 and found that hospital expenditures grew at a less rapid rate in markets with high HMO penetration than those with low penetration. Giving further weight to this perspective, the finding was mirrored in a 1985 to 1993 national sample.[52] The containment in high- over low-penetration markets in the California study was due largely to reductions in volume and service mix, but also to changes in bed intensity and bed capacity,[51] as confirmed in a later review by Miller and Luft.[53] The assertion has been made that greater HMO penetration leads to moving hospitals to the periphery of healthcare in lieu of non-hospital ambulatory services, with Miller and Luft[53] showing that increased penetration leads to more preventive activities but reduced access to uncompensated care and high-cost technology (such as magnetic resonance imaging).

Taking this work a step further, Bamezai et al.[54] examined national US data and found that expenditure growth in hospitals is related not only to HMO penetration but also to the degree of competition in the hospital market. It is not clear, though, if these results are explained by the effect of penetration on practice or due to a selection bias, with HMOs being attracted to areas with better hospital care. But taking this literature as a whole, HMOs, at least for a while, obviously intensified price competition between hospitals,[55] which can effect a significant reduction in hospital cost inflation.[56]

While it would seem that HMO plans do decrease hospitalisations, it is unclear if total costs are lowered,[57] and available evidence does not provide a clear answer on quality of care across plan type or between HMO and non-HMO plans.[53,58] Ultimately, as Kemper et al.[59] argue, it may be that HMO plans will appeal to some individuals but not others. Those in HMOs may receive more primary care and face lower out-of-pocket costs, but at the same time meet increased barriers to accessing providers, receive less specialist care and report less satisfaction of care overall. The debate is further complicated by apparently differing results for HMO and non-HMO plans depending on an individual's health state and income level.[60,61]

In the classic RAND Health Insurance Experiment (HIE), 1673 individuals were randomly assigned to one HMO or to an FFS plan in which care was provided free at the point of delivery.[62] Results demonstrated that outpatient visit rates from HMO enrollees were similar to those for people on the free care insurance plan, although expenditure per person in the HMO group was 72% of those on the free care FFS plan. This difference is a result of a markedly less hospital-intensive style of care in the HMO plan.[63,64] On average, those people assigned to the HMO suffered no adverse effects when compared with those in the 'free' FFS plan. However, health outcomes in the two systems of care differed for those individuals in both high- and low-income groups who began the experiment with health problems. For those in the high-income group who were initially sick, the HMO produced significant improvements in cholesterol levels and in general health ratings by comparison with the free FFS plan. Those in the low-income group (i.e. those in the lower fifth of the income distribution) who were initially sick, found that HMO care resulted in significantly more bed-days per year due to poor health, more serious symptoms and a greater risk of dying compared with free FFS care. Wagner and Bledsoe[65] disputed this evidence, claiming that such differences may be due to chance, as analyses of results by income group were based on small sample sizes and large standard deviations. Furthermore, it is not clear if such results were due to demand-side effects (HMO enrollees not presenting for care) or supply-side effects (with less effective care being provided), although, on balance, there is less reason to suspect the former than the latter.

A recent study comparing group and staff HMO elderly hip fracture patients to FFS patients found HMO enrollees had improved functioning and ambulation while utilising less physician services.[66] Others have found similar inpatient management levels but improved survival rates for HMO patients, as was the case for elderly patients with syncope.[67]

In contrast, Yelin et al.[68] compared utilisation and outcomes for rheumatoid arthritis patients in pre-paid group practice and FFS settings over an 11-year follow-up period and found no difference in quantity of services used and no differences on outcomes including symptoms, functional status and work disability. Baseline data did show the prepaid group to be more educated than the FFS group, introducing a bias likely to favour the HMO plan, at least in terms of outcomes. (Given similar educational levels, the prepaid group practice population may have fared worse than the FFS population.) Even so, others have found similar survival patterns between HMO and FFS plans, at least in the case of stroke patients.[69]

Ware et al.[61] found that elderly and poor, chronically ill subgroups in HMO plans had worse physical outcomes than in FFS systems, but that this difference was not observed for the average patient. Yet another study, which perhaps supports these results, found that HMO hospital readmission in the frail elderly was greater than that for patients in FFS plans.[70] In addition, a recent study found that those who are unhealthy are more likely to have greater satisfaction with FFS plans, while healthy individuals are more likely to report a higher level of satisfaction with HMO plans.[60] In essence, it would seem that those who need fewer services tend to favour HMO plans, which does fit with the evidence of lower utilisation rates in HMOs, and referring to Kemper et al.,[59] it would indeed appear that HMOs will appeal to some individuals and not others.

The suggestion from this evidence is that HMOs may have to select risks in order to achieve cost savings without adversely affecting health. This confirms results from other work on risk selection in HMOs,[71,75] although such results have recently been contradicted by Schaefer and Reschovsky[76] who show that the main attraction of HMOs is lower cost regardless of risk status. Whether HMOs select good risks or good risks select HMOs is not clear. Potentially sicker people may prefer to stay in an FFS system. (It should be noted, however, that such selection, or 'cream skimming', is consistent with what one would expect in a competitive environment.)

Finally, different models of HMO plan type may affect utilisation and quality of care. Group and staff models have rosters of patients and display similar characteristics to the 'gate-keeping' model used in general practice in the UK NHS. Independent practice associations (IPAs) use FFS remuneration, and practitioners see only some HMO patients. The latter are less restrictive and, in some plans, patients can even self-refer to specialists. A study in the early 1990s compared a random sample of 42 staff, group and IPA model HMOs, and found that group and staff model HMOs scored more favourably than IPA models on level of services provided, preventive care and various quality of care outcomes.[77] Interestingly, however, IPA models were found to result in better patient satisfaction and access. The lesson here, of course, is that not all HMO plans are alike, and thus caution must be asserted in making sweeping claims, in terms of service utilisation and quality, between HMO and FFS systems. Of note, a recent study by Reschovsky et al.[78] made a similar point in their more detailed investigation of managed care, as they delineated between FFS, PPOs, open-model HMOs and closed-model HMOs.

As mentioned above, selective contracting appeared in California in the 1980s as a means of fostering price competition among healthcare providers by encouraging the use of PPOs. An extensive review of the literature found selective contracting to have enabled managed care plans to obtain lower prices from hospitals, particularly when there is more competition in the hospital market.[79] However, limited evidence exists on the effect of selective contracting on health outcomes.

Early work by Robinson and Luft[80] demonstrated that the Californian strategy reduced hospital cost inflation by 10% over the period 1982 to 1986 compared with 43 control states, but that the effects were almost entirely confined to areas of high competition (i.e. local markets with more than ten competitors). These results were confirmed in a study which examined a large set of hospitals in California over a 14-year period (1983–97). Zwanziger et al.[81] found that hospitals in more competitive areas had a substantially lower rate of increase in both costs and revenues, which was attributed to the growth in selective contracting. However, it was unclear if the cost reductions were due to increased efficiency or reduced quality. In essence, with selective contracting, providers negotiate in advance with contractors to accept fixed payment rates. By excluding high-cost providers, and with the introduction of price competition, third-party payers' expenditures are reduced, the conclusion being that price competition, based on California's experience, can change provider behaviour.[82]

Despite these arguments in apparent favour of selective contracting, empirical evidence in California also suggests that costs escalated for over half the public hospitals through the 1980s as uncompensated burdens rose. As many counties were left without a public hospital by 1990, access to those hospitals by the poor diminished.[83] Not to discount this concern, Cubellis[84] did find that over a nine-year period (1984–92), selective contracting in a set of California hospitals had a beneficial effect on surgical outcomes for open-heart surgery. The key factors contributing to this effect were patient concentration (high volume resulting in high-quality outcomes) and contractor monitoring of patients in network hospitals.

So, where does all of this evidence leave us, specifically in terms of the efficiency of HMOs and PPOs as purchasers? From the studies reported here, the evidence is not completely clear. Reasons for the difficulty in deciphering clear effects of managed care on utilisation and outcomes are that, overall, there have been relatively few studies that have explicitly examined these issues, and those that have often use different methods and have varying scope.[53,58] Coupled with the different types of plan, the ability to make an overall assessment is limited. At issue is whether HMOs can lower total resource consumption while maintaining or improving health outcomes.[58] While the evidence, on balance, may suggest that utilisation rates with HMO plans are reduced, the cost advantages thought to be brought about by HMOs seem not to have materialised.[57] At the system level, evidence of this has been demonstrated recently by Altman and Levitt[85] who show that over the years no major reform of the US system, including managed care, has abated cost increases. Lee and Tollen[86] claim that healthcare premiums in the US rose by 11% in 2001 and are forecast to increase by 12.7% in 2002.

Concerns now seem to have switched to ensuring quality of care. Many states have passed legislation which prevents managed care organisations achieving cost savings (through, for example, introducing minimum lengths of hospital stay). Despite this, systematic reviews of the literature have shown that the concern with quality lying behind such legislation is unfounded.[87] It has been speculated that the mismatch between this type of finding and the public perception of substandard managed care performance (as embodied in the legislation referred to) could be due to the influence of the medical profession on such perceptions or the lead time between when recently published research was actually conducted and more recent assessments of market conditions.[87,88] Indeed, since Robinson's article,[87] studies have shown positive associations between improved health outcomes (both clinical and in terms of reduced mortality) and nurse staffing levels, backing up the legislation in some US states which raises staffing levels above those suggested by hospital providers.[89,90] A comprehensive programme for dealing with medical error has been laid out by the Institute of Medicine's Quality of Health Care in America Committee.[91]

Returning to how economists would look at these developments, if anything, it seems that on the demand side the market is simply segmenting in a 'natural' way, with consumers choosing the plans which suit them best. Indeed, Kwon[92] has shown theoretically and empirically that consumers will trade off 'quality' and premium level to select the combination desired, resulting in FFS plans being associated with both higher income (and, thus, willingness to pay) and higher severity of illness among enrollees. Indeed, other analyses have shown that the market is responding to such a situation with increasing enrolment in more traditional Blue Cross and Blue Shield plans since the mid-1990s, and, to compete with this, managed care plans are now offering less-restrictive and higher-cost packages.[93,94] This may be a good thing, but does counter any evidence that HMOs reduce, or even stabilise, costs overall.

Coupled with consumers opting into higher-cost plans has been a significant supply-side response, with a series of hospital mergers, initially aimed at combating aggressive managed care organisations by achieving greater efficiencies in production, but now leading to higher prices being charged back to consumers through their plans,[95] a result which is consistent with the predictions of economic theory.[96]

The evidence for managed care never was that strong. But now, with the combination of these demand- and supply-side effects and the related, and growing, concern for quality, it seems that rather than the revolution being sustained, a counter-revolution, comprising the dreaded alliance of providers and consumers, has occurred and managed care is now dead.[2,97]

Conclusions

It is easy to dismiss the UK internal market reforms of the early 1990s (and perhaps less so those in Sweden) due to political pyrotechnics which have avoided the use of evidence. However, these reforms had some positive effects, having displayed the potential to reconfigure services in a way that is more in line with population needs, e.g. resulting in more of an emphasis on primary care.

It has been claimed that reforms involving purchasing in the UK led to clearer roles being established for health authorities and providers, leading them to become more cost conscious and considerate about what to provide, to whom and at what standard.[98] Undoubtedly, in the UK, such reforms led to a change in the role of GPs, who, at least for a while, were more closely involved in many decisions about service provision than they had ever been previously.[98] It is claimed in other countries that both purchasers and providers have a preference for maintaining the split relative to returning to the old-style system.[11] Others might go even further and say that the reforms actually worked, but that the potential for purchasing to drive the system further in terms of efficiency was not fully exploited.

Contrary to recent developments, it seems that purchasing has a place in driving provider efficiency from a population health perspective in publicly financed healthcare systems, and that international experience reflects this. Part of the reason for it not working as effectively as some might hope is that such systems have objectives which go beyond efficiency, to equity. This gives the impression of purchasing being mission impossible; but, more positively, it is mission only partly possible!

Managed care organisations, it seems, can act more effectively to keep costs down. This may or may not be as a result of purchasing (and providing) more efficient care. However, the evidence seems to suggest that although cost control at the level of the organisation may be better achieved in managed care, the overall effects on the system may be minimal because of: (a) selection problems (i.e. costs are reduced because lower-risk people are attracted to managed care, and thus total system costs are not reduced at all); (b) squeezing consumers too much, with the consequent effect that some are now choosing higher-cost plans; and (c) squeezing providers too much as well, with the consequent effect that they, also, are biting back with mergers and, thus, higher prices. Such 'biting back' is not possible within the more highly regulated UK system, where, despite the existence of local monopolies, price increases cannot be fuelled by encouraging consumers to pay more by opting for higher-cost plans. Also, adverse equity effects arise under managed care in the US if hospitals are squeezed to the point where they cannot provide uncompensated care.

The demise of managed care seems to have left the US in a bit of a policy vacuum. Concerns for quality do exist and are seemingly being acted upon, but apart from that, more and more reliance is being placed on the consumer, taking us back to where we started this chapter. As Robinson[2] has pointed out, 'a purely consumer-driven healthcare system would be grossly inefficient as well as grotesquely inefficient'. We need to be mindful of such experiences, as well as our objectives, even when undertaking similar initiatives in the more protective frameworks offered by publicly funded systems, such as the 'patient choice' experiment in the UK NHS.

Some feel that Robinson's prediction is correct, but that that is due to the current structure of the US system, whereby, in the latter years of managed care, it was employers who chose the plan into which patients enrolled (or were herded!). Given that part of the managed care backlash has been shown empirically by Enthoven et al.[97] to have arisen because consumers were not given choice, a system of managed competition has been suggested, offering employees a wide variety of insurers and healthcare delivery systems.[99]

Purchasing within a more 'socialised' system may still be best for meeting the twin goals of equity and efficiency, dependent on objectives. The challenge for these systems is to strengthen the purchasing function so as to allow the purchasers to move resources around the system more in line with population need. The messages for the US system remain as always; strengthening purchasing will not do much in a system where 'missions impossible' seems to be: (a) to agree on objectives for the system; (b) to act accordingly in terms of broader healthcare system reform (whether in terms of going back to the original ideals of managed competition, as suggested above, or to a more socialised system); and (c) to accept that some amount of sacrifice (likely by better off members of society and also by healthcare providers) may be required to achieve such reform.

References

1 Evans RG (1987) Public health insurance: the collective purchase of individual care. *Health Policy.* **7**: 115–34.

2 Robinson JC (2001) The end of managed care. *Journal of the American Medical Association.* **285**: 2622–8.

3 Donaldson C, Gerard K (with Mitton C, Jan S, Wiseman V) (2005) *Economics of Health Care Financing: the visible hand* (2e). London: Palgrave Macmillan.

4 Evans RG (1984) *Strained Mercy: the economics of Canadian medical care.* Toronto: Butterworths.

5 McGuire A, Henderson T, Mooney G (1988) *The Economics of Health Care: an introductory text.* London: Routledge and Kegan Paul.

6 Donaldson C, Gerard K (1991) Minding our Ps and Qs? Financial incentives for efficient hospital behaviour. *Health Policy.* **17**: 51–76.

7 McGuire A, Hughes D (2003) The economics of the hospital: issues of asymmetry and uncertainty as they affect hospital reimbursement. In: Scott A, Maynard A, Elliott R (eds) *Advances in Health Economics.* Chichester: Wiley.

8 Laffont JJ, Tirole JA (1993) *Theory of Incentives in Procurement and Regulation.* Cambridge, MA: MIT Press.

9 Secretaries of State (1989) Funding contracts for health services. Working Paper 2. London: HMSO.

10 Minister of Health (1993) Your Health and the Public Health: Green and White Paper. Wellington: Department of Health.

11 Bergman S-E (1998) Swedish models of healthcare reform: a review and assessment. *International Journal of Health Planning & Management.* **13**: 91–106.

12 Scott CD (1994) Reform of the New Zealand healthcare system. *Health Policy.* **29**: 25–40.

13 Kent H (1999) New Zealand embraces a parallel private system – and a growing gap between rich and poor. *Canadian Medical Association Journal.* **161**: 569–71.

14 Enthoven A (1985) *Reflections on Management in the National Health Service: an American looks at incentives to efficiency in health services management in the UK.* London: Nuffield Provincial Hospitals Trust.

15 Enthoven A (1999) *In Pursuit of an Improving National Health Service.* London: Nuffield Trust.

16 Goodwin N, Mays N, McLeod H, Malbon G, Raftery J (1998) Evaluation of total purchasing pilots in England and Scotland and implications for primary care groups in England: personal interviews and analysis of routine data. *British Medical Journal.* **317**: 256–9.

17 European Observatory on Health Care Systems (2002) *Health Care Systems in Eight Countries: trends and challenges.* London: London School of Economics and Political Science.

18 van de Ven WMM (1989) A future for competitive healthcare in the Netherlands. Occasional Paper No 9. University of York: Centre for Health Economics.

19 van de Ven W, Rutten F (1994) Managed competition in the Netherlands: lessons from five years of healthcare reform. *Australian Health Review.* **17**: 9–27.

20 van Doorslaer E, Schut F (2000) Belgium and the Netherlands revisited. *Journal of Health Politics, Policy & Law.* **5**: 875–87.

21 Zweifel P (2000) Switzerland. *Journal of Health Politics, Policy & Law.* **25**: 938–44.

22 Jack W (2000) Health insurance reform in four Latin American countries. Theory and Practice. Policy Research Working Paper 2492. The World Bank Development Research Group, Public Economics.

23 Twigg J (1999) Regional variation in Russian medical insurance: lessons from Moscow and Nizhny Novgorod. *Health & Place.* **5**: 235–45.

24 Mays N, Mulligan JA, Goodwin N (2000) The British quasi-market in healthcare: a balance sheet of the evidence. *Journal of Health Services Research and Policy.* **5**: 49–58.

25 Ashton T (1993) From evolution to revolution: restructuring the New Zealand healthcare system. *Health Care Analysis.* **1**: 57–62.

26 Hughes D, Griffiths L, McHale J (1997) Do quasi-markets evolve? Institutional analysis and the NHS. *Cambridge Journal of Economics.* **21**: 259–76.

27 Raftery J, Robinson R, Mulligan JA, Forrest S (1996) Contracting in the NHS quasi-market. *Health Economics.* **5**: 353–62.

28 Appleby J, Smith P, Ranade W, Little V, Robinson R (1994) Monitoring managed competition. In: Robinson R, Le Grand J (eds) *Evaluating the NHS Reforms.* London: King's Fund Institute.

29 Audit Commission (1997) *Higher Purchase: commissioning specialised services in the NHS.* London: HMSO.

30 Gerdtham U-G, Rehnberg C, Tambour M (1999) The impact of internal markets on healthcare efficiency: evidence from healthcare reforms in Sweden. Working Paper Series in Economics and Finance. Centre for Health Economics, Stockholm School of Economics.

31 Tambour M, Rehnberg C (1997) Internal markets and performance in Swedish healthcare. Working Paper No. 161. Stockholm School of Economics.

32 Harrison MI, Calltorp J (2000) The reorientation of market-oriented reforms in Swedish health care. *Health Policy.* **50**: 219–40.

33 Ham C (1996) *Public, Private or Community: what next for the NHS?* London: Demos.

34 Petchey R (1995) General practitioner fundholding: weighing the evidence. *Lancet.* **346**: 1139–42.

35 Baines DL, Brigham P, Phillips DR, Tolley KH, Whynes DK (1997) GP fundholding and prescribing in UK general practice: evidence from two rural, English Family Health Services Authorities. *Public Health.* **111**(5): 321–5.

36 Whynes DK, Heron T, Avery AJ (1997) Prescribing cost savings by GP fundholders: long-term or short-term? *Health Economics.* **6**: 209–11.

37 Baines DL, Whynes DK (1996) Selection bias in GP fundholding. *Health Economics.* **5**: 129–40.

38 Wilson R, Buchan I, Walley T (1995) Alterations in prescribing by general practitioner fundholders: an observational study. *British Medical Journal.* **311**: 1347–50.

39 Coulter A, Bradlow J (1993) Effect of NHS reforms of general practitioners' referral patterns. *British Medical Journal.* **306**: 433–7.

40 Howie J, Heaney D, Maxwell M (1994) Evaluating care of patients reporting back pain in fundholding practices. *British Medical Journal.* **309**: 705–10.

41 Propper C, Wilson D, Soderlund N (1998) The effects of regulation and competition in

the NHS internal market: the case of general practice fundholder prices. *Journal of Health Economics.* **17**: 645–73.

42 Propper C, Burgess S, Green K (2004) Does competition between hospitals improve the quality of care? Hospital death rates and the NHS Internal Market. *Journal of Public Economics.* **88**: 1247–72.

43 Propper C (1998) Who pays for and who gets healthcare? Delivery of healthcare in the United Kingdom. Nuffield Occasional papers. London: The Nuffield Trust.

44 Le Grand J (2002) Further tales from the British National Health Service. *Health Affairs.* **21**: 116–28.

45 Goddard M, Mannion R, Smith P (2000) Enhancing performance in healthcare: a theoretical perspective on agency and the role of information. *Health Economics.* **9**: 95–107.

46 Scott A, Farrar S (2003) Incentives in healthcare. In: Scott A, Maynard A, Elliott R (eds) *Advances in Health Economics.* Wiley: Chichester.

47 Harris BL, Stergachis A, Reid DL (1990) The effect of drug copayments on utilisation and cost of pharmaceuticals in a Health Maintenance Organisation. *Medical Care.* **28**: 908–17.

48 Zwanziger J, Auerbach RR (1991) Evaluating PPO performance using prior expenditure data. *Medical Care.* **29**: 142–51.

49 Melnick GA and Zwanziger J (1988) Hospital behavior under competition and cost-containment policies: the California experience, 1980 to 1985. *Journal of the American Medical Association.* **260**: 2669–75.

50 Miller RH and Luft HS (1994) Managed care plan performance since 1980: a literature analysis. *Journal of the American Medical Association.* **271**(19): 1512–18.

51 Robinson JC (1996) Administered pricing and vertical integration in the hospital industry. *Journal of Law and Economics.* **39**(1): 357–78.

52 Gaskin DJ, Hadley J (1997) The impact of HMO penetration on the rate of hospital cost inflation, 1985–1993. *Inquiry.* **34**: 205–16.

53 Miller RH and Luft HS (2002) HMO plan performance update: an analysis of the literature, 1997–2001. *Health Affairs.* **21**: 63–86.

54 Bamezai A, Zwanziger J, Melnick GA, Mann JM (1999) Price competition and hospital cost growth in the United States (1989–1994). *Health Economics.* **8**(3): 233–43.

55 Dranove D, White WD (1994) Recent theory and evidence on competition in hospital markets. *Journal of Economics and Management Strategy.* **3**(1): 169–209.

56 Robinson JC (1991) HMO market penetration and hospital cost inflation in California. *Journal of the American Medical Association.* **266**(19): 2719–23.

57 Sullivan K (2001) On the 'efficiency' of managed care plans. *International Journal of Health Services.* **31**(1): 55–65.

58 Miller RH, Luft HS (1997) Does managed care lead to better or worse quality of care? *Health Affairs.* **16**(5): 7–25.

59 Kemper P, Reschovsky JD, Tu HT (1999) Do HMOs make a difference? Summary and implications. *Inquiry.* **36**: 419–25.

60 Dellana SA, Glascoff DW (2001) The impact of health insurance plan type on satisfaction with health care. *Health Care Management Review.* **26**(2): 33–46.

61 Ware JE, Bayliss MS, Rogers WH, Kosinski M, Tarlov AR (1996) Differences in 4-year health outcomes for elderly and poor, chronically ill patients treated in HMO and fee-for-service systems. *Journal of the American Medical Association.* **276**(13): 1039–47.

62 Ware JE Jr, Brook RH, Rogers WH, Keeler EB, Davies AR, Sherbourne CD, Goldberg GA, Camp P, Newhouse JP (1986) Comparison of health outcomes at a health maintenance organisation with those of fee-for-service care. *Lancet.* **1**: 1017–22.

63 Manning WG, Leibowitz A, Goldberg GA, Rogers WH, Newhouse JP (1984) A controlled trial of the effect of a prepaid group practice on use of services. *New England Journal of Medicine.* **310**: 1505–10.

64 Manning WG, Newhouse JP, Guan N, Keeler EB, Leibowitz A, Marguis MS (1987) Health insurance and the demand for medical care: evidence from a randomised experiment. *American Economic Review*. **77**: 251–77.

65 Wagner EH, Bledsoe T (1990) The Rand Health Insurance Experiment and HMOs. *Medical Care*. **28**: 191–200.

66 Coleman EA, Kramer AM, Kowalsky JC, Eckhof D, Lin M, Hester EJ, Morgenstern N, Steiner JF (2000) A comparison of functional outcomes after hip fracture in group/staff HMOs and fee-for-service systems. *Effective Clinical Practice*. **4**: 229–39.

67 Getchell WS, Larsen GC, Morris CD, McAnulty JH (2000) A comparison of medicare fee-for-service and a group-model HMO in the inpatient management and long-term survival of elderly individuals with syncope. *The American Journal of Managed Care*. **6**: 1089–98.

68 Yelin EH, Criswell LA, Feigenbaum PG (1996) Healthcare utilisation and outcomes among persons with rheumatoid arthritis in fee-for-service and prepaid group practice settings. *Journal of the American Medical Association*. **276**(13): 1048–53.

69 Retchin SM, Brown RS, Yeh S-C J, Chu D, Moreno L (1997) Outcomes of stroke patients in medicare fee for service and managed care. *Journal of the American Medical Association*. **278**(2): 119–24.

70 Experton B, Ozminkowski RJ, Pearlman DN, Li Z, Thompson S (1999) How does managed care manage the frail elderly? *American Journal of Preventive Medicine*. **16**(3): 163–72.

71 Berki SE, Ashcraft M, Penchansky R, Fortus R (1977) Enrollment choice in a multi-HMO setting: the roles of health risk, financial vulnerability, and access to care. *Medical Care*. **15**: 95–114.

72 Buchanan JL, Cretin S (1986) Risk selection of families electing HMO membership. *Medical Care*. **24**: 39–51.

73 Juba DA, Lave JR, Shaddy J (1980) An analysis of the choice of health benefits plans. *Inquiry*. **17**: 62–71.

74 Moser WL (1987) The evolution of healthcare delivery in American industry. *Geneva Papers on Risk and Insurance*. **12**(45): 297–307.

75 Porell FW, Turner WM (1990) Biased selection under an experimental enrollment and marketing Medicare HMO broker. *Medical Care*. **28**: 604–15.

76 Schaefer E, Reschovsky JD (2002) Are HMO enrollees healthier than others? Results from a community tracking study. *Health Affairs*. **21**: 249–58.

77 Burns L, Wholey D (1991) Differences in access and quality of care across HMO types. *Health Services Management Research*. **4**: 32–44.

78 Reschovsky JD, Kemper P, Tu H (2000) Does type of health insurance affect healthcare use and assessments of care among the privately insured? *Health Services Research*. **35**(1): 220–37.

79 Morrisey MA (2001) Competition in hospital and health insurance markets: a review and research agenda. *Health Services Research*. **36**(1 Pt 2): 191–221.

80 Robinson JC, Luft HS (1988) Competition, regulation, and hospital costs, 1982 to 1986. *Journal of the American Medical Association*. **260**: 2676–81.

81 Zwanziger J, Melnick GA, Bamezai A (2000) The effect of selective contracting on hospital costs and revenues. *Health Services Research*. **35**(4): 849–67.

82 Zwanziger J, Melnick GA, Bamezai A (1994) Costs and price competition in California Hospitals, 1980–1990. *Health Affairs*. **13**(4): 118–26.

83 Mobley LR (1998) Effects of selective contracting on hospital efficiency, costs and accessibility. *Health Economics*. **7**(3): 247–61.

84 Cubellis J (1997) *Selective Contracting and Hospital Quality under Managed Care: an empirical analysis of network open-heart surgery hospital in California over time*. Irvine, CA: University of California.

85 Altman DE, Levitt L (2002) The sad history of healthcare cost containment as told in one chart. *Health Affairs (Web exclusive* W83). Available at URL http://content.health affairs.org/cgi/

86 Lee JS, Tollen L (2002) How low can you go? The impact of reduced benefits and increased cost sharing. *Health Affairs (Web exclusive* W229–W241). Available at URL http://content.healthaffairs.org/cgi/

87 Robinson R (2002) Managed care in the United States: a dilemma for evidence-based policy? *Health Economics.* **9**: 1–7.

88 Robinson R, Steiner A (1998) *Managed Health Care.* Buckingham: Open University Press.

89 Aiken LH, Clarke SP, Sloane DM, Sochalski J, Silber JH (2002) Hospital nurse staffing and patient mortality, nurse burnout and job satisfaction. *Journal of the American Medical Association.* **288**: 1987–93.

90 Needleman J, Buerhaus P, Mattke S, Stewart M, Zelevinsky K (2002) Nurse-staffing levels and the quality of care in hospitals. *New England Journal of Medicine.* **346**: 1715–22.

91 Kohn LT, Corrigan JM, Donaldson MS (eds) (2000) *To Err is Human: building a safer health system.* Committee on Quality of Health Care in America, Institute of Medicine. Washington, DC: National Academy Press.

92 Kwon S (1997) Payment systems for providers in health insurance markets. *Journal of Risk and Uncertainty.* **64**: 155–73.

93 Draper DA, Hurley RE, Lesser CS, Strunk BC (2002) The changing face of managed care. *Health Affairs.* **21**: 11–23.

94 Cunningham R, Sherlock DB (2002) Bounceback: Blues thrive as markets cool towards HMOs. *Health Affairs.* **21**: 24–38.

95 Bond P, Weissman R (1997) The costs of mergers and acquisitions in the US healthcare sector. *International Journal of Health Services.* **27**(1): 77–87.

96 Town R, Vistnes G (2001) Hospital competition in HMO networks. *Journal of Health Economics.* **20**(5): 733–53.

97 Enthoven AC, Schauffler HH, McMenamin S (2001) Consumer choice and the managed care backlash. *American Journal of Law and Medicine.* **27**: 1–15.

98 Le Grand J (1999) Competition, cooperation or control? Tales from the British National Health Service. *Health Affairs.* **18**: 27–39.

99 Enthoven AC (2003) Employment-based health insurance is failing: now what? *Health Affairs (Web exclusive* W237–W249). Available at URL http://content.healthaffairs.org/cgi/

Endnotes

i In private (and, to a lesser extent, some public) systems an element of 'consumer power' still exists, or seems to be believed in, as on an annual basis, consumers choose which insurer or other collective purchaser will represent them. This may be more apparent than real, however, as when faced with rising healthcare costs in the late 1980s and early 1990s, many employers in the US have been described as having 'herded their employees into managed care'.[2]

ii Much of the evidence cited here stems from the work we have conducted in updating our book, *Economics of Health Care Financing: the visible hand*.[3] When first published, there was not much evidence and, therefore, ability to draw conclusions about purchasing innovations in healthcare. However, through the 1990s and early 2000s, much more research has been conducted on purchasing innovations in both public and private systems, allowing for slightly less tentative conclusions than before!

iii In New Zealand and Sweden, health authorities could purchase GP services.[11,12] This was not the case in the UK, where most GPs were eventually established as 'rival' purchasers to health authorities (see below). In New Zealand, GPs were given control over budgets for drugs and laboratory procedures.[13] A further innovation in New Zealand was that individuals could take their share of public funding and place it in a healthcare plan, thus establishing another sort of 'rival' purchaser to health authorities.[12] However, this last innovation did not really take off in any appreciable fashion, largely because of a lack of awareness among the public that it was a possibility and a general apathy towards it.

iv It is thought that the main proponent of HMOs, Professor Alain Enthoven of Stanford University, provided the stimulus to the UK reforms, when he reviewed the UK healthcare system in the mid-1980s.[14] In a more recent monograph, he (rightly) attributes the idea for GP fundholding to Alan Maynard (editor of this book and Professor of Health Economics at the University of York).[15]

v With FFS remuneration doctors are paid a fee for each item of service provided to patients. For example, for a surgeon, an 'item of service' may be defined as a particular operation carried out. A radiologist may receive a fee for reading a mammogram, and a GP for a consultation or for providing a more specific item of service like a vaccination. The more services provided, the higher the doctor's income.

vi Many of these people will not be poor enough to qualify for Medicaid, which means they would be left without public or private coverage.

Chapter 4

The public–private mix in the UK

Rudolf Klein

Introduction

One of the distinguishing characteristics of the British system of healthcare is the relatively high proportion of total spending that is publicly financed and, conversely, the relatively small share that is privately funded.[1,2 i] This characteristic is in common with most of Scandinavia and other countries that have tax-funded national health services, but in sharp contrast with those of European and other countries which have more pluralistic, social insurance-based systems, as well as that eccentric example of exceptionalism – the United States. The percentage ratio of public and private spending is 83:17 in the UK as against 69:31 in the Netherlands, 70:30 in Australia and Canada, and 76:24 in France and Germany. Indeed, if public expenditure on healthcare alone is considered, in 1998 the UK government was already close to achieving its target of matching the EU average level of spending, i.e. even before the Prime Minister, Tony Blair, committed it to a dramatic expansion in the rate of spending in January 2000. UK public spending on healthcare in 1998 represented 5.7% of gross domestic product (GDP) as against the unweighted EU average of 5.9%. Given the acceleration of public spending since then, the UK is not so far off the higher, weighted EU average of 6.4%. If Britain still appears to be a laggard in terms of healthcare expenditure, and if the funding issue dominated decisions and debate in the Chancellor of the Exchequer's budget in 2002, it is in large part because private spending remains conspicuously lower: 1.1% of GDP as against an EU average of 2.0% (unweighted) or 2.1% (weighted).

This statistical overture might suggest two rather different conclusions. The first is that the private sector is – in line with the spending figures – relatively unimportant in the wider context of healthcare provision in the UK. The second is that if Britain's health services are indeed inadequate as a result of decades of underfunding – a view that has come to be accepted by the Blair Government and is now the conventional wisdom – it is because of a policy failure to promote private spending on healthcare.

The facts, as we shall see, are more complicated: political significance cannot be read off the fiscal scale. For the story has its roots in the history of the National Health Service, which was created in 1948 in a national spasm of innocent idealism. The giant of Disease – like the giants of Want, Ignorance, Squalor and Idleness – was, in the words of the Beveridge report, to be slain.[3 ii] Moreover, there was a widespread feeling – reflecting not just the ideology of the Labour Party but a wider social consensus born of shared wartime experiences – that not only should healthcare be free at the point of delivery but that even to talk about money was to risk corrupting the principles of the NHS. Interest in the costs of the

NHS, and how to meet them, was conspicuous by its absence in the run-up to the launch of the service.[4][iii] There was no debate about the role of private spending or the private sector; why indeed should there be, given that the NHS was supposed to provide a free, universal and comprehensive service to the whole population? In effect, the NHS was born in a state of fiscal virginity and there were many determined to defend that state. The fiscal chastity of the NHS and of healthcare more generally has been compromised over time, but it has been compromised by inadvertence rather than by intent, which is why the public–private mix that has developed in the UK over the decades is the product of ideology, political expediency and professional self-interest, not of deliberate design or economic logic.

This chapter will, therefore, first set out the evolutionary history of the public–private mix in the UK healthcare system: the path taken in 1948 which still determines, to a surprisingly large degree, present policy markers.[5][iv] The following section will then examine the current situation in greater detail, while the final section will turn to more general policy issues raised by the co-existence of the NHS and a private sector as well as the changing government policies about the relationship between the two. In all this, we shall be discussing a peculiarly British compromise – one that has achieved a large degree of distributional equity but at the expense, it may be argued, of social solidarity.

The age of innocence

At the root of the 1948 settlement there was tension. On the one hand, private practice was institutionalised in the NHS, and on the other, the NHS's first article of faith was that the delivery of healthcare should be divorced from the ability to pay. This section explores the translation of both notions into policy and practice over time. We also distinguish, of course, between private payments for privately provided services (like consultant fees) and private payments towards publicly provided services (like prescription charges) – a conventional distinction in the analysis of spending on healthcare – leaving it to the next section to complete the picture by attaching figures to the different funding streams, including the public purchase of private healthcare. The flows of funding are set out in Figure 4.1.

		Funding	
		Public	Private
Provision	Public	A 63%	C 3%
	Private	B 19%	D 15%

Figure 4.1 The public–private mix of funding and provision: percentage of total spending on healthcare falling into different categories.

The principle enshrined in the NHS, from its launch, was that all doctors should have the right to engage in private practice. Commitment to the NHS, whether as a salaried hospital consultant or as a contracted GP, would not preclude private practice though in both cases there were and are (as we shall see) conditions limiting the exercise of that right. Given the difficulties Aneurin Bevan faced in persuading a suspicious, largely hostile medical profession to accept the NHS,[4,6] any other solution would have been one battle too many, endangering the whole project. After all, private practice had been the norm for most doctors and any attempt to circumscribe its exercise would most certainly have reinforced professional paranoia. However, there were worries, both among Bevan's Cabinet colleagues and among Labour backbench MPs, about the perpetuation of a two-standard system. As one Labour MP put it in the first debate on the NHS Bill: 'When everyone is entitled to free service, it is difficult to see why anyone should want to go to a doctor outside the public service unless he expects a better standard of service than that which the doctor usually gives to his public service patients'.[7] In the Cabinet discussions preceding this debate, Bevan's reply to similar points was that he appreciated 'the importance of avoiding any impression that better treatment might be obtained privately than within the National Service. The remedy was to provide and maintain a very high standard of treatment under the National Service',[8] a hopeful formula that was to be repeated many times by his successors. So, notwithstanding reservations, the 1948 settlement confirmed the marriage of public and private medicine.

The terms of cohabitation were also prescribed at this time. Consultants could opt either for whole-time contracts or for part-time contracts, which left them free to engage in private practice (while still collecting most of their NHS salary). At the inception of the NHS, three-quarters opted for the latter,[9] a figure that was to decline subsequently. GPs could treat patients privately, but could not commute between private and NHS treatment for the same patient (e.g. by writing NHS prescriptions for private patients). Also, as part of the 1948 settlement, hospitals set aside 'pay beds' where consultants could treat their private patients and collect their own fees. This risked, as Bevan conceded,[10] creating a 'two-tier system' but, he claimed, had the advantage of giving the consultants an incentive to carry out their private practice in NHS hospitals rather than taking themselves off to private nursing homes. These pay beds must be distinguished from the so-called amenity beds (usually in single-occupancy rooms rather than wards) where NHS patients paid for privacy but not for treatment, a facility that the NHS, in contrast to many other healthcare systems, never promoted or developed on any scale, possibly because of the lack of financial incentives to hospitals. In the event, some 6600 pay beds were designated in 1949 (just over 1% of all the NHS beds). Subsequently, with occupancy rates by private patients hovering around the 50% mark, the number of pay beds declined steadily and by the end of the 1960s it was down to 4350.[11]

Demonstrating the lack of symmetry between statistical and political trends, the decline in the number of pay beds was accompanied by an increase in the political salience of the issue of private practice within the NHS.[12] In 1972, the Employment and Social Services Sub-Committee of the House of Commons Expenditure Committee[11 v] listed the potential abuses inherent in the system of pay beds, though without the ability to quantify their scale. The report's conclusions are worth noting if only to underline how little has changed in the 30 years since it was written. Many of its criticisms were to be echoed in another Parliamentary report[13] published in the new millennium, and if the criticisms remain unchanged, so has the difficulty of establishing the scale of the abuse. The system, the Sub-Committee claimed, gave consultants an incentive to build up their waiting lists in order to divert patients to their private practices, leading to the neglect of their NHS responsibilities. It encouraged queue jumping and led to the exploitation of nurses, junior doctors and other hospital staff. Further, the Sub-Committee argued, the NHS had failed to develop any adequate mechanism for the identification and control of abuse. While stopping short of recommending the total expulsion of private practice from the NHS, it proposed a greater degree of control, changes in consultant contracts designed to provide incentives to engage in NHS rather than private work and, for the longer-term future, 'measures to establish a clear and comprehensive division between the two sectors'.[13]

Evidence on the extent of abuse may have been inadequate and inconclusive in 1972 and, indeed, remains so. However, this did not stop the advance of ideological militancy concerning the issue, reflecting the ever-increasing influence of left-wing radicalism (of the Marxist variety) within the Labour Party and the trade union movement. In 1974, as Harold Wilson's Labour Government took office, a series of rank-and-file strikes against pay beds broke out, most prominent in London and so assured of media attention. Prompted by this pressure Mrs Barbara Castle, the Secretary of State for Health, introduced legislation to phase out pay beds from the NHS. Justifying her policies, in response to the all-out opposition of the medical profession, she said, 'Intrinsically the National Health Service is a church. It is the nearest thing to the embodiment of the Good Samaritan that we have in any aspect of our public policy. What would we say of a person who argued that he could only serve God properly if he had pay pews in his church?'

Mrs Castle's position may have been ideological; so was that of the medical profession for whom private practice was a symbol of independence, reflecting their status as professionals as distinct from hired hands. However, strong self-interest reinforced ideology. Any threat to private practice was seen as a threat to income. Rough estimates suggest that at the time of the great pay bed battle, part-time consultants earned some 20% more than their full-time colleagues (while, in the case of general practice, private practice and other freelance activities added only some 10%). Further, the medical profession saw the pay beds issue in the context of a wider strategy by the government to limit the scope and attractiveness of private practice in negotiations about the consultant contract. Hence the mobilisation of the medical profession against Mrs Castle's proposals.

The details of the battle are of no concern here. Nor is the immediate outcome, which was a negotiated compromise: pay beds were to be phased out only to the extent that there was alternative provision in the independent sector of healthcare, with a new regulatory machinery for supervising both the phasing out and the construction of private hospitals. The legislation had hardly come into effect when Labour was replaced by Mrs Thatcher's Conservative Government, ideologically sympathetic to private practice, which immediately reversed the policies of its predecessor. Phasing out pay beds and regulating the mix of public and private facilities was abandoned. Instead of changing the consultant contract to strengthen incentives for full-time commitment to the NHS, the right to engage in private practice was extended to all consultants – whether on a full- or part-time contract. The only restriction was that full-time consultants were barred from earning more than 10% of the value of their NHS income through private practice.

The real significance of the confrontation between the Labour Government and the medical profession is rather different. First, it demonstrated that the result of institutionalising private practice in the NHS in 1948 was subsequently to create a strong professional self-interest in maintaining the status quo. Second, it showed that the combination of professional ideology and self-interest was a potent political force, strong enough to force a governmental retreat. Third, and of most importance, the confrontation was to have an unexpected – and from Labour's point of view perverse – result: it marked the beginning of an era of rapid expansion of private medical care throughout most of the 1980s. Pay beds, which had been so central in the 1970s, soon came to be seen as an irrelevant side issue as independent hospitals proliferated, private insurance boomed and private practice incomes for NHS consultants rose in the following decade.

The situation created will be analysed in the next section, but here it is worth noting a puzzle. Just why did private medicine expand? Government policies provide at best a partial explanation. Labour's strategy may have prompted the medical profession to take out an insurance policy by developing private hospitals as an alternative to their NHS facilities. Conservative changes to the consultant contract may have increased the number of doctors with an incentive to create a market for their goods. However, the main (speculative) explanations point to other factors. On the one hand, the rise in private practice can be interpreted as evidence of the NHS's failure to provide the 'very high standard of treatment' which Bevan saw as the best way of heading off the emergence of a two-tier healthcare system. On this interpretation, private practice provides a barometer of private satisfaction or dissatisfaction with the NHS, and dissatisfaction with the NHS[14] may have grown in line with rising expectations in a consumerist-orientated society, where not only the expectations but also the financial capacity to satisfy them was increasing. On the other hand, both income and tax policies gave employers an incentive to reward their workforce by providing them with private insurance coverage, in much the same way as they provided them with cars or other perks. This explanation is all the more plausible given that it was collective rather than individual insurance policies that increased most from the end of the 1970s onward.

But private practice was not the only element to be incorporated into the institutional structure of the NHS in 1948. More importantly and more significantly for the long-term future, was the notion that the NHS should be funded out of general taxation. While the social security system was to be financed, following Beveridgean orthodoxy, predominantly from national insurance contributions, the position was reversed in the case of the NHS. A specifically labelled 'NHS contribution' element was incorporated into the national insurance scheme. But this was a notional element, never perceived to be a source of finance for the NHS independent of the tax system by the public and by fiscal policy makers, although the latter flirted briefly with putting more reliance on contributions in the 1960s. At the start of the service, the NHS contribution accounted for 9.8% of total funding, rising to a peak of 17.2% in the early 1960s, and then gradually falling over the years to below the 10% mark.

That the method of funding inhibited the development of the service was acknowledged from the start. The NHS had to compete for resources with education, housing and other public services within budgets constrained by the desire of all governments to avoid losing elections by raising taxes and largely shaped by a series of economic crises in the 1950s, 1960s and 1970s. Further, the ability of Ministers of Health to argue for more generous settlements in the annual rounds of public spending negotiations was weakened by the experience of the years immediately after the launch of the NHS, when the budget set for the service was regularly and spectacularly exceeded. The 'spendthrift' image of the NHS took a long time to exorcise:[15 vi] expenditure fell in real terms throughout the 1950s and only gradually started to rise in the 1960s. Even so, it is worth noting that despite the parsimony with which the NHS was treated in the 1950s, Britain's public spending on healthcare in 1960 was the highest, at 3.4% of GDP, among OECD countries. Only Sweden matched Britain's record,[16] but the picture changed when it came to total expenditure on healthcare, taking private spending into account. Britain then emerged as a laggard (3.9% of GDP) compared to, for example, Germany (4.8%), Sweden (4.7%) and France (4.3%). In short, the future pattern had already been set in concrete by 1960, and Britain never deviated from its chosen path over the coming 40 years even while evidence accumulated that the NHS was no longer the envy of the world.

The evidence, in turn, prompted challenges to the existing fiscal foundations of the NHS. By the early 1960s, economists were quoting Bevan's dictum 'If we were rich enough, we would not want to have free medical services, we would pay the doctor' and arguing that Britain had reached a stage of affluence where individuals should be encouraged to make private provision for medical care.[17] Others sought to demonstrate that the system of public funding did not accurately reflect individual preferences, and that tapping people's willingness to pay directly would produce a more generous system of healthcare.[18] Even former Labour Ministers – witnesses of the annual blood bath of hopes involved in the public expenditure review – were suggesting that other forms of funding should be considered.[19] The British Medical Association (BMA), too, flirted briefly with the idea of moving towards an insurance-based system. A BMA panel recommended such a system,[20] but this never became official BMA policy. These notions, naturally enough, were most appealing to Conservative governments with a commitment to halting the rise in public expenditure. In 1970 the incoming Heath Administration set up a working group to examine possible alternative methods of financing health and welfare services. It concluded that any substantial switch from public to private provision 'would increase the cost and would reduce the effectiveness of public services', and that there was 'very limited scope for any changes whose benefits would outweigh the practical difficulties to which they would give rise'.[21]

Ten years later, with the arrival of the Thatcher Government, there was a brief flurry of interest in alternative sources of funding, but a tour of the European countries by an official produced a sceptical report, which denied the advocates of change any ammunition. And even Mrs Thatcher's review of the NHS in the late 1980s did not resurrect the notion, despite her ideological bias towards promoting market solutions – as demonstrated by her insistence, over the dead body of the Treasury, that private insurance contributions by the over-60s should be tax exempt.[6] This reluctance to contemplate any basic change in the method of funding healthcare was perhaps all the more surprising given that Mrs Thatcher did not shy away from a radical reorganisation of the NHS, introducing the so-called internal market in 1991. But while the reorganisation of the NHS aroused the ire of the medical profession and others working in the service, it did not directly affect the pockets of the population at large. In contrast, the earlier leakage of a report by the Central Policy Review staff setting out options for change in the financing of public services (including the replacement of part of the NHS by compulsory private insurance) had produced howls of outrage, not least among Cabinet Ministers, prompting a public repudiation of the proposal by the Prime Minister,[22] thereby closing off this option. Nor was there any pressure from powerful interest groups, as distinct from pamphleteers, to move in this direction. By the 1980s the BMA, whatever its earlier reservations about the NHS, had become a fervent defender of the status quo. Industry did not advocate radical change: the existence of a tax-funded NHS allowed them to offer their employees private insurance as an extra perk on the cheap (see below). In short, both the constellation of interests and electoral calculation argued against radicalism. Even incremental change would, given the high political visibility and salience of the NHS, be politically dangerous.

Amidst all this, there was a surprising continuity in the arguments deployed. Not only was tax funding an efficient way of raising the money but also much cheaper, it was frequently pointed out, than complex social insurance schemes, let alone private insurance as in the US. It was also more equitable than the alternatives. Moreover, as the 1978 Royal Commission on the NHS pointed out in 1979,[23] any radical change would 'mean a great deal of upheaval'. The onus, then, was on the advocates of change to demonstrate that benefits would outweigh costs. And much the same themes appeared in the 2001 report of an inquiry commissioned by Labour's Chancellor of the Exchequer endorsing the existing system of funding the NHS and rejecting any adoption of social insurance or other models.[1] Funding out of general taxation remained the preferred system even though, as the 2001 report argued, the NHS had always been chronically underfunded. That there might be a link between the method and level of funding was not considered. The fact that over the decades, as the report demonstrated, the year-by-year funding of the NHS had fluctuated erratically in line with political calculation and economic cycles was not seen as being in any way related to (far less a weakness of) the funding structure.

In the case of the Labour Government, rational argument buttressed an ideological position. In the case of Conservative governments, it might be said, that ideology was forced to submit to rational argument. But all this presumes that Britain had miraculously found the best way of funding healthcare in 1948; not a sustainable assumption. Other reasons for the persistence of the 1948 model have to be found. One such is, of course, the non-heroic but pragmatically sensible argument of the 1979 Royal Commission: once a particular system has taken root, the disturbance costs of change may outweigh potential benefits. While the costs of change are certain, the benefits may be problematic. In addition, any costs will be immediate, concentrated and highly visible, involving dislocation and possibly demoralisation in existing services, while future benefits will be dispersed among countless patients and taxpayers. So there is a rational case for preserving a less-than-ideal or second-best status quo: for making a virtue of path dependency.

More importantly, the 1948 model of funding the NHS served the interest of the most powerful department in British government: the Treasury. For the Treasury, the great enduring appeal of the 1948 model NHS was precisely that it was the most parsimonious healthcare system in the advanced industrialised world – an effective tool of economic management, where the tap could be turned on in good times and off in bad times. From the Treasury's perspective, complaints about inadequate funding represented a compliment rather than a criticism: they demonstrated that the Treasury was doing its job in controlling costs and squeezing more productivity out of the service. Conversely, from the Treasury's perspective, the arguments that different systems of funding would produce more money for healthcare represented a threat rather than a hopeful vision. It was only at the turn of the 20th century that the rising political costs of continued frugality forced the Treasury to accept that the economic costs of the NHS would have to rise.

Short of radical change to the funding model, there was another way of lessening the NHS's dependence on tax revenue: co-payment by the healthcare consumer. Here we encounter another of the foundation principles of the NHS, which continued to be part of Labour's ideological baggage into the 21st century: it should be free at the point of delivery. As Tony Blair put it during the general election of 2001: ' If you are paying for basic healthcare, you are in breach of fundamental principles of the health service . . . I don't believe as a matter of principle that the NHS should be charging'.[24] Nonetheless, successive Labour governments compromised their principles. In response to growing budgetary pressure in 1950 the Labour Government introduced charges for prescriptions, dental treatment and spectacles, precipitating the resignation of Bevan. Subsequent Labour governments came to office committed to abolishing charges but, persuaded that the cost of so doing would be at the expense of more urgent public spending priorities, came to accept them if only reluctantly and slightly shame-facedly.

Conservative governments had no ideological predisposition against charges. If anything, their bias was towards increasing them. And so they did. When Labour left office in 1951, charges accounted for less than 1% of the NHS's total budget. By the early 1960s, the figure had peaked at 5.6%. Thereafter followed a long decline initiated by Labour administrations but not substantially reversed by Conservative governments, apart from an upward hiccup at the turn of the 1980s. By the time Labour replaced the Conservatives in office in 1997, the figure was down to 2.3%.[23,25] Political expediency may provide one explanation: charges were, and remain, highly visible. But institutionalised notions of administrative feasibility, developed by successive generations of civil servants and policy makers in the NHS, may be a more important factor. There was general agreement that if charges were not to impede access to needed care, thereby not only discriminating against the poorest but also adding to the future burden of illness, there had to be a system of exemptions – whence flowed a dilemma. If a system of exemptions was fine-grained (i.e. relating the charges closely to the individual's capacity to pay), the administrative costs would be high. Conversely, if the system of exemptions was coarse-grained (i.e. applying to categories rather than individuals) the administrative costs would be low but so would be the revenue.

Early in the history of the NHS, the choice fell on exemption by categories. Wide swathes of the population – pensioners, those on social security and sufferers from certain chronic conditions – were automatically exempted from charges. Administratively, this appeared to be a neat and cheap solution, but once institutionalised, this system constrained future policy. First, it ensured that the yield would be low. By the turn of the century, 85% of all prescriptions were issued free of charge. Second, it meant that in order to generate more than trivial revenue, the charges would have to be relatively high for those who actually paid them – in effect, a steep marginal tax rate with a disproportionate impact on those on low incomes but not included in the exempt categories. Third, it led to the semi-automatic rejection of the regularly made proposals for extending charges to visits to GPs or stays in hospital (normal practice in many countries), partly because of the technical difficulties of devising a system that was both fair and capable of raising significant revenues, partly because of the political costs of any change. As with private practice in the NHS, or the service's dependence on tax revenue rather than national insurance, the system of co-payments is the product of a complex chemical interaction between ideology, administrative inertia, political expediency and economic imperatives.

Much the same is true of institutional long-term healthcare for the elderly, where there has been a largely unintended revolution in the balance between NHS and private provision. Originally, the NHS was the dominant provider of such care. As late as the mid-1970s, there were twice as many NHS geriatric beds as nursing home places (traditionally nursing homes have been run by either for-profit or voluntary providers). Twenty years later, there were four times as many beds in the private as in the public sector.[26][vii] The transformation came about as the by-product of an administrative tidying up of the supplementary benefit rules by the Department of Health and Social Security (as it then was) in 1983. In effect, though not in intent, a system of discretionary payments to those already in private homes was transformed into a system of entitlements for those looking for care.[27] The only test was financial: provided that the applicant met the social security system's criteria of financial need, support followed automatically. Individuals were given an incentive to go into residential care, whatever their state of health, as distinct from seeking help in the community. And more importantly, NHS authorities and hospitals were given an opportunity to decant the inhabitants of geriatric (and psychiatric) wards into nursing homes, switching the financial burden of long-term institutional care to the open-ended social security budget. There followed the run-down of NHS facilities and explosive growth in the private sector. If anything, the Conservative Government welcomed the growth of private provision as very much in harmony with its ideological bias. However, appalled by the runaway fiscal costs, it changed tack at the start of the 1990s and introduced a capped budget, administered by local authorities. Eligibility was to be determined not just by financial resources but also by clinical and social criteria of need. But by then there had been a decisive shift towards the private provision, albeit largely publicly funded, of long-term institutional care.

In summary, no consistent strategy or philosophy guided the evolution of Britain's mix of public–private provision and funding. It was, in fact, determined by the structure of interests created in 1948 and by institutionalised assumptions about what was economically desirable, administratively feasible and politically advisable. The next section analyses the results of this process of muddling through, setting the scene as it looked at the turn of the millennium.

Funders, providers and professionals: the picture now

As we saw in Figure 4.1, public funds are the dominant source of finance for healthcare in Britain (cells A+B). Not all the public funds are absorbed by the NHS itself: quite a high proportion (cell B) is channelled to private providers and private contractors of specific services. The figure of 19% is misleadingly exaggerated to the extent that general practitioners are included as private providers, since they are not salaried employees of the NHS but work on contract. As against this, the figures understate the public funds channelled to private providers of long-term nursing home care, since these come in large part out of either the social security or local authority budget. However, the relative unimportance of private payments for NHS services (cell C) – prescription charges, pay beds – is unambiguously confirmed by the figures. This section will analyse first the flows of funding from, and the relationship between, the NHS and the private acute sector, then examine the privately funded/privately provided sector (cell D) and the benefits flowing to the medical profession, before analysing the policy changes introduced by the Labour Government.

The level of spending in cells B and D reflects a series of developments that started in the 1980s under a Conservative government and were maintained, against all expectations, in the 1990s and thereafter under a Labour government. Some of these have already been noted in the previous section, e.g. the unplanned torrent of public funding of residents in private long-term institutions (included in cell B), subsequently restrained. Second, there was the largely spontaneous growth of the private acute sector (cell D), spontaneous in as far as it predated the only government policies aimed at promoting it (tax concessions for the over-60s as noted above) and was scarcely dented by the subsequent abolition of this subsidy. There were, in addition, some specific government initiatives, starting in the 1980s, designed to enlarge the role of the private sector – initiatives which reflected general governmental policy rather than being designed specifically for the NHS. Hospitals (like other public services) were encouraged to contract out specific, non-clinical services, notably cleaning, catering and laundry (also included in cell B). And in 1992 the Conservative Government's Private Finance Initiative (PFI) was launched in the NHS. This scheme was designed to circumvent Treasury restrictions on capital spending in the public sector by contracting out the building and non-clinical services of hospitals and other facilities to the private sector. PFI spending does not appear in Figure 4.1, since it involves capital rather than current spending. Suffice it to note that PFI continues to attract criticism,[28] and not just from those who see any involvement of the private sector in the NHS as an ideological affront to its principles. While in theory, PFI is designed to transfer risk to the private sector, in practice it is not clear that the NHS has the managerial capacity to make a success of the programme.

The most important change under the Conservative Government was the one which had the least immediate effect on the growth of the private sector but which ironically became increasingly significant under the successor Labour Government. The foundation stone of the 1991 reforms of the NHS – introducing the so-called internal market – was the separation of purchasing from provision. Purchasers, according to the rhetoric of reform, would be free to buy care from whatever source – including private providers. As with so many other aspects of the 1991 reforms, not much came of this: there was no dramatic switch of purchasing to the private sector. Subsequently, in another outburst of reform rhetoric, the new Labour Government 'abolished' the internal market. But the foundation stone remained in place. Purchasing and provider functions remained separate. And, as we shall see, it was a Labour government – performing an astonishing ideological somersault – which used purchasing from the private sector as an explicit tool of national policy. While at the end of the 1970s a Labour government had given an unplanned boost to the expansion of the private sector, at the beginning of the new millennium a Labour government deliberately sought to use it to promote the goals of public policy.

The growth of privately financed, privately provided acute healthcare (cell D), kick-started by the Labour Government in the 1970s, accelerated in the 1980s. Throughout the decade, spending on these services rose rapidly in real terms – by 29% in 1980 and over 36% in 1981, dropping to 16% the following year but never falling below 10% for the rest of the decade. In the 1990s, expenditure growth was sustained at between 4 and 7% a year,[29] and was mirrored in the growth of private hospital provision. This increased from 7000 beds (in 154 hospitals) in 1981 to a peak of 11 680 (in 227 hospitals) in 1995, declining thereafter. One reason for the decline may have been that NHS hospitals were exploiting the freedom they had been given to develop, and market energetically, profit-making private wings or wards. Throughout this period there has been much churning of ownership, with American and European for-profit chains moving in and out of the British market. But the net effect has been a change in the balance of ownership from non-profit providers to for-profit providers: the latter controlled 67% of beds in 2001, compared with 41% in 1979.[26]

Most of the private sector's acute activities are financed by insurance. The number of subscribers to private insurance schemes almost trebled between 1979 and 2000 – most of the rapid growth occurring in the 1980s, thereafter flattening out – rising from 1 292 000 to 3 685 000. The number of persons covered by these schemes increased from 5% of the UK population in 1980 to 11.5% in 2000.[26] Significantly, this upward trend reflected changing employment practices – i.e. the structure of reward packages for (mostly) the salariat – as much as individual demands for private healthcare insurance. Collective company schemes have driven the overall expansion, although self-financed private treatment remains significant. About a fifth of all treatment episodes in private hospitals are self-financed,[26] but this probably understates the scale of self-financed healthcare use. Information about payment for private outpatient consultations with doctors, let alone complementary or alternative practitioners (an expanding sector of activity), is conspicuously incomplete. Use of the private sector rises with social class and income,[30] and there is also a geographical bias. Even controlling for class and income, use of the private sector is highest in London and the South East and lowest in Scotland.

For the most part, private medical insurance (PMI) costs have run ahead of general inflation. Between 1991 and 2000, average annual real cost inflation was 2.5%[26] but the average annual PMI subscription remains, certainly by US standards, relatively modest. In 2000, it was £676 a year – rather less than the cost of buying a season ticket at a successful premiership football club. The figure, however, increases steeply with age and the reason for this is simple. Private practice is symbiotic with – it could even be said parasitic on – the NHS. The private acute sector is highly specialised, with elective surgery as its main business. For example, 20% or more of all varicose vein procedures, hernia repairs and hip-joint replacements are privately financed, while the proportion rises to nearly two-fifths for cosmetic operations.[31] It does not deal with medical emergencies – the kind of cases which fill NHS Accident & Emergency departments and beds. However, even those with private insurance coverage frequently use the NHS.[32] Those who have had a heart attack or suffered trauma after an accident will end up in an NHS hospital and, emergencies apart, will routinely consult their NHS GPs. In short, the insurance premiums are relatively modest because the private sector can rely on the NHS to pick up the tab for the most expensive procedures and patients, as well as most of the routine care.

The other reason for seeing the acute private sector as dependent on the public sector is, of course, that it relies on NHS consultants to do the work. Very few specialists work exclusively in the private sector, so the two-thirds of NHS consultants who engage in private practice have benefited handsomely from the expansion of this sector over the past two decades. In 1999, average net private income was estimated to be £75 000 for plastic surgeons and £59 000 for orthopaedic specialists at the top of the ladder, falling to less than £17 000 for psychiatrists and £8000 for pathologists. In the middle of the distribution, anaesthetists averaged £27 000 a year. There is much controversy about whether the fiscal attractions of private practice cause consultants to short-change their NHS employers. The evidence is clear that some do, but the unresolved question is the scale of abuse. As the House of Commons Health Committee recently concluded, lack of information makes it impossible 'to ascertain the extent to which consultants are failing to meet their NHS obligations because of their private practice'.[13,33,34 ix] To the extent that there is abuse, it reflects two more general NHS characteristics: poor information about the activities of clinicians and managerial timidity vis-à-vis consultants. There remains a reluctance, for example, to monitor why surgeons cancel NHS operating sessions (as likely to be because of an invitation to a conference in an attractive resort, funded by the pharmaceutical industry, as the lure of private practice). Similarly, poor information makes it difficult to determine whether consultants deliberately inflate their NHS waiting lists in order to encourage their patients to go private. Perverse incentives are undoubtedly inherent in the system but evidence about their impact is patchy and inconclusive.

Given the Government's decision to stake its reputation on bringing down waiting lists,[35] the private sector can be seen as either one of the causes of the problem or as a possible solution. It can be argued that if only consultants could be persuaded, bribed or compelled to devote their energies exclusively to the NHS, waiting lists would quickly dwindle: perverse incentives would be eliminated; more NHS operations would be carried out. The trouble with this argument is, of course, that consultant time is only one of the constraints on the output of elective surgery. Shortage of operating theatre time is another – the NHS is conspicuously inefficient in the way it uses existing facilities.[36] Add to that a strained bed capacity and it is not self-evident that diverting consultants from private to public practice, the Government's preferred strategy, would necessarily do the trick. In any case, this strategy has proved difficult to implement. At the end of 2002 consultants in England voted, by a two to one majority,[37] against a new contract with the profession which would have given managers both greater control over their working schedules and first option on any extra time they are prepared to work. (Interestingly in Scotland and Wales, where there is less private practice, the vote went the other way.) Subsequently, in October 2003, they accepted a much watered-down version of the contract,[38] the Government having retreated from the prospect of a head-on clash with the profession. However, even allowing for the constraint of competition for limited medical manpower, the private sector represents an opportunity to mobilise underused resources. Occupancy rates are low; many beds are empty; there is spare capacity in operating theatres.

Hence the dramatic reversal of policy by the Labour Government. After initially cold-shouldering the private sector on coming into office in 1997 (in line with traditional party ideology), the Government three years later enfolded it in a warm embrace. Having decided that extra billions of public funds would need to be poured into the NHS, the Government came up against the realisation that capacity, as much as money, was the main constraint on improving services in the short term (i.e. before the next General Election). Increasing the number of beds and recruiting more doctors and nurses into the NHS would take time. Meanwhile the private sector was beckoning. In line with New Labour's pragmatic philosophy – what counts is what works – Ministers embraced the private sector. The *NHS Plan*, published in 2000 soon after the Prime Minister's announcement of large increases in NHS funding, proclaimed a new era. 'For decades there has been a stand-off between the NHS and the private sector. This has to end', it asserted. 'Ideological boundaries or institutional barriers should not stand in the way of better care for NHS patients'.[39] Partnership was the new motto and a formal concordat was promptly signed between the Department of Health and the private sector, setting out a programme of cooperation on staffing and planning for the future.[40] As the Government's rhetorical commitment to promoting patient choice grew, so did its emphasis on using the private sector.[41] Patients faced with a last minute cancellation of their operation were given the option of choosing an alternative hospital, including a private one, for their treatment, as were heart patients who had waited longer than six months for their surgery. The Government not only encouraged the export of patients to private hospitals in Europe, but also proposed bringing overseas providers of healthcare to establish services for the NHS.[42] In 2002 an estimated 50 000–60 000 operations were being funded by the NHS in private sector facilities.[29] In effect, the Labour Administration was reinventing – in this as in other respects – the internal market that the party had in the past denounced bell, book and candle as a sign of the cloven foot.

The change was dramatic, but as Ministers rightly argued, it did not represent a threat to the founding principles of the NHS. Those principles, they stressed, required not a public monopoly of provision but public control of how tax-funded resources were used. Provided treatment continued to be free at the point of delivery, and that the same criteria were used in allocating patients to NHS or to private hospitals, no new issue of principle was involved. Whether, in fact, the NHS would prove more successful than in the past in contracting with the private sector – whether it had the necessary information about costs or the required managerial capacity – was, of course, another question, which remains to be answered. To date, the evidence as to whether the private sector provides value for money is inconclusive.[29]

The Government was not only moving towards a more pluralistic model of healthcare provision – though not funding – but it was also (for the first time since 1948) abandoning the identification of a principle with an institution. The various ministerial pronouncements represent a move towards thinking about a health-care system which embraces both the NHS and the private sector, though whether the consequences of so doing have been thought through is doubtful. However, in one limited respect, institutional fusion is already in train: there is to be a common regulatory regime for both the NHS and the private sector. The same agency – a beefed up version of the Commission for Health Improvement (CHI) – will be responsible for inspecting both sectors.[43] The logic is clear: public regulation, like public funds, will follow patients wherever they are treated. The new system will replace the very fragmented system of local regulation of private healthcare, whose effectiveness has frequently been questioned.[44] Unsurprisingly, this will leave unanswered questions about the regulation of the market for private health insurance, i.e. whether the existing system of consumer protection is adequate.[45] Unsurprisingly, because, for all the changes in the Government's thinking, it appears to have given little or no thought to what the proper role (if any) of privately financed private healthcare should be. The assumption appears to be, in line with Bevan's rhetoric, that if only the new, generously funded model healthcare system delivers the promised improvements, two-tierism will be a minor irritant rather than a major policy issue. The concluding section addresses this and other matters.

Issues and questions

In one respect, the NHS and the private sector have settled down to a successful, if unsanctified, partnership. The NHS does not threaten the private sector. The abolition of the private sector has never been on the political agenda; moreover, as already argued, the private sector would have to invent the NHS if it did not exist already. Conversely, the private sector does not threaten the NHS. There is little evidence in support of the notion that expanding opportunities for exit would undermine loyalty to the NHS – that growth of the private sector would undermine support for a universal service. Over the past 20 years the growth of the private sector has gone hand in hand with continued public endorsement of the principle of a health service for all, by something like four-fifths of the population, and rising support for more spending on the NHS.[46] Those with insurance coverage or using private care tend to be slightly – but only slightly – less supportive of the NHS than those who stick to the public sector. In one survey, 75% of the former opposed restricting the NHS to people with low incomes as against 81% of the latter.[32] Nor is there any evidence that the availability of the exit option weakens voice. The past 20 years have seen a steady upward trend in complaints and lawsuits: support for the argument that the possibility of switching from the NHS to the private sector empowers people to voice their grievances by removing the threat of retaliation.[47] Lastly, the NHS's success in keeping specialist salaries to a relatively modest level by international standards – thereby possibly saving billions over the decades – can be attributed, at least in part, to the ability of consultants to supplement their earnings by private practice – a benefit to set against the costs (in terms of perverse incentives and diverted energies).

But in one respect, the private sector undeniably poses a threat to the principles of the NHS: it represents a challenge to the notion that access to healthcare should be determined only by need. A considerable academic literature has grown up over the years, devoted to testing whether or not the NHS has achieved its equity goal in this respect. Overall, the evidence suggests that, in broad terms, it has done so. There remain methodological problems in interpreting the statistics; there are undoubtedly examples of a failure to match resources to need for specific procedures or communities.[48,49] Nevertheless, given that no healthcare system has achieved a perfect fit, the NHS is a remarkable success story by international standards. Hence, Britain's high ranking for fairness in the distribution of resources in WHO's (methodologically dubious in other respects but probably accurate in this case) assessment of health systems performance.[50]

In contrast to the NHS, privately financed healthcare appears to be inequitable by definition. Access is determined not by need but by the ability to pay. Its very *raison d'être* is to allow people to jump queues. If it did not enable people to queue jump and if it did not allow people to make sure that it is a consultant of their choice who operates on them, there would be very few takers, apart from those putting a high premium on hotel comfort. PMI is a way of buying privilege. If there is no privilege, why spend money on private healthcare? And we know that the ability to buy access through the private sector is, predictably, strongly associated with higher incomes and social class.[30] What we do not know – and there has been remarkably little discussion, analysis or research thereon – is the effect on the overall distribution of access, even though the direction of the effect is clear enough.

But equity is not an absolute value and neither is its definition self-evident. Not all inequalities are necessarily inequitable.[51] The private sector, as we have seen, deals predominantly (though not exclusively) with elective surgery rather than life-threatening conditions. Its activities are designed to improve quality of life rather than extending life. The same is true, of course, of many NHS activities. If it is accepted that disability may impose a cost on the individual concerned (earnings foregone, career disrupted) or on society (lost productivity), it might be argued that the NHS should give waiting list priority to those who require treatment in order to be able to go on working or to look after their families. Sometimes it does this, but the criteria used in managing waiting lists and deciding priorities are opaque. Contrariwise, if equity is defined to mean that the NHS must be blind to social or individual costs – if medically defined need is to be the only criterion – then some mechanism will be required to give weight to individual preferences and to social efficiency. In short, once it is accepted that there is a trade-off between competing values, it is possible to mount a principled case for a supplementary private market in healthcare alongside the NHS.

It is well beyond the scope (or purpose) of this chapter to make such a case. The aim has merely been to suggest that such a case could be made and indeed that it should be made as part of a debate designed to clarify the issues created by private healthcare. In particular, it is important to disaggregate both the notion of equity and the activities of the private sector: to ask which activities of the private sector raise specific issues of equity. For example, as noted above, over 38% of cosmetic operations are privately funded. In the case of gender reassignment, the proportion of privately funded operations rises to 70%.[31] These figures reflect the policies of NHS purchasers who have tended to exclude such procedures from their list of priorities,[52] and because they do so, they do not cause acute worries about equity. To the extent that the private sector is supplementary to the NHS – as distinct from providing a quicker route to the same set of services – so equity concerns appear to diminish. Again, the ability to buy access to complementary medicine, to turn to an osteopath or aromatherapist, is unequally distributed, as is the ability to buy over-the-counter medicines or heat pads for one's back. All these make a considerable contribution to the billions spent on privately financed healthcare, but they do not cause concern about equity, perhaps because there is no medically-sanctioned evidence about the effectiveness of such interventions. The moral may be that equity considerations about the distribution of access – whether in the NHS or in the private sector – do not arise in the absence of evidence about effectiveness: inequalities in the distribution of snake oil do not cause moral anguish. And to the extent that the NHS sets a limit on its activities – whether as a result of evidence about lack of effectiveness or simply as a response to an explosion of new therapies coming onto the market – so there may be a growing supplementary role for privately financed healthcare.

Such a growth would, in fact, be compatible with fiscal, as distinct from distributional, equity. Private spending on healthcare is highly progressive. Household expenditure on healthcare, as a proportion of the household income, rises from 0.9% for the lowest decile to 2.9% for the fifth decile and 8.4% for the highest decile.[44] These figures indicate both the generosity of the exemption system for prescription charges and the skewed nature of spending on private healthcare. Hence the conclusion that increased supplementary private finance would be progressive in terms of total payments for healthcare.[53]

But would it be compatible with social solidarity? Britain's healthcare system offers a paradox. As noted at the beginning, it is remarkable for the dominance of public funding and the comparative unimportance of private financing, but as we have seen in the course of this analysis, it is a segmented system: the private sector has high political and public visibility. Although the NHS has achieved a high degree of fiscal and distributional equity, the healthcare system as a whole tends to be seen as socially divisive – and indeed it is so. In contrast, other systems depend more on private financing of healthcare – by imposing more direct user charges (France) or making patients carry more of the pharmaceutical costs (Canada) – but offer fewer incentives or opportunities to the public to opt out of the national system. In other cases (the Netherlands) private healthcare insurance and provision is simply one element in the national system, bringing no special privileges. To the extent that supplementary private insurance covers costs or charges imposed by the public system in these countries – as distinct from offering entry into a segregated system – it may be more successful than the NHS in maintaining social solidarity. In short, the NHS may have paid a considerable price for its insistence on fiscal chastity. In doing so, it may not only have deprived itself of a source of funding but, partly as a result, inadvertently and almost by accident encouraged the growth of an alternative rather than supplementary private sector. Tony Blair's Labour Government may have begun to incorporate the private sector as a contract-producer of healthcare for the NHS. It has yet to decide how best privately financed healthcare can complement the activities of the NHS, as distinct from competing with it.

There is, therefore, considerable uncertainty about the future public–private mix of healthcare in the UK. There is the trend towards greater pluralism on the provider side, which can be expected to continue. For example, the Government is proposing to allow successful NHS trusts to become 'Foundation Hospitals', a hybrid status which would give them a greater if uncertain degree of autonomy while keeping them within the public sector. While this is a long way from privatisation, it could be a first step towards a syndicalist model of healthcare, i.e. provider-run hospitals or consultants operating from chambers.[54] But there is also the policy emphasis – if only at the level of rhetoric at present – on promoting patient choice. In the case of the Conservative Opposition, there is an explicit if undetailed proposal to allow patients to choose between treatment in the NHS or in the private sector (receiving, in the latter case, a public subsidy equivalent to 60% of the cost of the treatment in the NHS, while paying the rest themselves). In the case of the Government, there is no such commitment, although (as noted above) certain categories of patient have been granted the right to opt for treatment in a private hospital. However, in translating the rhetoric of consumer choice into actual policy, there is a fundamental dilemma. While the logic of putting consumers in the driving seat is a demand-led healthcare system, there is no sign that the Labour Government (or any other once in office) is prepared to sign an open-ended cheque. The paradox may be that the greater the degree of choice, the smaller the menu from which consumers can choose. In other words, the NHS may move towards defining more precisely what is or is not publicly funded, as argued above, thereby setting limits to its financial commitments. In the past this has happened implicitly, with decisions often taken locally: thus the NHS has abandoned responsibility for long-term care of the elderly while individual purchasers have excluded specific procedures or drugs from their packages of care.[55] In future, this process may become more explicit. The decisions of the National Institute for Clinical Excellence (NICE) may define the boundaries of the NHS's responsibilities, particularly if it adopts a cost-effectiveness approach. In which case, the prospect is continuing growth for both the private sector and private funding as a result of accommodating the overspill of demand from the NHS and a change in the balance between the two sectors.

References

1 Wanless D (2001) *Securing our Future Health: taking a long-term view* – Interim Report. London: HM Treasury.
2 Wanless D (2002) *Securing our Future Health: taking a long-term view* – Final Report. London: HM Treasury.
3 Beveridge, Sir William (1942) *Social Insurance and Allied Services*: Report Cmd. 6404. London: HMSO.
4 Webster C (1988) *The Health Services Since the War*, vol. 1. London: HMSO.
5 Tuohy C (1999) *Accidental Logics*. New York: Oxford University Press.
6 Klein R (2001) *The New Politics of the NHS* (4e). Harlow: Prentice Hall.
7 Hansard Official Report (1946) 5th Series, Vol. 442, 30 April.
8 His Majesty's Government (1946) Cabinet 3 (46) CAB 128. London: Public Record Office.
9 Stevens R (1966) *Medical Practice in Modern England*. New Haven: Yale University Press.
10 Foot M (1997) *Aneurin Bevan*. Brivati B (ed.) London: Victor Gollancz.
11 Expenditure Committee (1972) *National Health Service Facilities for Private Patients* – Fourth Report. Session 1971–72. HC 172. London: HMSO.

12 Klein R (1979) Ideology, class and the National Health Service. *Journal of Health Politics, Policy and Law.* **4**(3): 464–90.

13 Health Committee (2000) *Consultants' Contracts Third Report – Session 1999–2000.* London: The Stationery Office.

14 Mulligan J, Judge K (1997) *Public Opinion and the NHS.* Health Care UK 1996/1997. London: King's Fund, pp. 123–38.

15 Guillebaud CW (chairman) (1956) *Report of the Committee of Enquiry into the Cost of the National Health Service.* Cmd. 9663. London: HMSO.

16 Organisation for Economic Co-operation and Development (1985) *Measuring Health Care, 1960–1983.* Paris: OECD.

17 Jewkes J, Jewkes S (1963) *Value for Money in Medicine.* Oxford: Basil Blackwell.

18 Seldon A (1968) *After the NHS.* London: The Institute of Economic Affairs.

19 Houghton D (1968) *Paying for the Social Services.* London: The Institute of Economic Affairs.

20 Jones IM (chairman) (1969) *Health Service Financing: report of a BMA Advisory Panel.* London: British Medical Association.

21 Webster C (1996) *The Health Services Since the War*, vol. 11. London: The Stationery Office.

22 Lawson, Sir Nigel (1992) *The View from No. 11.* London: Bantam Press.

23 Merrison, Sir Alex (chairman) (1979) *Royal Commission on the National Health Service: Report.* Cmnd 7615. London: HMSO.

24 *The Independent* 24 May 2001, p. 7.

25 Glennerster H, Hills J (eds) *The State of Welfare* (2e). Oxford: Oxford University Press, Table 4.2.

26 Laing W (2001) *Laing's Healthcare Market Review, 2001–2002.* London: Laing & Buisson.

27 Challis L, Day P, Klein R (1984) Residential care on demand. *New Society.* 5 April, p. 32.

28 House of Commons Health Committee (2001) *The Role of the Private Sector in the NHS.* First Report HC 308–1, Session 2001–2002. London: The Stationery Office.

29 Burchardt T (1997) *Boundaries Between Public and Private Welfare.* London: Centre for Analysis of Social Exclusion, London School of Economics.

30 Propper C (2000) The demand for private healthcare in the UK. *Journal of Health Economics.* **19**: 855–76.

31 Williams B, Whatmough P, McGill J, Rushton L (2000) Private funding of elective hospital treatment in England and Wales, 1997–8: national survey. *British Medical Journal.* **320**: 904–5.

32 Burchardt T, Propper C (1999) Does the UK have a private welfare class? *Journal of Social Policy.* **28**(4): 643–65.

33 Yates J (1995) *Private Eye, Heart and Hip: surgical consultants, the National Health Service and private medicine.* London: Churchill Livingstone.

34 Light D (2000) The two-tier syndrome behind waiting lists. *British Medical Journal.* **320**: 1349.

35 Klein R, Maynard A (1998) On the way to Calvary. *British Medical Journal.* **317**(4): 5.

36 Audit Commission (2002) *Operating Theatres.* London: Audit Commission.

37 Kmietowicz Z (2002) Milburn refuses to renegotiate consultants' contract. *British Medical Journal.* **325**(9): 1053.

38 Kmietowicz Z (2003) Consultants vote in favour of revised contract. *British Medical Journal.* **327**(25): 945.

39 Secretary of State for Health (2000) *The NHS Plan.* Cmnd 4818-l. London: The Stationery Office.

40 Independent Health Care Association (2001) *For the Benefit of Patients: a concordat with the Private and Voluntary Health Care Provider Sector.* London: Independent Health Care Association/Department of Health.

41 Milburn A (2002) Redefining the National Health Service. Speech to the New Health Network. London: Department of Health, Mimeo. 15 January.

42 Secretary of State for Health (2002) *Delivering the NHS Plan*. Cmnd 5503. London: The Stationery Office.

43 Secretary of State for Health (2002) *Learning from Bristol*. Cmnd 5363. London: The Stationery Office.

44 House of Commons Health Committee (1999) *The Regulation of Private and Other Independent Healthcare: Report*. Fifth Report, Session 1998–99 (HC 281–1). London: The Stationery Office.

45 Keen J, Light D, Mays N (2001) *Public–Private Relations in Health Care*. London: King's Fund.

46 Mulligan J (1998) Attitudes towards the NHS and its alternatives, 1983–96. In: Harrison A (ed.) *Health Care UK, 1997/98*. London: King's Fund, pp. 198–210.

47 Birch AH (1975) Economic models in political science: the case of exit, voice and loyalty. *British Journal of Political Science*. **5**: 69–92.

48 Goddard M, Smith P (1998) *Equity of Access and Health Care*. York: University of York.

49 Dixon A, Le Grand J, Henderson J, Murray R, Poteliakhoff E (2003) Is the NHS equitable? A review of the evidence. Discussion Paper No. 11. London: LSE Health and Social Care.

50 World Health Organization (2000) *Health Systems: Improving Performance*. Geneva: WHO, Annex Table 1.

51 Klein R (2002) Babel of voices: values, policy-making and the NHS. In: New W, Neuberger J (eds) *Hidden Assets: values and decision-making in the NHS*. London: King's Fund, pp. 33–45.

52 Klein R, Day P, Redmayne S (1996) *Managing Scarcity: Priority setting and rationing in the NHS*. Buckingham: Open University Press.

53 Propper C, Green K (2001) A larger role for the private sector in financing UK healthcare: the arguments and the evidence. *Journal of Social Policy*. **30**(4): 685–704.

54 Klein R, Davies C (1984) Britain: possible futures for the National Health Service. In: de Kervasdoue J, Kimberley JR, Rodwin VG (eds) *The End of an Illusion*. Berkeley, CA: University of California Press.

Endnotes

i The two Wanless reports were used by the Government to justify the political decision, announced in the April 2002 budget, to inject further billions into the NHS – and to raise taxes – as distinct from turning to alternative sources of finance.

ii Note that Beveridge discussed a variety of funding options, including hotel charges for patients.

iii In contrast to Beveridge, Treasury officials seem to have taken surprisingly little interest in the likely economics of a national health service, contenting themselves with updating estimates of pre-war expenditure. My own searches have, in this respect, been confirmed by those of Charles Webster.

iv This chapter is not intended as a contribution to the theory of path dependency: a somewhat elastic tool of analysis. However, Carolyn Tuohy has shown how this theory can be made to earn its keep. I use the notion here in the sense that she developed: the creation of a structure of interests in time A that shapes or constrains policy options in time B.

v Note that the report of the Employment and Social Services Sub-Committee (with a Labour majority) was subsequently radically toned down by the Expenditure Committee (with a Conservative majority).

vi Despite the fact that much of the initial rise in NHS spending reflected inflation, as the

Guillebaud Committee subsequently demonstrated. Interestingly, in the light of the subsequent debate about the underfunding of the NHS, the Committee also concluded that if the service were to meet 'every demand that is justifiable on medical grounds' – for example, by tackling deficiencies in services for the mentally ill, the chronic sick and hospital outpatient departments – 'a greatly increased share of the nation's human and material resources would have to be diverted to it from other areas'.

[vii] Laing's invaluable source of statistics and information about the private sector has been drawn upon throughout this analysis.

[viii] Figures derived from Burchardt refer to the year 1995/6 and should thus be read as an order of magnitude estimate for later years, although there is no reason to think that there has been a major shift between the different categories. The overall ratio between the public and private funding 82:18, is very similar to the Wanless ratio of 83:17 using 2001 OECD data.

[ix] Income figures derived from Health Committee report of 2000, which also provides a useful summary of the evidence (or lack of it) about the effects of private practice on NHS performance. John Yates and Donald Light provide the case for the prosecution.

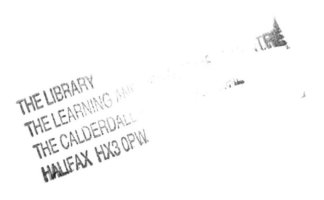

Chapter 5

UK healthcare reform: continuity and change

Alan Maynard

Introduction

During the past 15 years, the NHS has been subject to major reforms. However, while there have been continuing attempts to reform the supply side (providers) of the market, the demand side (funding) has remained largely unaltered. Patients have access to all secondary and tertiary care services free at the point of consumption and primary care is free, except for user charges for pharmaceuticals and the near privatisation of community ophthalmic and dental services.

While funding sources have remained practically the same since 1948, there has been continuous public conflict about the *level* of funding of healthcare in the UK. This 'underfunding' debate has been the product of frustration with long waiting times for elective procedures of relatively high cost-effectiveness, the poor quality of the equipment and capital stocks, and poor service provision for patients with chronic diseases. Some of these problems have been seen as the outcome not only of funding inadequacies and their perceived need to privatise finance to ensure 'proper' funding, but also as a symptom of the 'failures' of public provision.

The funding of the NHS will be discussed and will be followed by a critical appraisal of the reforms targeted at improving the efficiency of NHS provision since the Thatcher reforms in 1989. England will be the primary focus of this discussion.[i] The theme analysed throughout is the combination of regular and radical restructuring of the supply side of the English NHS, with bouts of increased funding, but with slow recognition and amelioration of efficiency and equity failures. After the abandonment of the Thatcher market reforms, similar structures and incentives are being reinvented and rebranded by the Blair Government. The market reform process has gone full circle, with the Government asserting that the 'constructive discomfort' of competitive challenges is essential to ensure the delivery of timely and efficient healthcare in the English NHS.[1]

The funding of the NHS

Revenue sources

The NHS is funded largely from taxation. In 2001, 86% of revenue was derived from general taxation, 12% from national insurance contributions and 2% from user charges. These percentages have shifted marginally since 1948 and the current share of national insurance contributions is rising as the Blair Government has opted for this proportional tax as a means of funding increased NHS expenditure.

The total UK NHS budget, 'the health vote', for the four constituent countries of the UK is divided by central government according to political agreements made in the past. As a result, Scotland and Northern Ireland are relatively overfunded, largely at the expense of England.[1,2] The overfunding in Scotland is associated with inferior performance indicators (e.g. longer periods in hospital for common procedures) and relatively poor health outcomes.[3] The Barnett formula that gives the Scots their relatively high levels of funding is to be altered to create greater equality.[4,5,6]

Each constituent country of the UK allocates national healthcare funding by an explicit budget formula, based on capitation weighted by 'need'. This is proxied by a standardised mortality rate and measures of deprivation. Variations on these formulae have been used since the late 1970s[7] and have mitigated differences in geographical capacity to fund hospital healthcare. The funding of primary care has been subject only to explicit formula finance incrementally in recent years, replacing a funding system that was demand-driven without an expenditure cap.

In England, about 75% of the public health budget is distributed by formula to local NHS purchasers (primary care trusts, PCTs). A considerable portion of the residue funds the NHS pension arrangements and the rest funds Departmental activity (some of which is being devolved to quangoes as the Department of Health is 'downsized') and central policy initiatives associated with the 'modernisation' of the NHS.

The private healthcare market is relatively small and specialised. Its largest element is elective surgery, with abortions, hernia repairs, hip and other orthopaedic procedures, and cataracts dominating the business. In 2001, Laing and Buisson estimated that there were 3.714 million subscribers with 6.656 million people insured, paying £2637 million in subscriptions and in receipt of £2006 million in benefits. According to their figure, just over 11% of the UK population have private health insurance.[8]

The growth in self-payment in the past decade is very marked, with the percentage of subscriptions paid as a total of private healthcare spending declining from 73% in 1993 to 52% in 2001. The total private spend on healthcare in 2001 was £5103 million, and the decline in the privately insured share was due to the increasing cost of insurance (and the relative lack of cost control by insurers).[8]

Expenditure

For many decades, healthcare expenditure in the UK has been relatively low compared to countries with similar levels of gross domestic product (GDP). In 2001, the UK spent 7.6% of its GDP on healthcare (Office of Health Economics, Table 2.3.[9]). Government funded 81% of this and 19% was privately financed (OHE, Table 2.5). By comparison with other OECD countries, UK public spending was high and its private spending was low (the OECD averages were 59% and 41% respectively).

Table 5.1 Change (per cent) in UK real NHS cost* and GDP in five-year periods

	Total NHS*	NHS per capita*	Real GDP*	NHS as a % of GDP
1977–82	15	15	5	10
1982–7	14	13	20	–4
1987–92	28	26	7	19
1992–7	14	13	17	–3
1997–2002	31	29	13	16

All figures include charges paid by patients. *At constant prices, as adjusted by the GDP deflator.
Source: OHE, 17 Box 2.

Table 5.2 Change in public health spending as a percentage of GDP in ten-year periods

	OECD	EU	UK
1970–80	42	39	29
1980–90	12	4	0
1990–2000	15	12	17

Figures for OECD and EU are based on weighted averages.
Source: OHE, 17 Box 3.

Expenditure on the NHS increased from 3.5% of GDP in 1948 to 6.5% of GDP in 2002. This rise disguises major fluctuations, as illustrated in Table 5.1, for the period 1977–2002. There are two periods (1982–7 and 1992–7) when NHS expenditure as a percentage of GDP fell, though both were times of rapid growth in GDP when NHS costs rose relatively modestly. The two periods in which total NHS costs rose rapidly were periods of more modest GDP growth (1987–92 and 1997–2002). The former was the period of the implementation of the Thatcher reforms and the latter, the period of the Blair Government when, after initial frugality, there was a rapid increase in NHS expenditure. Viewed internationally, UK expenditure on the NHS relative to GDP and by comparison with OECD countries grew less in the 1970s and 1980s, but more rapidly in the 1990s (Table 5.2).

Since 1999, the Government's *NHS Plan*[10] and subsequent annual Treasury statements[11] have set out its intention to raise public spending on the NHS by a significant amount. The current plan envisages a rise from £65 billion in 2002–3 to £105.6 billion in 2007–8.[12] By implication, this raises the share of the GDP spent on the NHS of 6.6% to 8.2%, with annual real planned increases in expenditure in excess of 7% each year. Such a revolutionary change in planned expenditure is a major challenge to the capacity of the healthcare system to absorb such increases efficiently when the supply of inputs such as labour (especially doctors and nurses) is difficult to increase in the short term.

The provision of healthcare

Introduction

Since 1989 there has been considerable change in the structure of the NHS, but the fundamental challenges of improving the efficiency with which care is delivered remain very similar. The delivery of healthcare at the local level is at the discretion of general practitioners (GPs) and their teams in primary care and of consultant specialists and their teams in the hospital sector. For most patients, the point of entry to the healthcare system is the GP's surgery or office. Over 90% of daily contacts with the NHS are managed there. Entry to the hospital system is determined either by the GP 'gatekeeper' in primary care, who can refer patients for outpatient investigation or inpatient care, or through the Accident and Emergency facilities of the hospital.

Organisational structure

The Thatcher and Major reforms 1989–1997

The Thatcher reforms separated the purchasing and the provision of healthcare. In England, funding passed though 14 regional health authorities to local health authorities and they contracted with secondary purchasers. Primary care was reformed with the introduction of GP fundholding and by changes in the GP contract in 1990, which introduced graduated fee-for-service payments for some preventive interventions and increased the percentage of capitation in the average GP's remuneration to 60% of income.[13,14]

The purchaser–provider contracting arrangements were innovative but weak, and not enforceable by law. The contracts were for packages of services and the element of per-case contracting was small and mostly related to the cold elective procedures that were purchased by the GP fundholders. However, the advantage of the purchaser–provider split was that for virtually the first time, managers began to scrutinise costs and activity rather than focus solely on balancing total income and expenditure. The new focus failed to incentivise the effective management of clinical practice variations or the measurement of success, by measuring and managing patient outcomes. Exchange between purchasers and providers was largely concerned with finance and slowly increasing specificity about aggregate volumes of activity.

The Thatcher reforms gave NHS hospitals a greater degree of independence and conferred the status of trust, though in reality the trust continued to be publicly financed. Nor was it able to access private capital markets because of Treasury fears that this would lead to inflation and asset creation which *de facto* would be a public liability and increase the size of the public sector borrowing. The trust's freedom to set local wages was used cautiously, because of the transaction costs of negotiating local wage deals. Any trust introducing short-term contracts soon abandoned them because it encountered professional opposition and recognised that such terms and conditions were generally more expensive.

Because government invested so little in investigating the effects of these radical reforms, evaluations and reviews were tentative and incomplete.[15–17] The opposition they created, as well as the parsimony of funding in the 1980s and the associated political pressure to demonstrate that 'the NHS was safe in the hands' of the Conservative Government, caused a considerable increase in public expenditure on the NHS. This created greater activity but appears to have had little effect on efficiency. Evidence is scarce to show that the creation of purchasing by health authorities and trusts had an effect on the quantity, cost and quality of healthcare delivery. Time may be one possible reason for this, as the acquisition of management skills and information systems is both costly, complex and time-consuming. The general political prejudice against 'grey suits' (managers) as opposed to 'white coats' (doctors) made it difficult to invest in reskilling managers and clinicians for their trading roles.

General practice fundholding was also poorly evaluated,[18,19] though this did not prevent the Conservative Government from making unsubstantiated claims of success for this and other aspects of the Thatcher reforms. The Labour opposition reached the opposite conclusions with a similar absence of evidence to substantiate its claims. Indeed, Labour's election pledge in 1997 was to abolish GP fundholding. Subsequent to its abolition, a retrospective study has demonstrated that GP fundholders reduced their hospital admissions significantly compared to non-GP fundholders.[20]

The Blair reforms 1997 to present

The Labour Government elected in 1997 deliberately chose to avoid specifics in its manifesto pledges on the NHS. Apart from rhetoric about the failure of the Thatcher reforms and a pledge to abolish the NHS internal market, it arrived in power with no detailed plans. In its first two years, the Government adhered to the parsimonious public expenditure plans of the outgoing Conservatives and focused on structural reforms, which varied widely in the increasingly autonomous parts of the UK. Scotland's new Assembly abolished the purchaser–provider split in 1999. In England and Wales, the split was maintained but with different organisational arrangements in the two countries.

English health authority purchasers were replaced by smaller entities, phased in with growing powers, initially titled primary care groups and now primary care trusts (PCTs). The English PCTs are smaller, covering average populations of 100 000 to 150 000, than the health authorities they replaced but have similar functions, holding the local budgets for both primary care and secondary care. They contract with local GPs and associated professionals providing primary care, and with local hospitals for diagnostic and therapeutic secondary and tertiary care. The transmogrification of health authorities into PCTs imposed high transaction costs on the NHS and led to difficulties in staffing the more numerous PCTs with managers of adequate skill and experience. Some of what the health authorities had learnt about purchasing (and in some cases the learning was limited!) was largely lost in the 'musical chairs' and early retirements associated with this 'redisorganisation'. As a consequence, the providers in general practice and hospitals, who were, for the most part, unaffected by these reforms, were able to maintain the status quo and the inefficiencies associated with the unmanaged nature of their practices.

In England, the Blair Government's simultaneous rejection of the Thatcher internal market and its reinvention, with some institutional change, involved some nice innovations. The first of these was occasioned by national scandals over poor-quality care involving individual practitioners, which had significant adverse effects on patients and were also of long standing, undetected by managers or, in cases where it appeared in routine data, ignored.

The Government responded to these problems by making the chief executives of hospitals responsible for the quality of patient care in addition to financial solvency. To facilitate quality improvement, elaborate and bureaucratic systems of clinical governance have been instituted to manage, *inter alia*, the measurement and mitigation of medical errors. The programme has been associated with considerable urging of change by central government and much organisational development. However, limited attention has been paid to the definition of quality (is it about processes of care and/or patient outcomes) systematic data collection and its use in quality processes.[21]

Clinical governance was augmented by intensification of inspection and regulation. One national body, created to set and inspect standards of care in local hospitals, was the Commission for Health Improvement (CHI). In 2004, this regulator changed into the Commission for Healthcare Audit and Inspection (CHAI), with responsibility for inspecting quality in the public and private sectors. A separate agency has been created for social care providers in the public and private sectors. Other new agencies include the National Patient Safety Agency and an agency to deal with poor quality doctors (National Clinical Assessment Authority, NCAA). These arrangements have strengths, in particular to increase the focus on quality and hopefully in time on patient outcomes. They also have weaknesses, such as their costs and the overlapping of activity between them and with established bodies such as the National Audit Office and the Audit Commission.

Another important quality-orientated reform was the creation of the National Institute for Clinical Excellence (NICE), with its aim of appraising new and old technologies and giving guidance to the NHS as to which they should adopt for particular subgroups of patients. Since 1999, NICE has been evaluating increasing numbers of technologies (www.nice.org).

The success of NICE in improving decision making is dependent on the quality of its science and its transparency in showing how that science is affected by political processes, e.g. applying a 'rule of rescue' and approving the use of some non-economic therapies where no other treatments exist (e.g. a treatment for amyotrophic lateral sclerosis[22]). However, its greatest challenge is to carry out the task for which it was created: rationing.[23]

It is a curious anomaly that while NICE guidance is mandatory and PCTs have an obligation to fund NICE decisions, there is no budget constraint. Consequently, NICE makes its recommendations and asserts that the Government or the NHS should determine whether its proposals are affordable. The upshot of this bizarre arrangement is that NICE is inducing considerable inflation and distortion of priorities in the NHS. Government ignores the issue of affordability, arguing that there is money enough in the system to fund NICE guidance, leaving the NHS as the *de facto* rationer, with local trusts making disparate decisions about implementation.

An alternative approach to this rationing problem would be to give NICE an explicit budget and require it to fully fund all of its decisions.[24] The organisation would then be obliged to recognise the opportunity costs of its decisions and prioritise its guidance to the most cost-effective interventions. At present, with a *de facto* cut-off for NICE approvals of £25 000 per quality-adjusted life-year (QALY), NICE decisions are inflationary and sometimes relatively inefficient. While its guidance often proposes the use of technologies only for specific subgroups of patients, this cut-off appears to be too lenient, with the result that some marginal technologies are being approved, driving out more cost-effective interventions that have yet to be considered by NICE but are parts of National Service Frameworks (NSFs) and access targets.

The NSFs are comprehensive and largely evidence-based programmes of service enhancement that have to be provided universally from the increased NHS funding. There are NSFs to raise the quality of patient care in cancer, heart disease, mental health, diabetes, renal medicine, for the elderly and for children. A good example of this is the elderly NSF that requires the progressive achievement of specialised stroke services (which have been shown to improve outcomes) and policies to reduce falls. This NSF is complemented with sharp new incentives to reduce the number of patients in need of social care who are delaying discharge from acute hospitals. Emulating Swedish policy, local government is now fined if delayed discharge targets are not met, a policy which enables hospitals to free up resources to achieve another important element of the NHS plan.[25]

Waiting times in the UK have traditionally been a source of national criticism and international shock. Often these reactions are not evidence based, e.g. elective patients are usually ranked by urgency and in many NHS hospitals 70% of people wait less than three months. But waiting experiences vary geographically and there is a long tail in the distribution, with some patients waiting much longer. Government policy has reduced this tail so that now very few wait over one year and by April 2004, none waited more than nine months. The Government's target is that by 2005, no one will wait over six months for elective procedures. If they do, at the end of that year they will automatically be given the choice of five alternative providers who can treat them.[26]

The scope and ambition of these proposed improvements in service delivery are impressive. The Government is investing heavily in the NHS and expecting that this will transform both the volume of activity, reducing waiting times, and the quality of care. These are noble aims that will hopefully have significant effects on the health of the population. As the first Wanless report noted in 2002, the traditional parsimony of NHS funding is undergoing a dramatic reversal in order to improve service delivery times and quality for all citizens.[27] What are the challenges created by this policy?

Challenges of meeting the Blair agenda

In early 2004, the OECD produced its annual review of the British economy and in its comment on the ambitious public sector reform programme of the Government, it warned about the capacity of the systems to absorb large and rapid increases in spending over a short period.[28] This concern has been expressed separately and on many occasions, with some arguing that rapid investment in the NHS is not necessarily the best way to improve the health of the population.[29]

The continuing need to prioritise

Increased NHS funding will be efficient in producing health gains only if it is targeted at investments of proven cost-effectiveness. Priorities must be set across the whole range of government policies, including waiting times, NSFs, NICE guidance and the myriad other targets accumulated by the Government dating from the introduction of *The NHS Plan*. In fact, priorities are being set in isolation with covert steering from politicians and the media as to which targets are the most important. This prioritisation process is made more difficult by the impossibility of costing the enormous and detailed agenda set by the Government. Even were costing and prioritisation across all sectors of the NHS possible, the Government still has difficulty confronting the dual realities that rationing will still exist and that variations in local investment will lead to new forms of politically sensitive differences in local access to services (known as postcode prescribing).

Capacity constraints

Even if priorities are defined clearly and pursued efficiently, there are significant capacity constraints in the NHS that will create pay and price inflation. As a result, increased investments in the NHS will create 'rents' or price increases for labour in particular, rather than fund increases in activity and quality. *The NHS Plan* established ambitious targets for timed increases in the numbers of GPs, hospital consultants, nurses and other professional groups. There is also an ambitious programme of creating a 'consultant-led' service with reductions in the hours of trainee doctors, who were previously important providers of patient care. With sharp financial penalties for those hospitals negligent in reducing junior doctors' hours, the pressure on consultant recruitment has been sharp. Furthermore, the Thatcher reforms of the GP contract and service pressures led to problems of recruitment and retention in primary care.

The policy response to these pressures has been to increase medical school intake by 30%, raise entry to training in nursing and other professions, and recruit from overseas. The latter raises ethical issues, as it involves attracting practitioners from low- and middle-income countries such as the Philippines and South Africa, as well as high-income countries such as Finland and Spain. With nurse shortages emerging in many developed countries, international competition for nursing skills is considerable.[30]

Efforts to raise capacity by increasing employment ignore the issue of whether existing staff are working efficiently. The work of Yates in the 1990s and Bloor *et al.* recently, has shown large variations in activity and some evidence of unused capacity.[31–33] Attempts to deal with such inefficiencies have been muted and usually based on exhortation rather than the incentivisation of providers with financial rewards and performance management.

Associated problems of the efficient use of existing physical capacity are difficult to resolve. The Thatcher privatisation of cleaning, catering and laundry services was a mixed success. It offered scope for cost cutting but subsequent problems of quality control, as epitomised by cleaning services, where private contractors pay low wages with few fringe benefits and the result is a high labour turnover and poor standards of cleanliness. The Government's regulatory response has been to implement external inspections and relate the results of this work to performance rating, in particular NHS hospital star classification. Not only does poor cleaning lead to patient dissatisfaction, it can also add to infection control problems.

The Government has sought to galvanise hospitals into offering cleaner facilities and better food by issuing directives and instituting reward systems. It has followed the Thatcher method, increasing physical capacity and using the private sector particularly for elective capacity. These efforts are associated with the choice directive to be implemented in 2005. The aim is to reduce waiting times for cataract removal to three months in 2005 and for other elective procedures by 2008. In north London, where the patient choice initiative has been evaluated, the threat of increased private capacity has induced the local NHS to develop public Diagnostic and Treatment Centres (DTCs). Only two of the 11 new DTCs are in the private sector!

Nationally, the Government has announced two waves of Independent Treatment Centres (ITCs) and is reported to have said that in the short term, the NHS might outsource 5% of elective surgery to the private sector, this figure rising to 15% in 'our lifetimes'.[34] Such organisations are being subsidised for four years with prices 15% above the national tariffs that are being introduced into the NHS. Once established, they will have an equity stake in the prosperity of the NHS and their development will lead to increased competition for staff.

In addition to DTCs and ITCs, the Government is funding additional hospital development out of taxation and with the Private Finance Initiative (PFI). PFI is very contentious, seen by some of its critics as both inefficient and as a means of privatising the supply of hospital care. The PFI was developed by the Conservatives and has since been expanded by the Labour Government. Macro-economically, it is a means by which public sector projects can be developed in ways that avoid the title 'public expenditure'. With PFI not adding to the Public Sector Borrowing Requirement, the size of the UK public sector is reduced and this is helpful for local politics and for international commitments that constrain the size of public activity.

PFI involves detailed contracting, with high transaction costs for the facility, and its funding obtained from private sources. An advantage of public borrowing is that commercial markets lend at low interest rates, deeming it impossible that the State will go bankrupt and be unable to repay a loan. PFI does not share this advantage, but commercial incentives may lead to greater efficiency in the design, execution and running of projects. It is hoped that this efficiency will compensate for the higher costs of private borrowing, but this is yet to be demonstrated.[35-38]

Pay and prices inflation

The large increases in the level of capital investment, both to renovate the poor quality of the equipment and facilities stock, and to increase them, is putting considerable pressure on the building industry. Similar investments in education, railways and other parts of the public and private sectors make for cost inflation.

However, the most significant problem for the NHS is labour market pay inflation. While UK pay for doctors was modest by international standards[39] and has remained much the same in structure since 1948, the Government aimed for a radical restructure of its nature and level. One goal of this reform was to improve the recruitment and retention of doctors. A second, more covert, goal was to improve the efficiency of medical practice.

General practice is largely data-free in terms of the availability and use of routine activity information. While individual practices, and in some cases groups of practices, have good data, there is no national system to provide robust comparators with which local practice can be evaluated. National data on prescribing practices of GPs are collected by the national Pharmaceutical Pricing Authority (PPA). These data can be used to identify and discipline extreme high prescribers, but the appropriateness of practice cannot be managed, as patient linkage is not possible and there are no diagnostic data on the prescription. When electronic patient records become the national norm, such information may be linked to prescribing activity to determine inappropriate use by individual patients and to identify cost-effective prescribing in relation to, for instance, NICE guidelines. Opportunities such as these have been available for decades but unexploited, with the PPA more concerned with the reimbursement of pharmacists than the delivery of cost-effective care to patients.

Unlike primary care, hospital practice could be illuminated by the use of available data. Hospital Episode Statistics (HES) are collected for each patient in NHS hospitals and returned to the Department of Health for collation and feedback. These processes cost millions of pounds each year but result in little use of the data, let alone information-based improvement in service delivery. The system includes the GP practice referring the patient, his/her postcode, the care given in hospital (with up to seven diagnoses and up to four procedures) and mortality outcomes. These data could thus point to variations in referrals by social class (using electoral ward deprivation data and postcodes), variations in GP practice referral rates, variations in the activity of consultants[40] and differences in mortality rates.[41,42]

The failure to exploit the potential of these data is a product of persistent poor incentives that may now be changing. Clinicians have rejected the HES as inaccurate or incomplete, despite the fact that the data are largely of their own reporting. They may now drive investment in its validation and use, as the Government has introduced a series of reforms raising awareness of the need to understand clinician practices more fully. Consultant appraisal is increasingly being informed by the HES and although the Royal Colleges are bureaucratising the reaccreditation process introduced by the General Medical Council, an element of this will have to be integrated data about NHS and private activity rates and outcomes. The increased awareness by the profession of the need for validation and use of the HES can be seen at the website of the Royal College of Physicians.[43]

Confronted by knowledge of practice variation, the availability of HES and uncertainty about GPs' activity rates, an attempt has been made to reform doctors' contracts. This not only addresses retention and recruitment but also the challenge of improving the workforce's productivity. Unfortunately, the success of these reforms may prove to be limited.[44]

The Department of Health failed to convince the British Medical Association (BMA) in 2003 that the introduction of a capped fee-for-service (FFS) system of payments for consultants with activity above the 40th percentile of the national HES distribution for surgeons would be efficient in shifting the mean of this distribution and increasing activity from the existing workforce. The avowed reason for this rejection was that it would lead to detailed management of clinical activity and this was unacceptable to the profession and its trade union, the BMA. However, the BMA has now realised that the combined effects of reduced NHS waiting times and private suppliers' attempts to reduce practitioners' fees will reduce private practice income for its members. As a consequence, it is likely that FFS payments for surgeons will be introduced into 30 NHS hospitals.

The final reform of the consultant contract has given practitioners a significant pay increase of £10–15 000 per annum, depending on age and experience.[45] The task of costing the contract involves a diary exercise in which consultants declare their working hours. This then has to be managed so that practitioners are working a basic 40 hour week of 10 four-hour sessions, with those who wish to do private work having to do an additional four-hour session (a total of 11 four-hour sessions or 44 hours per week for the NHS). This includes time for continuous medical education and administration, as well as patient contact.

Those groups with hours in excess of this could reduce their working hours and additional consultants may have to be employed to maintain cover and activity. The Departmental costing of the new contract, which was backdated to April 2003, was flawed and its eventual cost is much greater than anticipated. For instance one district general hospital in the North East anticipates an additional wage cost of £2 million and a teaching hospital in the same region anticipates a cost of £6 million for this new contract.

The hundreds of millions added to the consultant wage bill have been spent with little specificity in terms of *quid pro quo*. The variations in activity revealed by Bloor *et al.*[33] were the basis for Departmental endeavours to increase the activity of existing consultants by FFS, but the new contract will only facilitate better management of variations if there is a radical change in clinical and managerial attitudes and behaviour. And why should such a change be expected when unexplained and unmanaged clinical practice variations have existed for decades and could have been managed with the old contracts if there had been appropriate motivation? Without change, there is the risk that pay levels will have been increased with no beneficial effect on activity or outcomes: the NHS is merely paying more for the same service.

The GPs' new contract is also expensive and will have mixed and complex effects on activity and outcomes. At the heart of the contract, which was implemented in April 2004, is the 'quality framework', with a shift in contractual focus from the individual to the practice, building on the 1990 contract and extending the scope of FFS remuneration. There are ten quality targets with payment based on achievement, e.g. controlling the blood pressure of known hypertensives on the practice list.[46]

The new GP agreement is contracted not with the individual practitioners but with the practice, which is required to deliver varying levels of care: essential, additional and enhanced. Practices will normally provide, and be paid for, the first two categories, funded within a global sum. Separate contracts will be drawn up for enhanced services, between the practice and the PCT. The basic contract is for the period 8 am to 6.30 pm from Monday to Friday, with additional payments made outside those hours.[46] GPs who give up out-of-hours work will have their annual incomes reduced by £6000, but can then contract with PCTs to work selectively and, in all probability, for considerably higher rewards.

The contract poses several challenges for the NHS. With FFS payment systems, that which is not incentivised is marginalised, so while the new quality framework is generally evidence based it is not comprehensive. The mental health quality target covers the monitoring and care of the severely mentally ill, but does not cover depression, one of the main causes of patient consultation. Some argue that depression and activities such as services to patients with illicit drug problems and in receipt of methadone and other treatments should be reimbursed as enhanced services. However, funding for enhanced services in cash-strapped PCTs may be absorbed by the out-of-hours change in the contract.

The shift to 'normal' hours of work (8 am to 6.30 pm five days a week) may improve recruitment and retention in general practice, but it inflates the cost of out-of-hours cover sharply. PCTs can either buy back GPs at premium rates or invest in changes in skill-mix, and while a paramedic or nurse can be reskilled, their prowess in diagnosis may be less than that of a GP. A decrease in the use of the GP because of the high cost involved, and the resultant use of other skills, may encourage patients to go directly to hospital emergency departments. Were such a shift significant, it could increase hospital costs and also threaten the achievement of high-profile emergency service access targets.

Another potential impact of the GP contract on the hospital system is that improvement in performance in the quality agenda, which is highly likely given the incentivising effects of similar but more small-scale reforms in 1999, will increase the flow of patients being referred to hospital for diagnosis and treatment. This cost has not been modelled, neither has the increased cost of pharmaceuticals likely to arise from the identification of more needs in practice populations. Nurses can deliver much of the quality contract, e.g. all the FFS items in the 1990 contract. The new contract legislates that a practice must have one registered GP in order to contract with the local PCT and the NHS, so one GP could, in principle, have a number of practices with teams of nurses and others delivering the service. The quality and cost effects of such skill-mix changes are not well documented, as the propensity is for policy makers to alter skill-mix and assume this is cost-effective.[47,48]

The Government intends to raise the remunerated quality framework levels and consider incentivising new services in the future. The new contract raises major challenges for claiming payment and auditing performance. Predicted service delivery improvements will benefit patients, but only careful evaluation will determine which services, if any, are crowded out by the highly incentivised quality framework.

To claim PCT contractual payments, practices will need improved data capture and must be prepared for audit by the local PCT and the national Audit Commission. As these information systems are integrated, another element of a national information service for general practice may emerge, though it and the PPA system for drugs and the HES data on hospital referrals will still not give a full national picture of practice in primary care. Until such data are available, management will be based on empirical ignorance!

The Government and the NHS recognise the need to both cap primary care expenditure and incentivise economy and innovation in the delivery of care. The new GP contract offers the opportunity of skill-mix innovation and the Government is now permitting the purchase and sale of practice goodwill. This may lead to public and private for-profit groups evolving larger practice units and chains, with branding and quality control.

Such innovation is encouraging PCTs to develop budgeting agreements with practices. Retrospective analysis has demonstrated some beneficial effects from GP fundholding.[20] These incentives are being reinvented (and rebranded) by PCTs anxious to improve the efficiency of primary and secondary care by reducing hospital referrals and other economies and to achieve expenditure control. Practice budgets, as well as the integration of finance and provision in primary and secondary care systems of integrated care, will create organisations like US health maintenance organisations.

The final cause of pay inflation is the policy entitled *Agenda for Change*.[49] Currently, there are over 500 pay scales for different grades and specialisms in the non-physician workforce, which the Government plans to merge into 11 grades, covering these 500 groups and doctors. This process will begin in 2005. The transaction costs of these changes will be considerable and, if not well managed, the costs of grade inflation may be high. At the same time, as with any change in contracts or grading, there is a risk of damaging the morale of staff due to changing relativities.

Pay reform is potentially very threatening in terms of creating inflation with little effective micro-management of clinical practice and efficient incentivisation of economy in the use of resources. These threats are recognised and being dealt with by further market-oriented reforms of the incentive structure facing practitioners and their organisations. The issue is whether these reinventions and developments of the Thatcher reforms will be more successful than the original attempts. They are made essential by the ambitious targets of NHS modernisation but will require considerable political determination to sustain.

Equity

One objective of the NHS is to reduce inequalities in health. The Blair Government has tackled this aim in a crab-like fashion, avowing firm intent but making limited progress. The Acheson report[50] charted the nature and causes of inequalities in health and healthcare and made over 100 uncosted and unprioritised recommendations. But the report did little to resolve the issue of whether investment in healthcare or investment in income and other forms of redistribution is the most cost-effective means of reducing health inequality.

The Labour Government has adhered firmly to its undertaking not to increase direct taxation. Its limited successes in reducing poverty and social exclusion have been, at times, the negligible product of investments of unproven efficiency (e.g. health action zones) and investments in social security programmes (e.g. to lift children out of poverty). These programmes have been funded by 'stealth taxes', levied on almost everything except direct income, and by an increasing budget deficit.

By early 2004, competition had emerged between the Secretary of State for Health, John Reid, who announced a public consultation on improving the public's health, and Derek Wanless, commissioned earlier by the Chancellor of the Exchequer, to review public health programmes and the mitigation of health inequalities. Investing *outside* the NHS to improve the nation's health may be more cost-effective than investing *in* it. Investment in education raises lifetime earnings. This, in turn, is associated with reductions in smoking and the adoption of behaviours conducive to health improvement. Similarly, reduction in poverty leads to investment in human capital and behaviour changes that improve the long-term health of the poor and their children, helping to reduce health inequalities.[51] However, the exploitation of this potential remains elusive.

Inequalities still remain in the distribution of healthcare finance between the constituent parts of the NHS, and with Labour dependent on Scottish votes in the London parliament, there is unlikely to be radical change soon. While peace in Northern Ireland continues, since the Good Friday agreement in 1999, there is no questioning the rationale of the relatively high level of NHS funding there.

From their beginnings in England in 1976, the processes around devising, implementing and revising the budget allocation formula for hospitals have progressed, although amidst continuing academic debate about the appropriateness of the need indicators and statistical methods used.[52] Cash limiting of primary care has been achieved under the Blair Government and the budget is increasingly allocated by capitation and need, with the exception remaining that part of the primary care budget that funds GPs. Significant inequalities in the geographical distribution of GPs have been demonstrated for years, but continue to be avoided by NHS policy makers.[53,54]

The continuing focus on structure rather than performance

Continuing reform of NHS structures supports the enormous increase in NHS funding. Many of these changes are expensive, consume scarce managerial effort much needed to improve the performance of the system, and are evidence free. For decades, successive Conservative and Labour governments have changed the organisational framework of the NHS without defining the precise problems they are addressing, let alone allowing time and resources for their social experiments to be evaluated. This sad characteristic of healthcare reform, both in the UK and elsewhere, survives despite the advocacy of cautious evidence-based reform.[55]

Nice examples of evidence-free reforms, with no accompanying evaluation, are those of the GP and consultant contracts, the creation of overlapping and costly regulatory mechanisms to improve quality, restructure of purchasing with PCTs, introduction of a system of national tariffs and enforceable contracts, and creation of Foundation Trusts. Two of these current reforms demonstrate this problem well: Foundation Trusts and national tariffs (called diagnostic related groups or DRGs throughout the world).

The reader of Labour's proposals to introduce Foundation Trusts from April 2004 will be struck by the similarity to Thatcher's proposals to create Hospital Trusts in 1989:

> *The government is committed to devolving decision making in the National Health Service to the local operational level in order to make hospitals more responsive to the needs of patients, to secure local commitment and to achieve greater value for money. The next logical step in the process of extending local responsibility is to enable NHS hospitals to achieve self governing status.[13]*

Had the Conservatives evaluated their Hospital Trust experiment, Labour might have decided against repeating their mistakes.[56] Rhetoric about flexibility and local decision making remains, despite the fact that the NHS is a publicly funded service with central accountability through Parliament. Furthermore, evidence of the few real increases in freedom in labour or capital markets that the Tory experiment gave the Trusts would have been clearly identified. Foundation Trusts are required to engage their local populations in decision making, but if their Boards of Governors elect for policies, the Trusts' ability to develop them is very limited, as their contracts are with local PCTs and they will follow the dictates of central government targets.

Some believe that the emerging national tariff systems will make the funding of Foundation Trusts more flexible.[57] In the initial period, those Trusts with prices below the national tariff will have surpluses, most of which will be creamed off to cross-subsidise the high-cost Trusts. Since Trusts are contracted to fixed volumes by the local PCTs, which have no resources to pay for additional activity, surpluses cannot be spent in this way. As a consequence, surpluses will be spent on 'quality' aspects of care, such as increased recruitment of nurses and provision of crèches to improve staff retention. It is curious that one of the Government's flagship reforms will not contribute to increasing activity to reduce waiting times.

However, one advantage of national tariffs is that they will oblige managers to focus on the detailed activity of their staff, particularly of consultants. With the Trusts' incomes dependent on claiming for every unit of activity (FCE), the management of variations in individual activity and its total level will be essential for survival.

Such reforms are good examples of Government frustration with the conservatism of the NHS and their perception of its reluctance to 'act smarter' to ensure that the large new investments in the Service create value for money. Out of this frenzied reform activity, a clear preference for the use of market mechanisms is slowly emerging. What was rejected in 1997 is now being seen as the primary focus of change in the English NHS.[1]

Overview

Many characteristics of the NHS as it was created in 1948 still remain. Public finance of comprehensive healthcare for the whole population from the cradle to the grave, with little use of patient charges, has survived 55 years of ideological dispute. The focus of reform in the past 15 years has been on improving the efficiency of the supply side of the market, with various market-oriented experiments.

The Thatcher reforms emphasised the purchaser–provider split, but the Government's initial enthusiasm for the market was soon tempered by fears over its effects in a cash-limited system. With many hospitals being local quasi-monopolies, there was concern that price flexibility would lead to inflation and reductions in service quality with some controversial evidence that competition may have increased inpatient mortality in the early days of Thatcher's internal market.[58] The inexperience of purchasers, preserved by primitive information systems and poor incentive structures, led to providers dominating transactions.

The stresses and strains of reforms, many induced by vested interests such as the trades unions and the professions, led to increased public expenditure to 'smooth' the transition to the internal market. It is probable that this funding explains most of the consequent gains in activity observed in the NHS in the early 1990s.

The initial reforms of the Blair Government were naive – a product of the Administration deliberately entering power with no explicit agenda except the abolition of the allegedly failed internal market of the Conservatives. But instead of abolishing the internal market, Blair chose to rebrand it, and after some initial parsimony, he has provided the largest increase in healthcare funding ever experienced in the UK. Some change but also some waste are the result. The volume and scope of services is changing and patient waiting times are declining, but no sustained attempt has been made to reduce the volume of unused capacity exemplified by variations in clinical activity, and the measurement of outcomes remains primitive. Furthermore, as anticipated,[29] attempts to raise activity in the absence of short-term flexibility in the supply of labour and capital has led to hundreds of millions of pounds being absorbed into price increases without activity and outcome increases, e.g. the GP and consultant contracts.

Frustration with this has led the Government to pursue renewed forms in payment systems, with quietly developed systems of GP practice budgets and FFS incentives for some NHS surgeons. This is being complemented with efforts to achieve greater quantification in the micro-management of medical practitioners and experimentation with novel systems of patient outcome measurement. Emulating the example of BUPA, the private insurer,[60] the Department of Health has announced its intention to assess the use of health-related quality-of-life measures as a means of evaluating the success of NHS and independent diagnostic and treatment controls.[5]

The Blair agenda to 'modernise' the NHS is welcome and essential to achieve efficient and equitable delivery of healthcare to the UK population. Change has been produced but the Government has failed to learn from the policy evidence base and be cautious and deliberate in experimenting with the new forms of delivery. Instead, it has used valuable resources that could have been better spent on improving population health. Such behaviour is partly the product of an electoral system that induces 'quick-fix' reforms rather than the deliberate and cautious procrastination as seen in parts of Scandinavia (e.g. Denmark, *see* Chapter 9). However, it is also the product of an unwillingness to identify and better manage long-standing and well researched inefficiencies in the UK NHS, particularly clinical practice variations and the absence of measures that demonstrate improvements in patient health during the care and cure processes. These deficiencies are common to most healthcare systems and can only be mitigated by incentivising radical, evidence-based innovations in service delivery.

References

1 Stevens S (2004) Reform strategies for the English NHS. *Health Affairs.* **23**(3): 37–44.
2 Maynard A, Ludbrook A (1980) Applying resource allocation formulae to constituent parts of the UK. *Lancet.* i: 85–7.
3 Birch S (1986) The RAWP review: RAWPing primary care: RAWPing the United Kingdom. Discussion Paper 19. York: University of York Centre for Health Economics.
4 Scottish Executive Health Department (1999) *Fair Shares for All: Report of the National*

Review of Resource Allocation for the NHS in Scotland. [Online] [accessed March 2004]. Available from URL www.scotland.gov.uk/fairshares/default.htm

5 Edmonds T (2001) The Barnett Formula. Research Paper 01/108. London: House of Commons Library, Economic Policy and Statistics Section.

6 Twigger R (1998) The Barnett Formula. Research Paper 98/8. London: House of Commons Library, Economic Policy and Statistics Section.

7 Department of Health and Social Services (1976) *Sharing Resources for Health in England: Report of the Resource Allocation Working Party.* RARP1. London: DHSS.

8 Laing W (2001) *Laing's Healthcare Market Review, 2001–2002.* London: Laing & Buisson.

9 Office of Health Economics (2003) *Compendium of Health Statistics 2003/4.* London: OHE.

10 Department of Health (2000) *The NHS Plan: a plan for investment; a plan for reform.* London: Department of Health.

11 HM Treasury (2000) *Spending Review 2000: prudent for a purpose: building opportunity and security for all.* London: HM Treasury.

12 HM Treasury (2002) *2002 Spending Review. Opportunity and security for all: investing in an enterprising, fairer Britain.* London: HM Treasury.

13 Department of Health (1989) *Working for Patients.* Cmnd 555. London: HMSO.

14 Department of Health and Social Security (1995) *General Practice in the NHS: a new contract.* London: DHSS.

15 Robinson R, Le Grand J (1994) *Evaluating the NHS Reforms.* London: King's Fund.

16 Mays N, Wyke S, Malbon G, Goodwin N (eds) (2001) *The Purchasing of Health Care by Primary Care Organizations: An evaluation and guide to future policy.* Buckingham: Open University Press.

17 Smith PC (2000) *Reforming Markets in Healthcare: an economic perspective.* Buckingham, England; Philadelphia, PA: Open University Press.

18 Gosden T, Torgerson DJ (1997) The effect of fundholding on prescribing and referral costs: a review of the evidence. *Health Policy.* **40**: 103–14.

19 Gosden T, Torgerson DJ, Maynard A (1997) What is to be done about fundholding? *British Medical Journal.* **315**: 170–1.

20 Dusheiko M, Gravelle H, Jacobs R, Smith PC (2003) The effect of budgets on doctor behaviour: evidence from a natural experiment. Technical Paper No. 26. York: Centre for Health Economics.

21 Sheldon T, Maynard A, Watt I (2001) Promoting quality in the NHS. *Health Policy Matters.* **May (Issue 4)**: 1–4.

22 Freemantle N, Bloor K, Eastaugh J (2002) A fair innings for NICE? *Pharmacoeconomics.* **20**(6): 389–91.

23 McDaid D, Cookson R, Maynard A, Sassi F (2003) Evaluating health interventions in the 21st century: old and new challenges. *Health Policy.* **63**: 117–20.

24 Maynard A, Bloor K, Freemantle N (2004) Challenges for NICE. *BMJ.* **329**: 227–9.

25 The Community Care (Delayed Discharges, etc) Act (2003). London: HMSO.

26 Department of Health (2003) *The Health and Personal Social Services Programmes: the Government's expenditure plans.* Cmnd 5904. London: Department of Health.

27 Wanless D (2002) Securing our future health: taking a long-term view. Interim report. London: HM Treasury.

28 OECD Economic Surveys (2004) Organisation for Economic Co-operation and Development, January 2004.

29 Maynard A, Sheldon T (2002) Funding for the National Health Service. *Lancet.* **360**: 576.

30 Bloor K, Maynard A, Hall J, Ulmann P, Farhauer O, Lindgren B (2003) *Planning Human Resources in Health Care – Towards an Economic Approach: an international comparative review.* Toronto: Canadian Health Services Research Foundation. [Online] [accessed March 2004]. Available from URL www.chsrf.ca/docs/finalrpts/bloor_e.shtml

31 Yates J (1995) *Private Eye, Heart and Hip.* London: Churchill Livingstone.

32 Yates J (1987) *Why Are We Waiting?* Oxford: Oxford University Press.

33 Bloor K, Maynard A (2002) Consultants: managing them means measuring them. *Health Service Journal.* **112**: 10–1.

34 Laing & Buisson (2004) *Healthcare Market News.* viii(iii): 51. London: Laing & Buisson.

35 Dawson D (2001) The private finance initiative: a public finance illusion? *Health Economics.* **10**: 479–86.

36 Pollock AM, Shaoul J, Vickers N (2002) Private finance and 'value for money' in NHS hospitals: a policy in search of a rationale? *British Medical Journal.* **324**: 1205–9.

37 Pollock AM, Dunnigan M, Gaffney D, Macfarlane A, Majeed FA (1997) What happens when the private sector plans hospital services for the NHS: three case studies under the private finance initiative. NHS Consultants' Association, Radical Statistics Health Group, and the NHS Support Federation. *British Medical Journal.* **314**: 1266–71.

38 Pollock AM, Dunnigan MG, Gaffney D, Price D, Shaoul J (1999) The private finance initiative: planning the NHS: downsizing for the 21st century. *British Medical Journal.* **319**: 179–84.

39 Bramley-Harker E and Aslam S (2003) *Fees for Medical Specialists: how does the UK compare?* London: National Economics Research Association.

40 Bloor KE, Maynard A, Freemantle N (2004) Variation in activity rates of consultant surgeons, and the influence of reward structures in the English NHS: descriptive analysis and a multilevel model. *Journal of Health Services Research and Policy.* **9(2)**: 76–84.

41 Jarman B, Gault S, Alves B, Hider A, Dolan S, Cook A *et al.* (1999) Explaining differences in English hospital death rates using routinely collected data. *British Medical Journal.* **318**: 1515–20.

42 Dr Foster [Online] [accessed March 2004]. Available from URL www.drfoster.co.uk

43 Royal College of Physicians [Online] [accessed March 2004]. Available from URL www.rcplondon.ac.uk

44 Maynard A, Bloor K (2003) Do those who pay the piper call the tune? *Health Policy Matters.* **October (Issue 8)**: 1–8.

45 Department of Health (2004) *New Consultant Contract.* [Online] [accessed February 2004]. Available from URL www.dh.gov.uk/PolicyAndGuidance/HumanResources AndTraining/ModernisingPay/ConsultantsContracts/fs/en

46 NHS Confederation and British Medical Association (2003) *New GMS Contract: investing in general practice.* London: NHS Confederation and BMA.

47 Richardson GM (1998) Skill mix changes: substitution or service development? *Health Policy.* **45**: 119–32.

48 Sibbald B, Shen J, McBride A (2004) Changing the skill mix of the health care workforce. *Journal of Health Service Research and Policy.* **9**: 28–38.

49 Department of Health, NHS Modernisation Agency. *Agenda for Change.* [Online] [accessed February 2004]. Available from URL www.doh.gov.uk/agendaforchange

50 Acheson D (1998) *Independent Inquiry into Inequity in Health.* London: The Stationery Office.

51 Chalmers I, Sheldon T, Rounding C (eds) (2000) *Evidence from Systematic Reviews of Research Relevant to Implementing the 'Wider Public Health Agenda'.* York: University of York, NHS Centre for Reviews and Dissemination.

52 Carr-Hill RA, Sheldon TA, Smith P, Martin S, Peacock S, Hardman G (1994) Allocating resources to health authorities: development of method for small area analysis of use of inpatient services. *British Medical Journal.* **309**: 1046–9.

53 Birch S, Maynard A, Walker A (1986) Doctor manpower planning in the United Kingdom: problems arising from myopia in policy making. Discussion Paper DP18. York: Centre for Health Economics.

54 Gravelle H, Wildman J, Sutton M (2002) Income, income inequality and health: what can we learn from aggregate data? *Social Science in Medicine.* **54**: 577–89.

55 Maynard A, Sheldon T (1997) Health policy. Time to turn the tide. *Health Service Journal.* **107**: 24–6.

56 Department of Health (2004) *Foundation Trusts, 2004.* [Online] [accessed February 2004]. Available from URL www.dh.gov.uk/PolicyAndGuidance/OrganisationPolicy/SecondaryCare/NHSFoundationTrust/fs/en

57 Department of Health (2004) *National Tariffs.* [Online] [accessed February 2004]. Available from URL www.dh.gov.uk/PolicyAndGuidance/OrganisationPolicy/FinanceAndPlanning/NHSFinancialReforms/fs/en

58 Propper C, Burgess S, Green K (2004) Does competition between hospitals improve the quality of care? Hospital death rates and the NHS internal market. *Journal of Public Economics.* **88**: 1247–72.

59 Vallance-Owen A, Cubbin S (2002) Monitoring national clinical outcomes: a challenging programme. *British Journal of Health Care Management.* **8**: 412-17.

60 Department of Health (2004) *Policy Research Programme. Patient Reported Outcomes Measurement System in Treatment Centres.* [Online] [accessed February 2004]. Available from URL www.dh.gov.uk/ProcurementAndProposals

Endnote

[i] Healthcare policies in Scotland and Wales are now determined by national governments, even though their funding continues to be determined by allocations by the UK (London) government. The Scots elected to abolish the purchaser–provider split introduced by the Thatcher Government. Like the New Zealanders, the Scots now have an organisational structure very similar to that before 1989, with Health Boards having integrated systems of funding and provision. Funding in Scotland remains high relative to England, even after taking account of the greater health needs of its population.[5] In Wales, the purchaser–provider split continues, but the perfomance of the system (e.g. very much longer waiting times despite increased funding) remains poor. This is predicted as likely either to lead to mergers of existing small hospitals and purchase agencies or abolition, as in Scotland, of the Thatcher purchaser–provider structures. Thus, although the British NHS remains publicly financed, there are now three different NHS systems in England, Wales and Scotland. Comparative analysis of the performance of these systems offers a nice opportunity to determine the efficiency of the 'three paths in one system'.

Chapter 6

The mix of public and private payers in the US health system

Uwe Reinhardt

Introduction

The US health system arguably represents the most complex intersection between the private and public sector to be found anywhere in the world. It is managed, so to speak, with an equally complex administrative superstructure whose day-to-day operation defies even the legendary power of US information technology. The sheer complexity of the system, one must suppose, and its high cost, has consistently earned it among the lowest ranking in international opinion surveys on health systems – among patients[1] and also among physicians.[2]

Even so, at conferences on healthcare, in the political arena or in the media, Americans faithfully observe the etiquette, praising their health system as the best in the world. The belief rests on the fact that, by international standards, US healthcare typically is delivered in luxurious settings with highly sophisticated technology. At its best, the system can boast of stunning clinical achievements, even though the nation as a whole ranks remarkably low on customary aggregate health-status indicators such as age-specific life expectancy and infant mortality rates.[3]

The administrative complexity of the US health system can be traced to two mutually contradictory strands in US culture and politics. On the one hand, Americans believe widely that private enterprise is inherently more efficient at any task than government can ever be. In debates on public policy, that credo often is treated as axiom – perhaps because the empirical evidence for it is weak and the term 'efficiency' cannot even be meaningfully defined in abstraction from the social goal posited for economic activity.[i] On the other hand, government seems to be the only institution the US public ultimately trusts. When disaster strikes – be it wind, flood, fire or terrorist attack – Americans instinctively flock to their government for succour. When houses collapse during hurricanes, or corporate financial scandals come to light, or patients die from medical errors, Americans wonder how government could have allowed this lax state of affairs, invariably calling for tough new regulations.

Indeed, to this author's mind, the best analogy by which to understand the puzzling relationship between Americans and their government is the relationship between teenagers and their parents, whom teenagers generally view as an oppressive nuisance until the enterprising youngsters find themselves in dire straits and parents become a trusted source of fiscal and physical relief.

US health policy, and the health sector it has begotten, reflect these conflicting views on government. Although Americans fancy theirs to be the only market-based system in the industrialised world, it is not at all surprising that, over time, they also have come to finance close to 60% of their annual health spending with taxes.[4] At roughly 9% of gross domestic product (GDP), tax-financed health spending in the US now exceeds the percentage of GDP most nations spend on healthcare from all sources, public or private.[ii] Nor is it surprising that US physicians, hospitals and other providers of healthcare find themselves chafing under a body of government regulations so voluminous and intrusive as to astound their counterparts in other industrialised countries. So feared are the consequences of violating these Byzantine regulations that prudent US hospitals now rank full-time 'compliance officers' in their executive teams. These officers, in turn, hire a variety of outside specialists from a booming compliance industry, to train the rank and file in the arcane mystery of these regulations, to audit the hospital's adherence to the rules on behalf of management and to certify compliance formally, as pre-emptive protection against a possible indictment by government. To quote on this point Brookings economist Henry Aaron (2003, p. 802), who is not known for hyperbole:

> *Like many other observers, I look at the US healthcare system and see an administrative monstrosity, a truly bizarre mélange of thousands of payers with payment systems that differ for no socially beneficial reason, as well as staggeringly complex public systems with mind-boggling administered prices and other rules expressing distinctions that can only be regarded as weird.[5]*

As Aaron reminds us, the onerous government regulations imposed on US healthcare come atop an equally Byzantine set of strictures dictated by a myriad of private health insurance contracts, each with its own complex set of dos and don'ts, including distinct formularies for prescription drugs and requirements for referrals. In the words of the executive vice president of the American Hospital Association:

> *Most [American] hospitals have 10 000 or more items or services in their fee schedules, they typically have [distinct] contracts with 25 or 100 or more [private] insurers, and the terms of those [distinct] contracts are changing continually.[6]*

Naturally, this complex administrative structure absorbs an unusually large fraction of total US health spending – perhaps as much as 25%,[4,7] a high percentage by international standards. Although some economists (e.g. Danzon[8]) impute to these high overhead costs benefits not available in other countries – for example, choice of insurance carriers, of providers of healthcare and of therapy. It has never been established that these benefits can justify their extraordinarily high cost.

The political rhetoric within the US's two-party system may suggest that these regulations are mainly the handiwork of Democratic governments, because Republicans invariably profess to favour private sector solutions to social problems while Democrats are not shy about favouring government solutions. Rhetoric in this context, however, can be deceiving. Some of the toughest and most intrusive government regulations in US healthcare have come not from Democratic but Republican administrations.

Despairing of inflationary pressures in the US economy during the early 1970s, for example, Republican President Nixon imposed price controls on the entire US economy for over a year and on the health sector specifically for over two years. Despairing of inflationary pressures, specifically in the federal government's Medicare programme for the elderly during the early 1980s, Republican President Ronald Reagan in 1983 induced Congress to legislate for that programme a payment scheme for hospitals resembling nothing so much as a Soviet approach to centrally administered prices – the case-based payment system for diagnostically related groupings of cases (DRGs). Less than a decade later, in 1992, his successor, Republican President Bush the Elder, imposed similarly administered prices on physicians treating Medicare patients, coupling that administered-fee schedule with a strict, unilaterally imposed global, national budget for the total annual outlay by Medicare on physician services, called the Volume Performance Standard (VPS). If in a given year, the physician's total billings at prevailing Medicare fees exceed this global budget, then fees in a subsequent year will be reduced sufficiently below what they would otherwise be to recoup the earlier overspending.

The only predictable constant in US health policy has been a tendency by both political parties – Republicans and Democrats – to grant the supply side of the health system rather more market power, relative to the demand side, than is customary in other industrialised nations.[9] It can explain why the US health system now spends almost twice as much per capita on healthcare than do the next most expensive health systems of Switzerland and Canada, while leaving some 40 million Americans totally without the benefit of health insurance and millions more with very shallow insurance coverage.

The purpose of this chapter is to describe and assess in more detail the complicated interplay between the private and public sectors in the financing of US healthcare. The discussion starts with a broad overview of the financing of healthcare in the US. The following section explores, in greater depth, the role of the public sector in the payment system, then this exercise is repeated for the private sector. Because the mix of payers in US healthcare is so varied, these two sections cannot be styled as a pleasant read. It is worth slogging through their pages, however, to get a feel for the sheer complexity of the system and to appreciate why few US experts and statisticians, let alone foreigners, can ever get a good mental grasp of the system. The next section explores the sundry advantages one frequently hears claimed in the US for this payment system and the many conceptual and practical problems it begets. The chapter concludes with a review of the recently enacted Medicare reform law, which serves as an augury of a brewing battle over the distributive ethic that is to govern 21st-century US healthcare.

Financing the US health system: an overview

Unlike the financing of health systems in most other industrialised nations, the financing of US healthcare is based on an intricate mosaic composed of distinct categories of people each with a distinct health insurance contract, if they have insurance at all. Figure 6.1 provides a bird's-eye view of that system.

The main criteria for categorising Americans by health-insurance status are:

	The poor	The near poor	The broad middle class	The rich
Children under age 18	A	B	C	D
Adults of working age	E	F	G	H
Persons aged 65 and over	I	J	K	L

Figure 6.1 The categorical basis for US health insurance.

- age (children under age 18, persons of working age and persons aged 65 and over)
- income (typically defined by the percentage their family income represents of the official federal poverty level)
- health status (e.g. the 'blind and disabled', persons afflicted with renal failure, women, if they are pregnant, and so on).

From a worm's eye view, the system can have many subclasses within the major cells in Figure 6.1, once again each with its own health insurance contract. The near-poor elderly in cell J, for example, are broken down into five distinct subcategories, each entitled to a different set of subsidies from the federal government, in addition to the general federal Medicare programme for the nation's elderly. Americans in cell J also have a myriad of private insurance contracts (many of them provided by former employers) that supplement whatever government assistance is available to them. It follows that the cost of any particular medical intervention rendered a particular elderly in cell J can come from a variety of sources, including the patient's own funds.

Table 6.1 provides a rough numerical overview of the health-insurance status of Americans. Because, as noted, the healthcare received by a particular person may be financed with a variety of private and public insurance plans, along with out-of-pocket payments at time of service, tabulations of Americans by their insurance status typically do not add up to 100%, as is apparent from Table 6.1. But the following rules of thumb describe the system in rough and ready fashion.

- Close to 70% of Americans have private insurance as their primary coverage for healthcare costs, the bulk of it provided by private and public employers through group health insurance. Less than 10% of the population is covered by insurance policies purchased directly from private insurers.
- About 13% of Americans are covered by the federal Medicare programme for

Table 6.1 Health insurance status of Americans, 2002

Total population (millions)	286	100%
Privately insured	199	69.6%
Employment based	175	61.3%
Direct purchase	27	9.3%
Government insurance	74	25.7%
Medicaid (mainly for low-income families)	33	11.6%
Medicare (mainly for the elderly)	38	13.4%
Military healthcare	10	3.5%
Uninsured	44	15.3%

Source: US Department of Commerce.[44]

    persons aged 65 and over and for certain special categories of younger persons afflicted by renal failure or on Social Security Disability Insurance.
- About 12% of Americans are covered by the Medicaid programme, which is administered by the state governments and financed jointly by the states and the federal government according to a progressive formula that provides more federal support to low-income states than to high-income states. Covered by the programme are low-income children and their mothers if their family income falls below thresholds set by the state governments, persons who are blind and disabled, and pauperised Medicare beneficiaries who can no longer cover with their own income outlays for healthcare not covered by the federal Medicare programme.
- Finally, about 15% of Americans have no health insurance whatsoever at any given point in time.[iii] The bulk of these belong to working families in the bottom third of the nation's income distribution whose employers choose not to offer them health insurance on the job or who are unwilling or unable to pay for their share of the premiums for such policies.

This breakdown of Americans by insurance status has changed only gradually over time during the past two decades. It will shift somewhat more rapidly towards Medicare once the Baby Boom generation begins to retire after 2010, although the fraction of persons aged 65 and over will not exceed about 21% even by 2040.

    Figure 6.2 illustrates how the shares of the public and private payers for US healthcare have changed since 1965. The graph measures share at the nexus between payer and provider of healthcare and not at the nexus of the household paying into the system with taxes, premiums or out-of-pocket payments. It is seen that there was a rapid increase in the public sector after the introduction of the Medicare and Medicaid programmes in 1965. Thereafter, the shares among payers have changed at a glacial pace. Over time, the fraction of healthcare paid out-of-pocket has shrunk somewhat while that of both private and public third-party payers has increased somewhat.

    In 2002, payments made by governments at all levels accounted to the providers of healthcare amounted to about 45% of total national health spending.

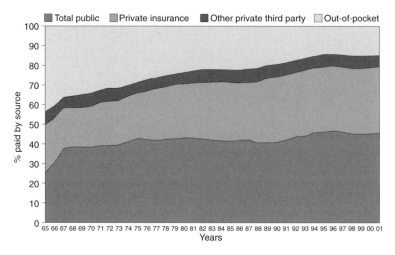

Figure 6.2 Sources of financing US healthcare, 1965–2001. *Source*: Centers for Medicare and Medicaid Services (www.cms.gov).

That figure, however, understates the role of government in the financing of healthcare, because governments at the state and federal level recycle some tax funds through private health insurers by means of vouchers toward the purchase of private health insurance. All federal civil servants and members of Congress, for example, have private health insurance coverage, which they purchase with tax-financed vouchers that cover the bulk of the premium.

If one measures the role of government in healthcare financing not by who paid the providers of healthcare, but in what form these funds have originated from private households (the ultimate payer of all healthcare in any nation) then, according to a recent estimate by Woolhandler and Himmelstein,[4] close to 60% of all health spending in the US can be said to be tax financed – or about 9% of GDP. The thrust of US public health policy at this time is to recycle more and more of the funds now flowing to the providers of healthcare through public health insurance programmes through the private insurance system, for reasons to be explored further on in this chapter.

Health spending by the US public sector

As in many other countries, the public sector's role in financing healthcare in the US is shared by the various levels of government according to complex formulae that change only gradually over time in a constant process of negotiation. Figure 6.3 illustrates the composition of the public sector's share in financing since 1965.

Federal health spending

Figure 6.4 shows that the federal Medicare programme for the elderly now constitutes by far the largest component of total federal spending on healthcare. The remainder of federal health spending, shown as the bottom segment of Figure 6.4, represents the US Public Health Service, the health system for the active military and their families, and the large healthcare system for veterans operated by the US Department of Veterans Affairs (the VA).

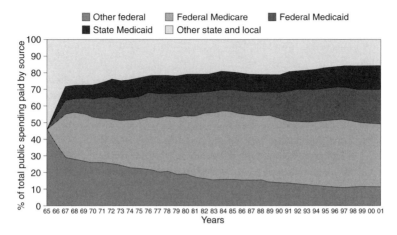

Figure 6.3 Composition of total public spending for US healthcare, 1965–2001. *Source*: Centers for Medicare and Medicaid Services (www.cms.gov).

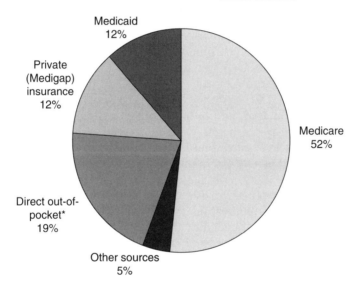

Figure 6.4 Sources of payment for Medicare beneficiaries' health services, 1999. *Source*: US Department of Health and Human Services, Centers for Medicare and Medicaid Services (CMS), *CMS Facts & Figures*, Section III.B.5, p. 2. Powerpoint presentation found at website http://cms.hhs.gov/charts/default.asp. *Beneficiary out-of-pocket spending does not include their payments for Medicare Part B premiums, private insurance premiums, or HMO premiums.

Medicare

The federal Medicare programme is a classic single-payer, government-run health insurance programme built on strictly egalitarian principles. Persons are eligible for the programme if they are 65 years of age or older and if they or their spouses are citizens or permanent residents of the US and have worked and contributed to the programme through payroll taxes for at least 40 quarters. Persons under age 65 are eligible for the programme only if they have received Social Security

Disability Insurance for at least two years, or if they have renal disease requiring dialysis. Of the roughly 40 million Americans covered by Medicare, about 82.5% are aged 65 and older and 12.5% are under age 65.[10] Under certain circumstances, persons not meeting these qualifications may be allowed to buy into Medicare at actuarially fair premiums.[10] Persons enrolled in Medicare pay a small monthly premium (now about $50) towards the programme out-of-pocket.

Under the traditional, government-run, fee-for-service programme, Medicare pays the providers of healthcare throughout the country roughly the same fees for particular services, regardless of the patient's socioeconomic status, although there are regional adjustments for local practice costs and malpractice premiums. Medicare permits physicians to charge patients up to 15% of the scheduled fees, plus the 20% of the fees that patients must pay as co-insurance. Other providers of healthcare, however, may not bill patients any additional fees other than whatever cost-sharing patients must absorb under the law.

The benefit package covered by Medicare is spotty and shallow by international standards, and also by the standards of employment-based private health insurance in the US. Even after full implementation of the recently passed *Medicare Prescription Drug, Improvement, and Modernization Act of 2003*, the programme will cover only about a quarter of the cost of prescription drugs used by the elderly. It does not cover chronic long-term care, and it visits heavy cost-sharing on patients for physician services (20% of allowable fees) and hospital care, for which beneficiaries pay out of pocket $840 per hospital episode and, beyond a stay of 60 days, $210 per day for the next 30 days, $420 per day for the following 60 days and all costs for hospital stays exceeding 150 days. In insurance parlance, Medicare provides better protection against lower levels of health spending than against truly catastrophic healthcare costs.

Because of its limited benefit package and the heavy cost sharing it imposes on patients, Medicare itself covers only slightly more than half of the total healthcare costs incurred for its beneficiaries (*see* Figure 6.4). About 12% of the total is covered by private supplementary insurance, which is either purchased by the beneficiaries themselves or provided by their former employers. Another 12% of total spending is covered by the state-administered Medicaid programme for pauperised Medicare patients unable to cover with their own resources expenditures not covered by Medicare. Finally, close to a fifth of the total is paid by the beneficiaries themselves, in the form of out-of-pocket payments, which, for beneficiaries living at or near the official federal poverty level, averages about 30 to 34% of their already meagre household budgets.[11]

In spite of Medicare's spotty benefit package, opinion surveys of both young and old Americans have consistently shown Medicare to receive the highest mark among all US private and public health insurance products for 'serving the consumer well'.[12] The high satisfaction level may reflect the fact that, relative to most private insurance products, Medicare has two important features not found in other US health insurance products. First, from the patient's perspective it is relatively simple. Second, it is permanent rather than temporary (the case with all other US insurance contracts). Basically, Medicare offers guaranteed insurance coverage on items in its benefit package for the rest of the insured's life. Proponents who pushed for the programme's enactment in 1965 naturally saw it as the first phase of an inexorable march towards a fully-fledged national health

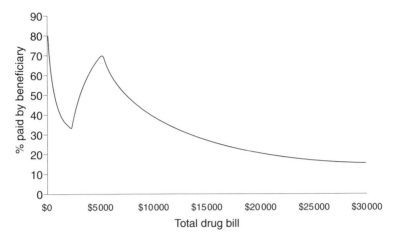

Figure 6.5 Percentage of drug bill to be paid by Medicare beneficiary under Medicare Reform Law of 2003.

insurance system for the US. It is exactly what its opponents feared at the time and have successfully prevented in the intervening years.

Under the recently enacted *Medicare Prescription Drug, Improvement and Modernization Act of 2003*, President Bush's administration and the Congress have sought to fill in one of the most glaring gaps in Medicare's benefit package: lack of any coverage for prescription drugs. The coverage provided by the bill, however, is far from generous – certainly by international standards. Figure 6.5 shows the fraction of their total annual drug bill that Medicare beneficiaries must still pay after the bill is fully implemented after 2006.

The peculiar shape of the cost-sharing curve in Figure 6.5 is driven by the equally peculiar parameters of the reform bill. They, in turn, were driven by an arbitrary, projected budget cap for tax-financed subsidies of $400 billion for the first eight years of the programme's existence. Medicare beneficiaries are to pay the first $250 of their annual drug bill out-of-pocket. Then, Medicare will pay 75% of the drug bill, but only up to an amount of $2250. Thereafter, to keep within the arbitrary budget cap, Medicare coverage stops entirely, until the beneficiary has paid $3600 per year out-of-pocket, a point reached when the total annual drug bill is $5100. Medicare will then pay 95% of drug spending that exceeds $5100. The uncovered gap between $2250 and $5100 is popularly known as the 'doughnut hole' of the bill.

It would be an intellectual challenge to defend these programme parameters with appeal to either clinical or economic science. Indeed, it would be hard to imagine that any nation other than the US would ever enact such a bill. The marvel is that the President of the US and Congress take genuine pride in this dubious construct, which they view as generous toward the elderly!

In keeping with the nation's traditional respect for the wishes of the supply side of the health system, the bill includes in its 700+ pages, the express provision that the government itself may not negotiate prices with drug manufacturers under this programme, and that the new benefit is to be administered and managed by private health insurance companies or by private pharmaceutical benefit management companies (PBMs). An additional provision forbids Medicare beneficiaries from purchasing private insurance coverage for the 'doughnut hole' left in the bill. This stricture illustrates, once again, a point made in the introduction to this chapter, namely, that Republican legislators do not hesitate to become remarkably intrusive in their regulation of private behaviour if that suits their purposes.[iv]

Privatisation of Medicare through Medicare+Choice

Since about the mid-1980s, Medicare has allowed beneficiaries to opt out of the government-run programme in favour of a qualified, private health maintenance organisation (HMO) or similar qualified health plans that agree to provide beneficiaries at least the Medicare benefit package, in exchange for a prepaid annual capitation payment from Medicare, plus, in many instances, additional premium payments by the beneficiaries. Since 1997, this programme has been known as 'Medicare+Choice' (M+C). In the recently enacted *Medicare Prescription Drug, Improvement and Modernization Act of 2003* is has been renamed 'Medicare Advantage.'

During the 1980s and 1990s, private health plans appear to have been able to attract more favourable risks from the overall pool of Medicare beneficiaries, which allowed the plans to offer the (relatively healthier) beneficiaries richer benefits – typically prescription drugs – for the capitation payments the plans received from Medicare.[13][v] In the latter half of the 1990s, however, that financial advantage appeared to shrink, just as the cost of prescription drug coverage began to soar. At the same time, in 1997, Medicare began to limit the annual increases in the capitation payments paid to the private plans in the high-cost areas to 2%, in an attempt to compress these payments, which varied by a factor of three across the US. The convergence of all of these unfavourable factors led many of the M+C plans to leave the business in areas that had become unprofitable.

To reverse this trend, the *Medicare Prescription Drug, Improvement and Modernization Act of 2003* provides for substantial increases in the payments Medicare makes to M+C plans, explicitly allowing tax-financed spending for beneficiaries enrolled in private health plans to exceed spending for similar beneficiaries under the government-run programmes.[14] One may view this gesture as the tacit recognition on the part of Congress that private health plans are unlikely to reduce the healthcare cost of the elderly below what is now being spent on them, which is not really surprising. First, it is unlikely that private health plans will, with any degree of consistency, be able to negotiate lower fees with the providers of healthcare than are set by the government-run Medicare programme. Second, private health plans require a much larger fraction of the premium they receive for marketing, administration and profits than does the government-run Medicare programme, which has neither marketing costs nor a need for a profit margin, and which has very low administrative costs. In 2001, Medicare used less than 2% of its total spending for administration.[15] In the same year, private health plans allocated between 14 and 19% of their premium income to marketing, administration and profits, a range that rose to 17 to 20% in 2002.[15] To overcome just this cost disadvantage, the private plans would have to make a substantial reduction in the volume of health services used by their Medicare enrollees, through managed-care techniques. There is no reason to assume, however, that elderly Americans, accustomed as they are to a government-run health insurance programme that gives them completely free choice of provider and therapy, would take any more kindly to these managed-care techniques (more limited choice of provider and therapy and direct utilisation controls) than did younger Americans who responded to these techniques with what has come to be known as the 'managed-care backlash'.

The capitation payments paid to private health plans by Medicare for beneficiaries in a given county are currently pegged on the actuarially 'adjusted average per-capita cost' (AAPCC) of beneficiaries under the government-run, fee-for-service programme. Because the proponents of privatising Medicare invariably hold out the prospect of greater efficiency through competitively bid premiums, Medicare attempted to field several local experiments with competitive bidding during the 1990s. As Dowd *et al.* report on these efforts, in each instance these experiments were vehemently opposed by the health plans and sundry other constituents, leading Congress to prohibit them in the end, in spite of having called for them initially.[16] As if to underscore a point made in the introduction to this chapter – that rhetoric about markets by Republican politicians often is just that, rhetoric – the authors write:

> *Also ironic is the fact that in three of the four attempted demonstration sites during 1996–1999, Republicans led the charge to halt Medicare's most sweeping test of market-based pricing.* (p. 24)

Part of the health plans' objection to the experiments was that the traditional, government-run, fee-for-service Medicare programmes at the experimental sites were not forced to compete for beneficiaries on the same terms as the private health plans,[17] which is a fair critique.[vi] On the other hand, one should never overestimate the enthusiasm of private sector entities for truly competitive bidding on government business under any circumstance. There is something intellectually twisted in the idea that competitive bidding for Medicare's beneficiaries will reduce the cost of their healthcare, or to expect that the supply side of the healthcare system – which books 'health spending' as 'healthcare revenue' – will heartily embrace that approach. As Nichols and Reischauer[18] observe on this important point:

> *In the end one overriding question remains: does Congress really want Medicare to use its potential buying power to become a more efficient purchaser? [Medicare] is an important source of income for providers and health plans. Senators and Congressmen represent local and immediate interests first and foremost. The gains from competition are distant and diffuse, and they come in small increments spread across many beneficiaries and taxpayers.* (p. 43)

In a nation that allows powerful, moneyed interest groups to become, effectively, equity holders in the legislative process, these observations do not augur well for the prospect of competitive bidding by private health plans for Medicare's enrollees.

The Federal VA health system

Many nations do not operate a separate health system specifically for veterans. Instead, their veterans are folded into the general national health insurance system and share the same healthcare delivery system as everyone else. In this regard the US represents an oddity. Although many US veterans do rely on a mixture of private health insurance or Medicare for their primary health insurance coverage, they look upon the VA health system as their own trustworthy fail-safe system, in case they lose their private insurance coverage or need items not covered by their private insurance. Currently, many veterans flock to the VA to obtain virtually free coverage for prescription drugs for which Medicare does not pay.[19]

That US veterans, who more often than not are politically conservative, would safeguard as jealously as they have the purest form of what would otherwise be decried as 'socialised medicine' – that is, a healthcare delivery system owned, financed and operated by the nation's central government – stands as powerful testimony to the brittleness of the nation's private health insurance system and to the trust that Americans of all political stripes ultimately repose in their government. Even more ironic, but perfectly understandable, is the visible solicitude that the staunchest conservative members of US Congress show towards this system of purely socialised medicine, all the while thundering against the inherent evils of socialised medicine in, say, the UK.

State and local governments

In 2001, state and local governments in the US paid directly for about 30% of total *public* health spending and about 14% of total national health spending from all sources. Roughly half of that fraction represented the state governments' share of the federal–state Medicaid programme for the poor, which since 1996 also includes a newly established federal–state programme specifically for children (the State Children's' Health Insurance Programme, known by the acronym S-CHIP). The remainder of state and local health spending covers the budgets of publicly owned inpatient facilities, community health clinics, and other state and local health programmes, including public health departments.

Medicaid

It is seen in Figure 6.3 that the combined federal and state spending on the Medicaid programme now closely rivals total federal outlays for the Medicare programme for the elderly. At the federal level, Medicaid is administered by the Centres for Medicare and Medicaid Services (CMS) of the US Department of Health and Human Services, the same agency that also administers the federal Medicare programme. In 2001, the programme enrolled 42.3 million Americans and spent a total of $226 billion. About a quarter of that total was spent on pauperised Medicare beneficiaries, mainly elderly persons in nursing homes or requiring home care. Close to 40% was spent on the blind or disabled and another quarter on children and non-disabled and non-elderly adults.[vii]

Unlike Medicare, which is an entitlements programme fully independent of the beneficiary's income, Medicaid is a means-tested programme into which or out of which enrollees tumble as a function of year-to-year changes in their economic circumstances. This lack of stability makes the programme highly complex from the perspective of both beneficiaries and administrators. It also makes it very difficult to help low-income Americans better manage their own health through long-term preventive strategies.

When the US Congress established Medicaid in 1965, the broad intent had been to grant federal financial assistance to states that chose to establish a health insurance programme for the medically needy. The federal government determines the minimum benefit package, which has remained remarkably comprehensive and does not yet call for any cost-sharing by patients (although that may change before long). The state governments, on the other hand, are free to decide whether to establish a Medicaid programme at all and, if so, how eligibility thresholds for the programme shall be determined, as well as the fees it pays the providers of healthcare under the programme. Within this framework, the federal government shares the costs experienced by the states in inverse proportion to the states' per-capita income. In 1998, the federal share, averaged across all states, was 56.5%.[20] It ranged from a minimum of 50% to a maximum of 76%, although the theoretical maximum is 83%.[21]

Because the states are free to determine the fees paid to healthcare providers, fees for the same procedure vary considerably across the states, although they are uniform within them. In general, they tend to be much lower than those paid for patients enrolled in Medicare and certainly much lower than those paid by commercial insurers. For that reason, many physicians refuse to accept any Medicaid patients at all. Hospitals, on the other hand, accept all Medicaid patients, even though, on average, Medicaid pays them less than their fully allocated costs of treating such patients.

During the past decade or so, many states moved their Medicaid populations into private health plans, to gain better control over the volume of services used by the beneficiaries. Some of these private health plans serve a wider mix of enrollees; others specialise in managing healthcare for the Medicaid population. Unlike Medicare beneficiaries, who can elect to remain in traditional Medicare or join a private health plan, Medicaid enrollees usually have no choice when state governments decide to move them into privately managed care. By 2002, 58% of the nation's Medicaid population had been moved to private health plans, a number that is expected to grow in the future.[22]

Federal–state relations

Over the past several decades, the relationship between the federal and state governments has gradually changed, as US Congress altered the requirements states had to meet to receive federal cost-sharing. For example, Congress has mandated that states enrol certain categories of patients, e.g. pregnant women, or parents of children already enrolled in Medicaid, with incomes below specified levels, or cover certain additional services. From the states' perspectives, these edicts amount to 'unfounded mandates', because they mandate the states to spend additional money on Medicaid with only partial reimbursement by the federal government. Unfunded federal mandates are a constant source of friction in federal–state fiscal relations in the US.

Since the early 1990s, Congress has allowed the US Department of Health and Human Services to approve applications from states for waivers from the strict requirements for federal cost-sharing under the programme. The idea was to let the states experiment with a great variety of approaches for Medicaid benefici-aries. A major problem with these incremental changes to the programme is that, over time, Medicaid's administrative superstructure has become so complex that few experts now have a clear overview. Worse still, many low-income families whose members are eligible for the programme either do not know it or do not have the capacity to overcome the myriad bureaucratic hurdles put in place by legislators and regulators to control the influx of ineligible enrollees. Of the roughly ten million children currently without any health insurance coverage, for example, close to seven million actually are eligible for either Medicaid or S-CHIP coverage but, for one reason or another, have not yet found their way into these programmes.[23]

The growing administrative complexity of the Medicaid programme has given rise to a new industry of Medicaid consultants who make a living trying to understand and explain it to the state bureaucracies. It has also given birth to ever more ingenious fiscal entrepreneurship of the sort that brings to mind the much-mouthed slogan: 'Only in America'.

In one such clever scheme, state governments milk the federal Treasury through a series of fake, intra-state transfers.[21] To illustrate, a municipal hospital within the state makes a so-called intergovernmental transfer of, say, $20 million to the state government. In return, the state's Medicaid programme raises the fees paid to the municipal hospital for Medicaid patients from the state's currently low levels to the maximum allowed by the federal government – the level that would be paid by the federal Medicare programme. The tactic might yield the municipal hospital an additional payment of, say, $22 million in Medicaid payments from the state, so that it is $2 million ahead. If the state's per-capita income is such that the federal government absorbs 70% of the state's outlays on Medicaid, then the federal government will send the state an additional cheque for 70% of the $22 million paid to the municipal hospital, that is, for $15.4 million. The net result of these fiscal transfers is that the health facility gains an additional $2 million, the state government gains an additional $13.4 million ($20m – $22m + $15.4 m) and the federal government loses $15.4 million. Worse still, the federal government effectively has little control over exactly how the state government will use that extra $15.4 million of federal money. With only a little legerdemain in its budget accounting, a clever state government could spend that federal money for a different purpose entirely, e.g. to build highways. Even so, the federal government will report its outlay as an outlay on Medicaid that accrued to the poor. Finally, the consultant's fee for inventing and implementing this negative-sum game[viii] will be counted as part of the nation's 'valuable output' – its GDP.

There is little disagreement that, since its enactment in 1965, the Medicaid programme has been a major blessing for the US's low-income families, and also for the providers of healthcare who otherwise would be besieged by these families for charitable care. As it has evolved over time, however, Medicaid now represents a nexus within federal–state fiscal relations at which, on the one hand, the federal government can saddle the state governments with unfunded mandates over which the states have little say while, on the other hand, the state governments can use clever intra-state transfers and other strategies to suck into the state additional federal funds over which the federal government has no control. For all of its many contributions to the life of poor Americans, then,

Medicaid is not really a shining example of the division of labour within the public sector or of federal–fiscal relations.

Health spending by the private sector

Private sector spending on healthcare in the US by patients and their insurers currently accounts for about 54% of total US health spending (*see* Figure 6.2). About 15 percentage points of these 54% represented out-of-pocket spending by patients and 35 percentage points was spending by private insurers. The remainder represents spending by third parties other than private insurers.

Private health insurance

As was seen in Table 6.1, close to 70% of the US population has private health insurance, of which the bulk is provided by private and public employers by means of group health policies that cover employees and their families.

The provision of health insurance to employees is entirely voluntary on the employer's part. As a highly prized fringe benefit, it is an attractive component of an employee's total compensation and, therefore, offered by most large employers and almost always to highly skilled and well-paid employees. By law, health insurance coverage must be offered to all employees in a firm, if it is offered to any employees. On the other hand, employees within the firm may be covered by a variety of different insurance products, ranging from tightly managed HMOs to open-ended fee-for-service products (the latter mainly for executives). Individual employees may elect not to accept insurance coverage from their employer, thereby saving the explicit out-of-paycheque contributions to the premium they might otherwise have to make. Employees do this when a working spouse has better family coverage or when their take-home pay is low and they would rather keep the money for other purposes.

Traditionally, employees have paid only a small fraction (around 20% or so) of the total cost of their employer-provided health insurance. They have done so by means of explicit deductions from their paycheques. The contribution varies across industries, depending on conditions in their respective labour markets, and it may also vary by the type of insurance product the employee chooses from the menu of options offered by the employer. It may even vary by the age of the employee. Other things being equal, the contribution is much higher for policies that cover the employee's entire family than it is for policies covering only the individual employee. Indeed, many small employers offer health insurance only to their employee, and not to other family members. Yet others, mainly small business establishments with low-wage workers, do not offer their employees any health insurance at all.

Employers may purchase insurance coverage for their employees from private insurers or they may self-insure. If the policies are purchased from insurers, they take the form of group policies whose premiums are 'experience rated' (actuarially fairly priced) over the employer's entire pool of employees (and family members). In that case, employers transfer the financial risk of illness among employees to the insurance carrier, at least for the duration of a year, before premiums can be raised in the following year. By law, such an arrangement is subject to regulation by state governments.

If employers self-insure, they usually use private insurance carriers only to administer the coverage, without shifting to them any financial risk for the employees' illnesses. In that case, the employees' insurance policies are not regulated by the state governments, but by the US Department of Labour under the *Employee Retirement Income Security Act of 1974 (ERISA)*. Because regulation by the insurance commissioners of states typically is stricter and more burdensome than regulation by the US Department of Labour (whose relatively small staff simply cannot supervise the entire business community effectively), most large employers have preferred to self-insure. That tendency has been a constant irritant in federal–state relations, and also among employees who would prefer the stricter state regulation of their insurance coverage.

By European standards the annual premium increases routinely tolerated by US employers for their group insurance policies may appear unimaginable. In the late 1980s, for example, these annual increases reached 18% for large firms, but were much higher for smaller firms. During the 1990s, the increases declined to virtually zero (by 1996), apparently with the help of the managed-care techniques then tried by private health plans but ultimately rejected by US employers and employees alike. By 2003, the average annual increases for large employers have been reported to be close to 14%,[24] although there is a high variance around this average. At the time of this writing, it is not clear what might constrain the growth of these private sector premiums in the future.

Implicit, regressive public subsidies to employment-based insurance

The private and public sectors interface at the nexus of employment through a tax preference that is one of the more ethically and economically perverse components of the US health system – at least in the eyes of economists.

Employers may deduct their share of the cost of health insurance that is not deducted explicitly from the paycheques of workers as a normal business expense. On the other hand, that part of an employee's total compensation is not viewed by the tax code as part of the employee's taxable income. Furthermore, the employee's own explicit contribution toward health insurance is deducted on the paycheque prior to calculating taxable income, which means it is not treated as taxable income either. The total revenue loss to the public sector resulting from tax preferences has been estimated to be about $110 billion or 9% of total national health spending in 1999.[25] Because this revenue loss must be made up by other taxes, the public sector indirectly subsidises the private health insurance of employed Americans. Under a progressive income tax system, the incidence of that tax preference is apt to be regressive.

Even more dubious on both economic and ethical grounds is the so-called 'Flexible Spending Account' (FSA) into which employed Americans (although not self-employed Americans!) may annually deposit specified sums out of their *pre-tax* income, to pay for health spending not covered by their employer-provided health insurance. Unspent balances at year's end, however, revert to the employer; they cannot be carried over into the next year. This stricture sets off an annual year-end rush to spend unused FSA funds – literally funny money by that time – on spectacles, needless tests or other care of dubious merit. One would wonder about the intellectual acumen of a Congress that has enacted this inflationary programme, were it not for the fact that, as noted, US Congress is unusually and steadfastly beholden to the interest groups who call health spending 'income'.

Even more dubious is the ethical precept built into the FSAs. Under the nation's progressive income tax system, the implied public subsidy toward the employee's healthcare increases directly with that employee's income, as marginal tax rates rise. In plainer English, the US Congress sees fit to ensure that the *after-tax* cost of services such as prescription drugs not covered by insurance, cost-sharing required by private insurance policies, teeth cleaning, massages and so on should be *lower in absolute dollars* for high-income Americans, if they are not self-employed, than it should be for low-income, employed Americans. It would be hard to defend this arrangement on ethical precepts other than, perhaps, a twisted version of the Calvinist doctrine of predestination, according to which well-to-do employees might be judged to deserve cheaper healthcare than their poorer brethren.

The recently enacted *Medicare Prescription Drug, Improvement, and Modernization Act of 2003* effectively has converted the FSAs into Health Savings Accounts (HSAs) whose unspent balances can be carried forward by their owners year after year and from employer to employer. This change eliminates at least the inflationary incentives inherent in FSAs, although the regressivity of the measure remains. The catch in HSAs is that to qualify for their tax preference, employees must be covered by a catastrophic health insurance policy with an annual deductible of at least $1000 per individual and $2000 per family. Both employers and employees can make deposits out of pre-tax income into these accounts, which accumulate interest, and are free of capital gains tax. These deposits cannot exceed the deductible *(excess)* of the catastrophic policy or (currently) $2250 per individual and $4500 per family. As in the case of the FSAs, these new HSAs will effectively make healthcare cheaper for high-income families than for low-income families. Some major commercial health insurance companies are ready to offer HSAs to their clients; but it remains to be seen how popular these policies will become among employers and employees.

The strengths and weaknesses of the US public–private sector mix of financing healthcare

In most of the industrialised world, the flow of funds from households to the providers of healthcare is gathered somewhere along the way into one or a few major pipes that can be relatively easily coordinated with one another and whose throughput can be relatively easily manipulated by government for two major purposes: (a) cost control, and (b) the provision of access to healthcare on egalitarian principles. The first is achieved through greater bargaining power[ix] and the latter by paying the providers of healthcare the same prices for a given service, regardless of the patient's socioeconomic or demographic status.

By contrast, the US health system relies for its financing on a myriad of fiscal tributaries of various sizes whose throughput is not easily controlled by any one authority. This system gives the supply side of the system a considerable market power vis-à-vis the fragmented demand side. Furthermore, it literally invites price discrimination, whereby large payers with some market muscle are able to pay much lower prices than smaller and weaker payers, among them the uninsured.

Although in its origin this system is a product of mere historical happenstance rather than of deliberate health policy,[x] the seemingly haphazard architecture it has developed over time also reflects the quite deliberate design of politically powerful groups of healthcare providers who see in that fragmented system the means of maximising the fiscal transfer to them from the rest of society.

Indeed, over the past four decades these groups have consistently and success-fully battled attempts to introduce national health insurance in the US, fearing that it would amass too much market power on the payment side of the health system and, with that monopsonistic power, reduce the money transferred to the providers of healthcare per unit of real resource that the latter transfer to society. The success of the strategy can be inferred from cross-national comparison of health spending, which shows that per-capita health spending in the US in purchasing power parity US dollars far exceeds that in other nations with much older populations, even after adjustment for the high GDP per capita in the US (*see* Figure 6.6).

Although a part of the higher US health spending, unexplained by higher GDP per capita, reflects the higher administrative costs of the US system, another substantial part is likely to reflect the higher prices paid for healthcare in the US.[9] In a cross-national analysis of health spending several years ago, Mark Pauly[26] found that government-run health systems with monopsony tended to use more real resources per capita in healthcare than did the US healthcare system but, by virtue of their monopsonistic power on the demand side, they cede less GDP to the providers of care in return. Subsequent research by the McKinsey Global Institute (1996) of the consulting firm McKinsey & Company yielded similar findings.[7] Using a highly sophisticated tracer analysis of real resource use for four common diseases, the McKinsey researchers were able to distinguish real re-source transfers from money transfers in the treatment of these diseases in the US,

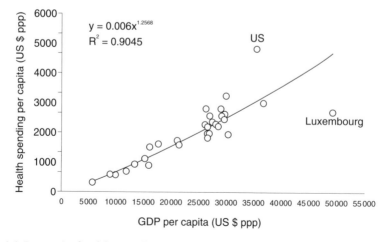

Figure 6.6 Per-capita health spending and per-capita GDP in 32 OECD countries, 2001. *Source*: OECD Data, 2003.[45]

Table 6.2 Decomposition of differential per-capita health spending in Germany and the United States, 1990 (US dollars, in purchasing power parity)

Per-capita spending in Germany	$1473	100%
Less use of real medical inputs in the US	($390)	−26.5%
Plus higher prices in the US	$737	50.0%
Plus higher administrative costs in the US	$360	24.4%
Plus 'other' higher costs in the US	$259	17.6%
Total additional costs per capita in the US	$966	65.6%
Per-capita spending in the US	$2439	165.6%

Source: Baily and Garber,[46] Figure 10.

the UK and Germany. Table 6.2 presents the gist of their analysis in the comparison of US with German healthcare.

McKinsey researchers estimated that, with Germany as the baseline and using US dollar purchasing power as the monetary yardstick, US patients actually used $390 worth *fewer* real resources per capita than did Germans, but transferred $737 *more* per capita to the providers of healthcare in generalised claims on the GDP, by means of higher money prices for the same services. In the comparison with the UK as the baseline, the researchers found that US patients received $388 worth more real resources than did patients in the UK and that US providers of healthcare received $686 more generalised claims on the GDP than did their colleagues in the UK.[7]

The preceding discussion suggests that, within the boundaries set by the willingness of the providers of healthcare to release real resources to the health sector, the size of the claim on the GDP that the providers of healthcare are allowed to take per unit of real resources is largely a political call on which economists have little to say objectively. Through their political process, Americans are inclined to be – or forced to be – rather generous on this score, certainly by international standards.

The advantages claimed for the US payment system's luxury and technical sophistication

Abstracting, for the moment, from the opportunity costs that the US health system visits on the rest of the US economy, the generous flow of funds it begets has supported the development of a highly luxurious and technically sophisticated health system that is accessible without undue delay to anyone who has good health insurance coverage or ample financial means. The US generally ranks at the very top in terms of the availability of expensive, cutting-edge medical technology and per-capita use rates of these technologies.[27]

Generally, this splendid healthcare delivery system is accessible also to low-income persons without health insurance, albeit mainly for tertiary care, when they are critically ill. Indeed, many of the uninsured then have access to the nation's prestigious academic health centres[xi] and teaching hospitals, which jointly care for a disproportionate number of the uninsured with funds drawn from paying patients or obtained from government through direct grants.[xii]

In short, it can fairly be claimed that, at its best, this richly endowed healthcare delivery system is unrivalled in the world. It is what Americans have in mind when they claim, as is their wont, that theirs is the best health system in the world. It is also what the many foreign patients have in mind when they flock to the US in search of treatments that they cannot find at home.

Innovation

The myriad of fiscal feeders into the US health system and the supply side's disproportionate control over the fiscal throughput of the system also has made the US health system hospitable to technical and organisational innovation – often before these innovations have proven their value. To be sure, the US health system dominates in these facets in part by virtue of the sheer size of that system; but the lack of central control over the funds flow in healthcare and over the configuration of the delivery system also enables experimentation.

Much of the technological progress in US healthcare is forged in the nation's academic health centres, which represent a fascinating confluence of diverse fiscal flows from both the public and private sectors. Many of these centres are part of state universities and, as such, are part of the public sector. Others belong to privately endowed universities, while still others, such as Mount Sinai in New York City, are privately endowed, free-standing academic health centres. Whatever their ownership may be, however, they all rely on a steady stream of federal financing to support their clinical research, the graduate medical education of physicians and their charitable healthcare. Traditionally, these centres also have been able to charge private insurers higher prices, on the tacit understanding that any profits they earn will be recycled into these centres' underfunded social missions, including basic biomedical research. In recent years, however, the centres have also engaged in joint ventures with investor-owned, for-profit producers of healthcare products, such as devices, pharmaceuticals or biotech products.

This nexus between the public sector, the private non-profit sector and the private for-profit sector remains controversial, because it is a double-edged sword. On the one hand, the joint ventures draw private capital venture capital into the biomedical research enterprise and, along with it, the powerful motivator of profits. On the other hand, however, these joint ventures trigger new conflicts of interest among researchers and thereby may hinder the hitherto free flow of information within the research community that has been the hallmark of the US's flourishing research enterprise. In this regard, nations that have not yet gone down this path can learn much from the US experience.

Responsiveness to patients

In its report on the performance of health systems around the world published in 2000, researchers at the World Health Organization (WHO) had ranked the *overall* performance of the US health system as 37 out of 191 countries, right after Dominica[35] and Costa Rica[36] but ahead of Slovenia and Cuba, which ranked in 38th and 39th place, respectively.[28][xiii] The overall performance index for this ranking was a highly controversial synthetic construct, one of whose components was an index of the health system's 'level of responsiveness'. On that index, the US health system ranked first worldwide, with a score of 8.14, ahead of second-place Switzerland with a score of 7.44 and much further ahead of seventh-place Canada, with a score of 7.44, and 26th place UK with a score of 6.51. Anyone sampling the nation's typically well-appointed and customer-oriented community hospitals, academic health centres or medical practices probably would not find that ranking surprising.

As Robert Blendon and his colleagues have pointed out,[1] however, the WHO rankings were based on responses of small samples of public health experts in each country, rather than larger, representative samples of citizens who experience their health system on a routine basis. Drawing on a variety of surveys of citizens, the authors find little correlation between the WHO rankings on either 'overall systems performance' or 'the responsiveness index', on the one hand, and the satisfaction scores citizens would give their country's health system in response to the question: 'In general, would you say that you are very satisfied, fairly satisfied, neither satisfied nor dissatisfied, fairly dissatisfied or very dissatisfied with the way healthcare runs in your country?' Among the 17 OECD countries selected by the authors for their study, 12 European countries and Canada scored higher than the US on the citizens' satisfaction index. While only 40% of American respondents declared themselves 'fairly or very satisfied' with the US health system, 57% of the UK respondents answered thus, although the UK ranked only 14th on the WHO responsiveness index.[1]

Choice among insurance products

One advantage frequently claimed for the US health insurance system is that, in comparison with the more uniform health insurance systems in other countries, the US system affords the individual so much more choice among different health insurance products.[8] The assumption is that individuals would like to have freedom of choice not only among the providers of healthcare and the therapies the latter may use, but also demand choices among the insurers who administer the payment system for that care.

The reasons for such a preference could be twofold. First, if a health insurance system actively involves patients in the processing of insurance claims – as it does in the US – then there is merit in allowing the insured to opt-out of one insurance-claims processing of insurers that displease them in favour of more congenial ones. Competition on this dimension among insurers ought to enhance the quality of that process and also its cost. Second, younger or healthier individuals and families may find it advantageous to drop out of higher-risk health insurance pools that force them to pay high cross-subsidies to relatively sicker and costlier members of that pool, in favour of insurance pools with lower actuarial risks and lower premiums. With modern information technology, the US health insurance industry is now poised to respond to that preference with what is called 'mass customisation', that is, insurance policies whose benefit packages and rules are tailored ever more closely to the insured's economic circumstances, family situations and health status of the insured individual.

An assessment of the value of choice among health insurance products cannot be made independently of the social role one posits for health insurance. If one sees health insurance mainly as a mechanism for smoothing out the individual's (or a family's) spending on health over time, on an *actuarially fair* basis,[xiv] then choice among insurance products and the ever finer segmentation of the health insurance pools into risk classes through the mass customisation of insurance policies can be viewed as a positive feature of a health system.

On the other hand, if health insurance is seen primarily as a social mechanism to finance the healthcare of individuals in a nation *collectively*, on the basis of the individual's ability to pay, and to distribute healthcare according to criteria other than ability to pay, then choice among diverse health insurance products and the mass customisation of insurance policies will be scored as a disadvantage.

In theory, of course, one could combine social solidarity in the financing of healthcare with the mass customisation of actuarially fairly priced private insurance products by distributing to individuals perfectly risk-adjusted vouchers for the purchase of private health insurance in a transparent, competitive insurance market. When pressed on the issue of social solidarity, the defenders of mass customisation usually fall back on this theory. Unfortunately, in practice such a system is not easily implemented and has not yet been made properly operational anywhere in the world.

The disadvantages attributed to the US payment system

While the ample flow of funds drawn into the US healthcare system has begotten many a splendid healthcare facility, the sheer size of that flow and its projected growth is now viewed as a nearly intolerable burden on the budgets of households, employers and governments at all levels.

Unsustainable spending trends

In 2003, an employment-based health insurance policy of a typical US family cost about $9000 a year.[24] If these premiums continue to rise at a rate of 10% per year (below recent experience), such a policy will cost at least $23 000 per year a decade hence. Unless Americans situated in the upper third of the nation's distribution of family income are prepared to subsidise more heavily than they have the healthcare of families in the lower third – as they show no inclination to do[29] – the US's low-income families will find themselves systematically priced out of the US health system.

In the longer run, the currently projected spending trends may not be sustainable even for the nation as a whole. As Chernew *et al.* have shown,[30] the US economy most probably could absorb health spending that grows one percentage point faster than the rest of the GDP throughout the next seven decades and still have real non-health GDP per capita growth throughout that period. On the other hand, a growth rate differential of two percentage points would keep non-health GDP per capita rising until about 2040, whereafter it would begin to decline at an ever more rapid rate. The actuaries at the Centres of Medicare and Medicare Services (CMS), however, project this growth differential to be 2.9 percentage points,[xv] which could be accommodated for the longer term only if Americans are willing to tolerate an absolute decline in their non-health GDP per capita even before 2040.

Enormous administrative overhead

As was noted in the introduction to this chapter, the more complex the payment system that pumps money from households to the providers of healthcare, the more of that money flow will leak out of the medical system proper into administrative expense.

In the previously cited research by the McKinsey Global Institute (1996) researchers found that, other things being equal, the US spent $360 more per capita in 1990 than did Germany's health system and an extra $259 per capita on 'other' items, which are costs not directly identified by the researchers, but may well include administrative burdens (*see* Table 6.2). The US was estimated to devote 24% of its total per-capita health spending that year ($2439) to administrative overhead, and Germany 13% of its total per-capita spending of $1473. In the comparison of health spending in the UK and the US, it was found that the US health system in 1990 spent $437 more per capita on administration than did the UK. Administrative overhead in the UK was estimated to be 16% of total costs, compared to 24% in the US.

These estimates, however, include only direct outlays of money on administration by insurers and providers. To get a more comprehensive measure of the administrative costs for the US, Woolhandler et al.[25] estimated that the combined administrative costs for insurers, employers, and the providers of healthcare in the US health system were 'at least $294.3' billion, in 1999, or about 24% of total national health spending.[xvi] The authors estimate that, on a per-capita basis, in purchasing power parity US dollars, administrative costs were $1059 in 1999 in the US versus only $307 under the administratively much less complex Canadian health system, a differential of $752.[xvii]

In a commentary on Woolhandler et al.'s paper, Henry Aaron argues that for a variety of methodological reasons the actual differential in US and Canadian administrative expense may be smaller than the authors find.[xviii] On the other hand, Woolhandler et al.'s estimate does not include the value of the considerable time US patients spend annually on choosing their preferred health insurance options and, more importantly, on the cumbersome task of the processing and adjudication of insurance claims, chores not usually faced by citizens in other countries.

Price discrimination

Price discrimination is the practice of selling identical goods or services, associated with identical production costs, to different classes of customers at different prices. It is widely practised in American healthcare, with several serious consequences.

First, the pluralism built into the payment system makes the payment even for particular medical treatments for particular patients a confluence of funds from several sources, creating difficulty for anyone in the system to appreciate the full cost of any treatment. It takes the government's large staff of actuaries one to two years to estimate roughly what the total national healthcare bill may have been two years earlier, and even those published totals can be viewed merely as guestimates based on numerous arguable assumptions. While in Canada, Germany and many other health systems, age-specific per-capita spending can be known with a high degree of accuracy from the underlying insurance records, in the US those figures must be cumbersomely composed as a pastiche of estimates from many diverse sources. It takes extraordinary effort and ingenuity to reconcile the estimates of total national health spending reported by two different government agencies within the same Department of Health and Human Services.[31]

Second, because every provider of healthcare charges a vast array of different prices for the same service to different payers, there is little price transparency in the US health system, making a mockery of the image proffered so often by the advocates of 'consumer-driven' healthcare, of the 'savvy healthcare consumer' (formerly patient) expected to shop around smartly for cost-effective healthcare. So far, the more appropriate image of the US healthcare 'consumer' is that of a blindfolded person groping about in a department store, knowing little about what items he or she grabs off the shelves and even less about their prices. For some 20 years, price transparency in US healthcare has remained the development just around the corner.

Third, price discrimination in healthcare raises serious ethical questions. On the one hand, patients without health insurance – who typically have low incomes – commonly are charged the highest prices for health services and prescription drugs, for no other reason than that they lack market power to resist those prices. As has been reported in *The Wall Street Journal*, some hospitals hound low-income families indebted to them through professional bill collectors who garnish the debtors' wages and take possession of their bank accounts.[32] On occasion, these hapless debtors are roused, arrested and jailed for failing to show up at court proceedings initiated by hospitals.[33] How typical these harsh collection practices are of the US hospital industry in general is not known; that they occur at all is troublesome.

On the other hand, the prices paid to the providers of healthcare can also be much too low. The state-run Medicaid programmes, for example, pay the providers of healthcare fees that are only a fraction of those paid by Medicare and private insurers, signalling to these providers that society's valuation of healthcare for the poor is commensurately low. Understandably, fully grasping these relative valuations of their work beamed at them by US society, many physicians have long refused to accept Medicaid patients altogether.

Barriers to information technology

In its use of information technology (IT) in healthcare, the US health system represents a paradox. On the one hand, much of the hardware and software for modern information infrastructures in healthcare is developed in the US. At the same time, the system's reliance on a highly complex payment system, coupled with the nation's enthusiasm for 'individualism' and 'pluralism', has made it difficult to develop national standards for the codes, fee schedules and other nomenclature that form the basis of a good platform for the full exploitation of IT's potential.

As the US Department of Health and Human Services[34] recently observed, '400 different formats exist today for healthcare claims', and that may well be an underestimate. The plethora of different claims forms, each with its own rules and nomenclature, makes it difficult for providers to submit what insurers call 'clean claims', that is, forms that have been properly completed by providers, with all the requisite information demanded by a particular insurer. As a result, it is not uncommon for providers to wait 100 days before being paid whatever the claims process ultimately determines to be the proper amount. In the meantime, claims travel back and forth between insurer and providers. Much of that traffic follows the old-fashioned route of mailed or faxed paper, rather than electronic interchange. To this day, paper remains the chief communications vehicle in the private insurance sector.

The IT industry specialised in healthcare and the health sector it serves perform an unhelpful *pas de deux*. The more sophisticated and cheaper modern IT processes become, the more readily they support ever-more-cumbersome administrative processes dreamt up by government or private insurance bureaucrats including, now, the mass customisation of private insurance policies to ever smaller firms and even the family.[35] As was noted earlier, a physician or hospital may work under several dozen insurance contracts, and hospitals under even more. Each contract will have its own rules on eligibility, coverage, regulations on prior authorisation and formularies for pharmaceutical products. To cope with this vast array of distinct contracts, the providers of healthcare have no choice but to enlist outside consultants, whose huge memory banks have captured most of the myriad of outstanding insurance contracts and whose specialised software is able to identify the particular contractual parameters attached to the particular insurance policy of particular patients. These outside consultants measure their success by three statistics:

- the fractions of submitted claims that are treated as 'clean' by the insurer
- number of days by which they can help reduce the provider's 'days accounts receivable outstanding'
- ultimately uncollectible billings as a percentage of total original billings. For each provider individually, these consultants can produce high benefit cost ratios.

For the health system as a whole, the complexity giving rise to this new consulting industry represents what economists call a 'deadweight loss' no less than that associated with taxation.

There is the distinct possibility that other nations, with their simpler health systems and their high tolerance for national standardisation, may leapfrog the US in the productive application of IT developed in the US. A recent cross-national Harris Poll found that 'European physicians, especially in Sweden, the Netherlands and Denmark, lead the US in the use of electronic medical records'[36] (p. 1 and Table 1). Only 17% of US general practitioners in the survey reported the use of electronic medical records in their practice. The comparable number was 90% for Sweden, 88% for the Netherlands, 62% for Denmark, 58% for the UK, 55% for Austria and 48% for Germany. Processing of claims through electronic data interchange also lags in the US insurance system relative to the more uniform social insurance systems in other countries or Canada's government-run system.

Recognising that the private sector is unlikely to produce an information infrastructure for 21st century US medicine and that such a system is, indeed, largely a public good, in 1996 the US Congress passed the *Health Insurance Portability and Accountability Act (HIPAA)* which mandated, in a section entitled 'Administrative Simplification', national standards for the electronic data interchange (EDI) of clinical, administrative and financial healthcare information.[37]

The act also mandated strict standards for protecting the privacy of patients' medical records. So far privacy has been sorely lacking in the private US healthcare sector, which in many instances has left the medical records of patients as open books accessible to insurers, employers and many other persons not directly involved with patient treatment.

Barriers to universal coverage

A peculiar feature of the US's complex private–public sector mix of paying for healthcare is that it has created a built-in inertia against any kind of reform, including attempts to achieve universal health insurance coverage through small, incremental steps. To be sure, many groups with a vested economic interest in the status quo will score the inertia built into America's health system as a decided advantage, not to be listed under the system's shortcomings. Few Americans, however, take delight in the plight of the uninsured and would score barriers against assisting them as one of the system's shortcomings, as it is here.

After the spectacular demise of President Clinton's ambitious attempt at health reform in 1994, Americans raised to an immutable axiom the erstwhile adage that major reforms of the health system are not feasible in the US. Since then it has become an article of faith among policy makers that any move towards universal health insurance coverage in the US must proceed in small, incremental steps.

Under that approach, someone in the public sector develops a novel health insurance programme for a narrowly targeted group of hitherto uninsured Americans. These objects of compassion (hereafter OCs) may be women, but only if they are pregnant and have an annual income 175% below the official poverty line. They may be children in some well-defined socioeconomic category. They may be unemployed, uninsured individuals, and so on. The proponent of the new programme calculates the budget cost of the programme per OC and, judging it affordable, introduces the requisite legislation.

At that moment, the nation's burgeoning health services research community – notably economists – jumps into action to estimate the number of persons who are not among the OCs of the moment who will somehow manage to crowd into the newly proposed public programme. Next, the researchers will estimate the total budget cost of this 'crowding-in' effect, add it to the projected budget cost of serving the original OCs, and divide the sum by the number of original OCs, to arrive at a usually daunting budget cost of the programme per original OC which may be enough to cause the programme's sponsors to demur.

To illustrate this dynamic concretely, in his 'Income-Based Subsidies Won't Work', Harvard economist and NBER President Martin Feldstein argued strongly against the health-insurance proposals then being proposed by Congressman Jim Cooper (D, Tennessee) and by Senator John Chaffee (R, Rhode Island). Both legislators had proposed income-based subsidies toward the purchase of private health insurance policies. It is instructive to quote Professor Feldstein at length:

> *Such income-based subsidy plans would be a terrible mistake. They would unnecessarily create a vast new welfare programme for more than 50 million people who already have health insurance. They would raise the marginal tax rates of 34 million taxpayers, typically by 20 to 30 percentage points, causing millions of lower-income taxpayers to face marginal tax rates of more than 65%. And they would be unconscionably expensive, costing more than*

$6000 of taxpayers' money to provide health insurance to each currently uninsured individual above the poverty level – more than $18 000 for a family of three. The total cost to taxpayers at 1994 levels of income and health spending could exceed $170 billion a year.[38]

To protect newly proposed incremental expansions of health insurance, its proponents sometimes seek to erect around them sophisticated bureaucratic fences designed to deter the threatening non-OC crowds. Alas, these hurdles may be so formidable that they also act as an effective barrier against the original OCs. For example, the previously cited State Childrens' Health Insurance Programme (S-CHIP) Congress enacted in the mid-1990s for children of near-poor families not entitled to Medicaid entailed so many bureaucratic hurdles that even now, over half a decade after the programme's enactment, some seven million children entitled to it remain uninsured.[39]

It may be mentioned in this connection that the 'crowding-in' effect raises fears not only because of its budget implications. Among private health insurers the phenomenon is known as the 'crowding-out' effect, as they fear that any new government-run insurance programme will crowd out of their book of business persons hitherto privately insured that might then crowd into the subsidised public programme. It is one reason why the champions of the uninsured may have to countenance the previously discussed recycling of tax moneys through the private health insurance sector, to still the opposition to their programme from private health insurers by giving them a financial stake in assistance to the poor – a tax-financed side-payment to private insurers, so to speak.

Alternative visions for the private–public payer mix of US healthcare

The heated political debate preceding the recently enacted *Medicare Prescription Drug, Improvement, and Modernization Act of 2003* is an augury of the battle likely to be fought over healthcare in the US during the next decade or so. Although, in the end, the actual legislation produced a minimalist and almost comical compromise that will make thoughtful persons blush in the international community, it contains the seeds for a brewing battle over the distributive ethic that is to drive 21st century US healthcare.

One of the warring parties, staffed predominantly by Democrats, would like to have seen the bill offer Medicare beneficiaries a much more generous prescription drug benefit folded into the traditional Medicare programme, which would administer the benefit and bargain directly with drug manufacturers over prices. That ideological camp is adamant that the financing of healthcare in the US should elicit from the healthcare delivery system a roughly egalitarian distribution of healthcare. Inspired in good part by the experience abroad, that camp believes that only a government-run programme paying the same prices for the same service, regardless of the patient's socioeconomic status, can guarantee such a distribution and control costs at the same time.

The opposing ideological camp, staffed primarily by Republicans, had envisaged a new division of labour for the Medicare programme. Government would continue to use its power to collect taxes for the programme, but it would delegate management of the benefits to private health insurance companies, each of which would offer Medicare beneficiaries a wide range of choice among different insurance products – ranging from tightly controlled Health Mainte- nance Organisations (HMOs) to completely open-ended and unmanaged fee-for- service plans. As before, the dream is that the economics of this construct will be driven by competitive premium bids by the participating health plans, in spite of the sorry history of that approach described earlier in this chapter.

To facilitate their choice of a private health plan, Medicare's beneficiaries would be endowed by Medicare with risk-adjusted, defined contributions towards the purchase of these private insurance policies, although all but the poorest beneficiaries would have to supplement these defined contributions with their own funds to cover the premiums of their chosen policy. Beneficiaries who elect expensive plans thus would pay a higher premium out-of-pocket than those who elected lower-cost plans. To the extent that the content and quality of the benefits offered by the competing plans were positively correlated with the premiums bid by the plans, there might emerge some tiering by income class of the benefici- aries' healthcare experience. The degree of tiering would depend, of course, on the difference between the defined contribution and the full premium charged by the private insurers. This is the outcome to which the opposing camp objects.

From the din of the recent debate over Medicare reform it is not easy to discern the prime motive for this proposed privatisation of Medicare. Several alternative objectives come to mind:

1 Reduction in *total* health spending per Medicare beneficiary, from all sources, however it may be split between taxpayers and Medicare beneficiaries.
2 Reduction only in the taxpayer's exposure to Medicare spending, even if it increased total health spending per Medicare beneficiary.
3 Obtaining better value for the healthcare dollar, whatever the source, and whatever Medicare reform does to total health spending per Medicare beneficiary, from whatever source.
4 Rescuing the private health insurance from a slow death march caused by the ever-finer risk segmentation that occurs under mass customisation of private health insurance.

To the author's knowledge, there is no body of empirical evidence to suggest that privatisation can achieve the first of these goals. On the contrary, there is every reason to believe that it would drive up the total annual cost of healthcare of the elderly,[xix] as is evidenced by the fact that, as part of the recently enacted Medicare reform bill, Congress is now willing to pay more, overall, per capita to the HMO chosen by Medicare beneficiaries under the existing Medicare+Choice pro- grammes than those beneficiaries would have cost government in the traditional Medicare programme.[14]

The second goal is most likely the primary one actually pursued by the proponents of privatisation, although it may yet be politically incorrect to state that goal explicitly. In effect, the traditional, government-run Medicare pro- gramme has been a defined-benefit programme, guaranteeing beneficiaries a defined set of healthcare benefits, whatever they might cost, forcing taxpayers to bear the risk of healthcare cost inflation. Under privatisation of Medicare, with a defined, tax-financed contribution toward the beneficiary's purchase of private health insurance, Medicare becomes a classic defined-contribution programme.

Changing Medicare from a defined-benefit to a defined-contribution programme would eventually enable Congress to shift more and more of the cost of healthcare for the nation's elderly from the shoulders of working-age taxpayers to the elderly themselves, unless the latter have the political muscle to force up the defined contribution in step with future healthcare cost inflation.

On first blush it may seem that the third goal – better managed care in private health plans – is realistic, if one believes that government-run health insurance programmes could never become the prudent purchasers of cost-effective healthcare that the private health insurance plans of the future will be – even though they have not previously functioned that way. On further thought, however, it is not clear why government-run insurance could not function in this way as well, particularly as single-payer insurance schemes furnish the ideal institutional platform for the sophisticated information infrastructure that the cost-effective procurement of healthcare presupposes.

Finally, the fourth goal is purely political. Imputing it to anyone may appear cynical; but in a nation that chooses to finance its political campaign in the US style, that goal may be more realistic than political innocence may lead one to believe. As Vladeck[40] has argued and others (Nichols and Reischauer[18]) have concurred, Medicare has long functioned as an income maintenance programme. Private insurers are part of the system's income facet and represent a highly influential interest group before Congress.

In the end, the minimalist compromise that was struck in the *Medicare Prescription Drug, Improvement, and Modernization Act of 2003* left the battle over the privatisation of Medicare for another day, settling instead for the vague promise of a yet another set of selected regional experiments with competitive bidding among private health plans, starting in 2010 and ending in 2016. How the ongoing battle over this idea will ultimately tilt will depend crucially on which party captures the White House and Congress in 2008.

The outcome will determine whether public financing of healthcare in the US in the future will be used as an instrument to force upon the delivery system a more or less egalitarian distribution of healthcare – the ideal still inculcated to all US students in health professional schools and still sought by governments in other countries – or whether government financing in the US is to be used merely to guarantee every US citizen access to a relatively bare-bones package of health benefits, letting the rest of the system develop into an officially sanctioned, fully-fledged multi-tiered healthcare delivery structure in which the healthcare experience of citizens is viewed as essentially a private consumer good, whose content and quality can be allowed to vary substantially with their ability to pay, just as it does for other basic goods such as food, clothing and shelter.

The coming decade will tell.

References

1 Blendon RJ, Kim M, Benson JM (2001) The public versus the World Health Organization on health system performance. *Health Affairs.* **20**(5): 10–20.

2 Blendon RJ, Schoen C, Donelan K, Osborn R, DesRoches CM, Scoles K, Davis K, Binns K, Zapert K (2001) Physicians' views on quality of care: a five country comparison. *Health Affairs.* **20**(5): 233–43.

3 Anderson GF, Poullier J-P (1999) Health spending, access and outcomes: trends in industrialized countries. *Health Affairs.* **May/June**: 178–92.

4 Woolhandler S, Himmelstein DU (2002) Paying for national health insurance – and not getting it. *Health Affairs.* **21**(4): 88–98.

5 Aaron HJ (2003) The cost of health care administration in the United States and Canada – questionable answers to a questionable question. *New England Journal of Medicine.* **349**(8): 801–2.

6 Pear R (2003) Some health care providers may face payment penalty. *The New York Times.* 28 December: A1.

7 McKinsey Global Institute, McKinsey Health Care Practice (1996) *Health Care Productivity.* Los Angeles, CA: McKinsey & Company.

8 Danzon PM (1992) Hidden overhead costs: is Canada's system really less expensive? *Health Affairs.* **11**(1): 21–43.

9 Anderson GF, Reinhardt UE, Hussey PS, Petrosyan V (2003) It's the prices, stupid: why the United States is so different from other countries. *Health Affairs.* **22**(1): 89–105.

10 National Academy of Social Insurance (1999) *Medicare and the American Social Contract.* Washington, DC: National Academy of Social Insurance.

11 Moon M (1996) *Medicare Now and In the Future* (2e). Washington, DC: The Urban Institute.

12 Henry J. Kaiser Family Foundation (1998) *National Survey on Medicare: the next big policy debate?* (accessed August 2002). Available from URL www.KFF.ORG/content/archive/1442/

13 Physician Payment Review Commission (United States Government Policy and Supporting Positions): 1996 Edition. Committee on Government Reform and Oversight. US House of Representatives 104th Congress, 2nd Session.

14 Congressional Budget Office (2003) *How Many People Lack Health Insurance and For How Long?* Washington, DC: Congressional Budget Office.

15 Centers for Medicare and Medicaid Services. US Department of Health and Human Services, CMS Programme Operations. CMS Facts & Figures, June 2002 Edition, Section II, Slide II.6. Available from URL http://cms.hhs.gov/charts/default.asp

16 Dowd B, Coulam R, Feldman R (2000) 'A tale of four cities: Medicare reform and competitive pricing'. *Health Affairs.* **19**(5): 9–29.

17 Ignani K (2003) Putting principles first: a better way to carry out a demonstration. *Health Affairs.* **September/October**: 44–8.

18 Nichols LM, Reischauer RD (2000) Who really wants price competition in Medicare managed care? *Health Affairs.* **September/October**: 30–43.

19 Stacom D (2004) Drug prices draw vets: rush swamps VA hospitals. *The Hartford Courant.* 24 August (accessed August 2002). Available from URL www.ctnow.com/news/health/hc-vets0822.artaug24.story? coll=hcpercentDheadlinespercent2Dhome

20 Henry J. Kaiser Family Foundation (1999) *The Medicaid Programme at a Glance.* Available from URL www.kff.org/medicaid/loader.cfm?url=/commonspot/security/getfile.cfm&PageID=14725.

21 Coughlin TA, Zuckerman S (2002) States' Use of Medicaid maximization strategies to tap federal revenues: programme implications and consequences. Urban Institute Discussion Paper (pp. 2–9). Available from URL www.urban.org/ViewPub.cfm?PubID=310525

22 Centers for Medicare and Medicaid Services (2003) *Health Care Industry Update: managed care.* Available from URL http://cms.hhs.gov/reports/hcimu/hcimu_03242003.pdf

23 Henry J. Kaiser Family Foundation (2002) *Health Insurance Coverage in America: 2000 data update.* Available from URL www.kff.org/uninsured/loader.cfm?url=/commonspot/security/getfile.cfm&PageID=14103

24 Henry J. Kaiser Family Foundation and Health Research and Educational Trust (2003) *Employer Health Benefits 2003 – Annual Survey* (accessed December 2003). Available from URL www.kff.org/insurance/loader.cfm?url=/commonspot/security/getfile.cfm&PageID=21185

25 Woolhandler S, Campbell T, Himmelstein DU (2003) Costs of health care administration in the United States and Canada. *New England Journal of Medicine.* **349**(8): 768–75.

26 Pauly MV (1995) US health care costs: the untold story. *Health Affairs.* **14**(3): 152–9.

27 Reinhardt UE, Hussey PS, Anderson GF (1999) Cross-national comparisons of health systems using OECD data. *Health Affairs.* **21**(3): 169–81.

28 World Health Organization (2000) *Health Systems: improving performance, World Health Report 2000.* Geneva: Switzerland.

29 Reinhardt UE. Is there hope for the uninsured? *Health Affairs (Web exclusive 082307).* Available from URL www.healthaffairs.org/WebExclusives/Reinhardt

30 Chernew ME, Hirth RA, Cutler DM (2003) Increased spending on health care: how much can the United States afford? *Health Affairs.* **22**(4): 15–25. (Exhibit 1)

31 Selden TM, Levit KR, Cohen JW, Zuvekas SH, Moeller JF, McKusick D, Arnett III RH (2001) Reconciling medical expenditure estimates from the Medical Expenditure Panel Survey and the National Health Accounts. *Health Care Financing Review.* **23**(1): 161–78.

32 Lagnado L (2003) Twenty years and still paying. *The Wall Street Journal.* 13 March: B1.

33 Lagnado L (2003) Hospitals take extreme measures to collect their overdue debt. *The Wall Street Journal.* 30 October: A1, A8.

34 US Department of Health and Human Services (2001) *Administrative Simplification: transactions and code sets.* Updated 2 November 2001 (accessed August 2002). Available from URL http://aspe.hhs.gov/admnsimp/bannertx.htm and http://aspe.hhs.gov/admnsimp/faqtx.htm#whynational

35 Robinson JC (1999) The future of managed care. *Health Affairs.* **March/April**: 7–24.

36 Harris Interactive (2002) *Health Care News.* 2(16). Available from URL www.harrisinteractive.com/news/newsletters/healthnews/HI_HealthCareNews2002Vol2_Iss16.pdf

37 US Department of Health and Human Services, Centers for Medicare and Medicaid Services (2002) *Electronic Health Care Transactions and Code Set Standards Model Compliance Plan.* 16 May 2002. Available from URL http://cms.hhs.gov/hipaa/hipaa2/ascaform.asp

38 Feldstein MS (1999) Prefunding Medicare. National Bureau of Economic Research Working Paper No. W6917.

39 Henry J. Kaiser Family Foundation (2002) *Trends and Indicators in the Changing Health Care Marketplace.* Available from URL www.kff.org/insurance/loader.cfm?url=/commonspot/security/getfile.cfm&PageID=14967

40 Vladeck BC (1999) The political economy of Medicare. *Health Affairs.* **January/February**: 22–36.

41 Reinhardt UE (2001) Can efficiency in health care be left to the market? *Journal of Health Policy, Politics and Law.* **26**(5): 967–92.

42 Heffler S, Smith S, Keehan S, Clement MK, Won G, Zecca M (2003) Health spending projections for 2002–2012. *Health Affairs (Web exclusive 020703)* [accessed December 2003]. Available from URL www.healthaffairs.org/WebExclusives/Heffler

43 Heffler S, Levit K, Smith S, Smith C, Cowan C, Lazenby H, Freeland M (2001) Health spending growth up in 1999; faster growth expected in the future. *Health Affairs (Millwood).* **20**(2): 193–203.

44 US Department of Commerce, Bureau of the Census (2003) *Health Insurance Coverage in the United States: 2002.* Table A-1.

45 Organisation for Economic Co-operation and Development (2003) *OECD Health Data 2003. A comparative analysis of 30 countries.* Paris: OECD.

46 Baily MN, Garber AM (1997) Health care productivity. In: Baily MN, Reiss PC, Winston C (eds) *Brookings Papers on Economic Activity: microeconomics.* Washington, DC: Brookings Institution, pp. 143–214.

Endnotes

i For an elaboration on this proposition, see the author's 'Can efficiency in health care be left to the market?' *Journal of Health Policy, Politics and Law.* **26**(5): 967–92.[41]

ii Total national health spending as a percentage of gross domestic product was about 15% in 2002. *See* Heffler *et al.* (2003), Table 1.[42]

iii There are various ways to count America's uninsured. In a recent study, the Congressional Budget Office (2003) estimated that between 21 to 31 million Americans were uninsured for the entire year 1998, and between 56.8 and 59 million were without health insurance at some point in 1998. In between is the number of Americans who tend to be uninsured at specific points in time during the year (when the survey was taken). In 1998, that number was estimated to range between 39 and 42.6 million, depending on the survey.

iv The bill was designed and pushed through the Republican Congress at President Bush's behest. The stricture on purchasing coverage for the 'doughnut hole' is intended to lower the probability that a beneficiary's drug bill will exceed $5100.

v The Physician Payment Review Commission (1996) compared expenditures incurred for beneficiaries who elected to join a private HMO six months prior to enrolling in the HMOs with expenditures for beneficiaries who remained in the government-run programme and found spending for the former group 63% lower than that for the latter group. The study also found that beneficiaries who had joined HMOs but then disenrolled to return to the government programme subsequently had expenditures in the government programme that were 60% higher than spending for beneficiaries who had never left the government programme. The Commission reports numerous other studies showing a selection bias in favour of HMOs, although not always of the magnitude detected by the Commission.

vi A health plan with a bid premium above the benchmark bid accepted by Medicare would have to charge enrollees the excess as an out-of-pocket contribution. The health plans complained that traditional Medicare could keep its out-of-pocket premiums to the elderly at the constant, legislated level.

vii Medicaid also spent about 9% of its budget on grants to so-called disproportionate-share (DSH) hospitals that treated a disproportionate share of low-income uninsured Americans.

viii Negative, because real resources are burned in the process.

ix That bargaining power, of course, can easily be abused by government, in which case society may have available to it fewer real healthcare resources than it would wish.

x The employment-based health insurance system, for example, traces its origin to wage and price controls imposed by Congress during World War II. Because fringe benefits were excluded from the wage caps, employers competed for scarce workers by paying fringe benefits rather than the controlled cash wages.

xi The institutions, of course, thereby gain access to what sometimes goes by the technical jargon 'teaching material', i.e. patients willing to let medical students and residents participate in their treatments in return for charity care.

xii Most academic health centres receive so-called 'disproportionate share' (DSH) monies from the federal and state governments, because they treat disproportionately large numbers of poor, uninsured patients.

xiii The overall performance score was driven by the system's estimated shortfall from a theoretical maximum potential performance, which in turn was a function strictly of per-capita health spending and educational attainment in the country.

xiv Actuarially 'fair' means that the premium charged the individual reflects on that individual's expected future health expenditures.

xv Calculated from Heffler *et al.*[43]

xvi Woolhandler *et al.*[25]; Heffler *et al.*[43] After excluding from health expenditures those categories of spending for which they could not estimate administrative costs, the authors conclude that administrative costs amounted to as much as 31% of total healthcare expenditures. Using their approach to estimating total administrative costs, the actual percentage is likely to lie between 24 and 31%.

xvii That differential is not inconsistent with a similar estimate of administrative costs in the German and American health systems published by the McKinsey Global Institute in 1996.[7] Considering the time span of a decade and the fact that Germany's multi-payer health system is administratively more complex than is Canada's, the per-capita spending differential for administrative expense estimated by Woolhandler *et al.*[25] appears at least plausible. *See* McKinsey Global Institute,[7] Executive Summary, Exhibit 5.

xviii Woolhandler *et al.*[25] estimated that Americans in 1999 spent PPP US$209 billion more on administrative costs than they would have, had they adopted Canada's single-payer approach. Using an alternative approach, Aaron estimates that the differential might be only PPP US$159 billion. *See* Aaron,[5] Table 1.

xix For an elaboration of this argument, see the author's *Primer for Journalists on Medicare Reform Proposals* (mimeographed, July 2003), available from the author in electronic form.

Chapter 7

Political wolves and economic sheep: the sustainability of public health insurance in Canada

Bob Evans with Marko Vujicic

Ingenuity: sustaining ourselves in an unfriendly world

In its simplest terms, 'sustainability' refers to nothing more than a comparison of rates of change. If a resource stock – a fishery, a forest, an aquifer, a bank account – is being drawn down faster than it is being replenished, then that stock, or better, that pattern of rates is not indefinitely sustainable. Continuous accumulation is equally unsustainable – the trees do not grow to the sky. Human nature being what it is, however, the latter form of unsustainability typically presents as some form of pollution or accumulating 'bad', while the former involves running out of 'goods'.

While the simple arithmetic of trend projection is beyond dispute, its relevance in any particular situation is not. The time horizon is critical. Economists, in particular, tend to be congenitally suspicious of mechanical projections, for reasons well illustrated in the controversies over the 'limits to growth' in the 1970s.[1] Computer models of resource use and pollutant generation used in the study commissioned by the Club of Rome showed rigorously that the world was approaching, in the relatively near future, absolute limits to economic growth. Worse, even then-current levels of output and income in rich countries were unsustainable in the long run. But critics emphasised that the very definition of a 'resource' depends on the tastes and technology of the day, and that the latter, at least, was endogenous.

Natural resources do not 'run out', they simply become increasingly expensive to locate and extract. But rising prices create powerful incentives to innovate around the tightening constraint, using an increasingly costly resource more efficiently and finding substitutes. Accordingly, depletion of any one resource need not constrain the whole complex economic system. Successful innovation will be

Note: Since this paper was originally submitted to the editor, both the Canadian Institute for Health Information (CIHI) and Finance Canada have revised and updated the data series from which most of the figures (7.2a,b, 7.3, 7.4, 7.5a,b and 7.7a,b) were originally drawn. The figures have thus been revised to incorporate (calendar year) health expenditure data from *National Health Expenditure Trends, 1975–2004* released by CIHI in December 2004 (2003 and 2004 data are forecasts), and (fiscal year) provincial government revenue and expenditure data from the Fiscal Reference Tables maintained on the Finance Canada website, updated in October 2004. The text, however, has not been revised.

reflected in stable (or falling) prices for the commodity that was previously 'running out'. Long-run resource price data seem to support this view; the economist Julian Simon, for example, challenged exponents of 'limits' models to find any natural resource whose price, over the long run, has risen in real terms.

More recently, however, students of sustainability have developed a broader, 'neo-Malthusian' perspective. The environments to which human societies adapt tend to become more hostile over time, sometimes from natural changes but especially from the activities of humans themselves – Malthus' point. On the other hand, human societies have always been ingenious in finding ways to advance their purposes even in the face of this deterioration. Successful societies generate a 'supply of ingenuity' sufficient to meet the challenges thrown up by both the external environment, and the consequences of their own (or others') activities.[i] But an 'ingenuity gap' can open up, with potentially serious consequences, if the supply fails to keep pace with the demand.[2]

This concept of ingenuity includes but goes far beyond advances in technical capacity, to include most importantly the institutional frameworks within which economic and social activity take place – and which also serve to mobilise ingenuity itself. Fiduciary currency, double-entry bookkeeping and limited liability corporations were fundamental advances in ingenuity. Price systems and markets are powerful institutional mechanisms, operating automatically to create incentives for technical innovations – or behavioural changes – to relax the constraints of any particular depleting resource. Pollutants become a problem when no institutional framework motivates a corresponding supply of ingenuity to limit their accumulation. 'Pollution markets,' in which rights to pollute could be traded at varying prices, have been suggested as such a possible framework.

Markets are only one form of social mechanism for mobilising ingenuity – or indeed for promoting any other social objective. Public regulation, for example, is more typically used for pollution control. The most appropriate institutional choice will depend on the context, and is ultimately an empirical question. There is no one 'right' institutional response to every social challenge.[ii] Nor, most importantly, is there any God-given guarantee that the supply of ingenuity itself will be sufficient to deal with emerging social problems. In the idealised world of economic theory, automatic, self-equilibrating mechanisms always take a society to the 'best of all possible worlds' (so long as they are not perturbed by misguided government interventions). But in the real world, societies may not find a satisfactory institutional answer to their problems, becoming more or less 'failed' societies with increasing suffering and misery and, in extreme cases, dissolution.[iii]

Societies split by deep tribal, ethnic, religious or economic divisions and having weak or non-existent unifying institutions, are at particular risk. A deteriorating environment may increase internal conflict, both diverting and dissipating the supply of ingenuity. The incentive to innovate is weakened when there is little security of reward; worse, plundering one's neighbours may become the most profitable application of ingenuity. In the most extreme cases, external challenges to deeply divided societies generate a vicious circle of violent internal conflict, deepening divisions and further deterioration. Unable to hang together, the population hang each other separately.

These extreme observations heavily underline the critical importance of political ingenuity as an essential basis for other forms of advance, in designing and

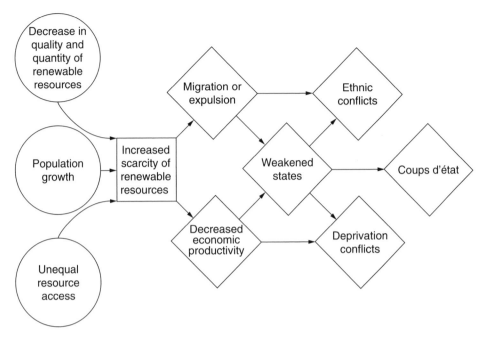

Figure 7.1 Some sources and consequences of renewable resource scarcity. *Source*: Homer-Dixon, Boutwell, Rathjens (1993) *Scientific American.* **268**(2): 38–45.

maintaining institutions for mitigating internal conflict and bridging fissures in the body politic. Absent these, and a whole society can become 'unsustainable'. Figure 7.1[3] provides a compact representation of the dynamics of violent conflict over renewable resources within rather than between states.

States do not generally collapse in high-income countries with highly developed, more or less democratic political systems and massive resources of ingenuity.[iv] Conflicts are typically political and legal rather than military; dramatic transfers of power and shifts in priorities take place not through coups d'état but by the election of a Margaret Thatcher or a George Bush. Nevertheless, the general framework seems to have very broad applicability. Social advance in the most general sense requires a sufficient supply of appropriate ingenuity to meet the challenges of a deteriorating environment. And that supply is threatened by internal divisions that divert ingenuity from promoting collective advantage into escalating political conflicts among competing interests. In particular, this framework seems to provide an interpretation for the seemingly endless conflicts over healthcare policy in high-income countries.[4] In this chapter we address the recently reignited debate over the 'sustainability' of the current system of universal public health insurance in Canada, showing that certain anomalous features of that debate can be readily understood within the neo-Malthusian framework.

Financing Canadian healthcare through fat and lean

The long-run economic environment in Canada has deteriorated significantly since the early 1980s. Figure 7.2a plots Canadian GDP per capita (adjusted for

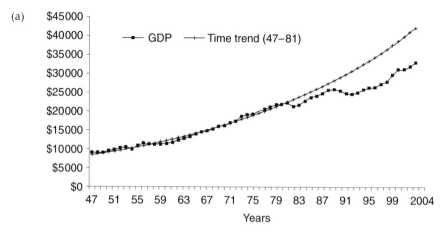

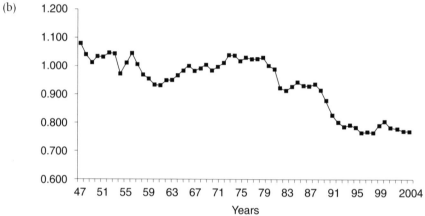

Figure 7.2 (a) Real GDP per capita $1992, 1947–2004; (b) Real GDP per capita over trend $1992, 1947–2004.

inflation) since World War II, fitting a log-linear trend to 1947–81 and projecting it to 2002.[v] Figure 7.2b shows the ratio of actual to fitted or projected values over this 55-year period.

The closeness of actual experience to this trend prior to 1982 is remarkable, with a discrepancy greater than 5% in only four years out of 35, and never reaching 10%. Recessions in 1954 and 1957–61 were followed not only by resumption of growth but also by recovery to the previous path – making up the lost ground.

The recession of 1982 was different. Real income per capita not only dropped sharply, but also failed to recover. Growth resumed in 1983 on a trend line parallel to that of 1947–81, but nearly 10% lower and after the even more severe recession of 1989–92, was along a still lower path. Canadians are not poorer now than in the past; average GDP per capita in 2002 was higher than ever before, and growing (between recessions) at roughly the same rate as in earlier decades. But that average is now more than 20% below where it would have been if the last two recessions had each been followed by real recoveries. For whatever reasons, the ground lost in recent recessions appears permanently lost.

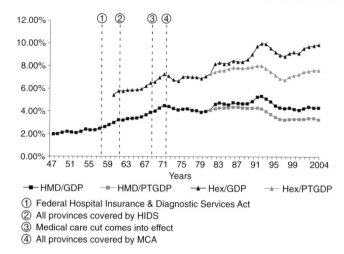

① Federal Hospital Insurance & Diagnostic Services Act
② All provinces covered by HIDS
③ Medical care cut comes into effect
④ All provinces covered by MCA

Figure 7.3 Total health, and hospital and physician expenditure over GDP and trend GDP projected, 1947–2004.

This implies, among other things, a permanent reduction in the income base from which to meet the demands of an expanding healthcare system. Figure 7.3 displays the ratio to GDP of Canadian expenditure (public and private) on hospitals and physicians' services from 1947 to 2002, and of total healthcare expenditure after 1960. It includes hypothetical lines showing what these ratios would have been, after 1981, if GDP had continued to grow along its pre-1982 trend while health spending had evolved as it did.

The hospital and physician data are of particular relevance because only these sectors are covered by the federal–provincial public insurance programmes – Medicare – whose 'sustainability' has been challenged. Administered by provincial governments, according to federal standards and with federal financial contributions, these provide universal comprehensive coverage without deductibles or co-insurance. Other components of healthcare, such as drugs, dentistry and long-term care, are covered through various mixes of out-of-pocket payment, public and private insurance, and direct public delivery.

Perhaps the most striking feature of Figure 7.3 is the remarkable stability of the share of national income devoted to the public insurance programmes. Provinces introduced these in different years, but coverage for hospital care was nationwide by 1961 and for physicians' services by 1971. The latter date was marked by a sharp break in the previous pattern of continuing cost escalation. Universal, comprehensive coverage was not more expensive than the previous fragmented mix of public and private insurance coverage and out-of-pocket payment. Consolidation of expenditures in the hands of a single payer made possible the control of rates of escalation, through a variety of different mechanisms.[5] From 1970 until 1981, the share absorbed by the Medicare services fluctuated in a narrow band between about 4% and 4.25% of GDP.

Nor was the Canadian experience unique. By the 1970s public universal and comprehensive health service or health insurance systems were in place in all the high income countries of the OECD. All developed, at some time during the 1970s or early 1980s, more or less effective mechanisms of cost control.[6] The pattern is sufficiently consistent that White[7] refers to it as 'the international standard'. The one exception, on both counts, is the US, and even there the federal Medicare programme for those 65 and older has been more successful than private insurers in controlling hospital and medical costs over the long term.[8] Single-payer public financing creates an institutional environment, encouraging the supply of ingenuity to contain costs. These are higher in multi-source funding systems where ingenuity is diverted into shifting costs onto someone else.[9]

The early 1980s increase in the Canadian ratio was largely a denominator effect. Health spending stayed on its trend path through the recession, but national income fell. Since the previous income trend was never regained, the share of income spent on hospitals and physicians remained permanently higher. Had there been no recession, or a full recovery, the hospital and medical spending share would have remained in the neighbourhood of 4.25–4.33% for another decade.

The ratio began to follow the same pattern in the next recession, rising sharply to 1992 but again maintaining a constant share of the pre-1982 GDP trend. This time, however, the fiscal exigencies faced by both provincial and federal governments forced a quite dramatic response. Public expenditures were frozen or cut across the board after 1992, including, for the first time, actual cuts in hospital spending. By 1997, hospitals and physicians' services were absorbing the same share of GDP as they had in 1971; if it were not for the persistent effects of the two recessions that share would have been back to early 1960s levels.

The pattern for total healthcare spending is roughly similar, but with a long-term upward trend. Shares of national income devoted to total healthcare expenditure in 1971, 1982, 1992 and 2002 were 7.2%, 8.1%, 10.0% and 9.9% respectively, while hospitals and physicians' services accounted for 4.5%, 4.6%, 5.3% and 4.3%. The year-to-year movements are strongly influenced by the general business cycle, but the 30-year trend indicates that cost containment has been much more successful in the Medicare programmes than in the other healthcare sectors.

Expenditures on prescription drugs, in particular, which are outside Medicare and reimbursed through a combination of public and private insurance and out-of-pocket payment, have been growing very rapidly over the past two decades, more than tripling their share of national income since 1980 (Figure 7.4). This pattern of rapid growth parallels the experience of the whole Canadian healthcare system prior to 1971 (and the American experience prior to 1992 and the 'managed care revolution'), again illustrating the link between fragmented funding sources and rapid cost escalation.[vi]

Adapting to adversity: public success, private failure

The deterioration of the Canadian economic environment after 1982 posed a challenge for the financing of healthcare. That challenge was met initially by allocating a larger share of national income to the healthcare system. The still larger shock of the early 1990s, however, triggered unprecedented reductions in public funding. Controversy has focused, then and subsequently, on the extent to which this mobilised ingenuity to provide care more efficiently and effectively, or whether it simply reduced the level and standard of care provided and left real needs unmet.

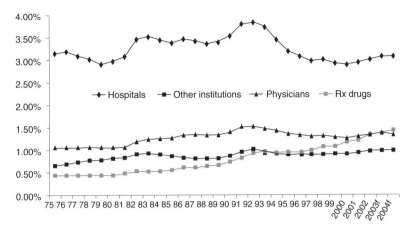

Figure 7.4 Health expenditures: selected components as a percentage of GDP, 1975–2004.

We will bypass this question here, except to note that however one interprets their impact on the health of Canadians, reductions in expenditure must necessarily correspond, as a matter of elementary accounting, to a reduction in total payments to those working in or otherwise supplying resources to the healthcare system. There is an inevitable element of conflict of interest between those who are paid for providing care and those who pay for it. Mobilising ingenuity to improve efficiency, if it lowers total expenditure, threatens the interests of the former even as it benefits the latter. The deterioration of the overall economic environment has tended to widen this division, intensifying the political and rhetorical conflict and clouding efforts to establish – and communicate – what actually happened.

For better or worse, however, the Canadian public insurance programmes did (have to) adapt to the general fiscal circumstances after 1992. Coincidentally, and through different mechanisms, so did US healthcare. The projection by the US Congressional Budget Office[10] that by 2000 the US would be spending 18% of its GDP on healthcare was spectacularly falsified; that percentage flattened in 1992 and remained between 13% and 14% until 2001.[11] As with the 'limits to growth' modelling of the 1970s, linear projections that fail to take account of the adaptability of complex systems are likely to be misleading. The trick is to create the institutional environments that most effectively mobilise the ingenuity necessary to support that adaptation.

Indeed, Canada's experience at the beginning of the 1970s makes the same point. At the end of the 1960s there was growing concern among policymakers (though not, apparently, the public) in both Canada and the US, about the continuing rapid escalation of health costs. The completion of universal public medical coverage in Canada coincided with the immediate flattening of the previous trend; the failure to achieve national health insurance in the US was associated with a continuation of their previous trend. Considerable ingenuity was applied in Canada, as later in other OECD countries, to achieve this result; even more ingenuity was expended, in the US, in frustrating it.

Yet American opponents of national health insurance have claimed for over 30 years that national health insurance would be 'unaffordable'. The counter-evidence, extending from Canada across the OECD world and now to Taiwan,[12] has made no impression on these arguments. Similar concerns were urged in Canada prior to the inception of the Medicare programmes, though perhaps with more excuse, in the 1960s.

Their resurgence in recent years, however, presents us with an obvious anomaly. Why would those alleging the financial unsustainability of Canadian healthcare focus on the public insurance programmes, on Medicare? Why would any rational person, concerned about cost escalation, advocate transferring costs from government budgets back onto patients, either directly or through increased private insurance contributions? On all the available evidence, accumulated across nations and decades, such a shift would almost certainly lead to more rapid escalation.

As the Yale political scientist Ted Marmor reminds us, 'Nothing that is regular is stupid'. If apparently intelligent and well-informed people (in Canada and the US) continue, in the face of the evidence, to revive the argument that universal public health insurance is 'unsustainable' and to advocate diversifying funding sources to increase private payments, then presumably they are either looking at different evidence, or have objectives other than cost control.

(a)
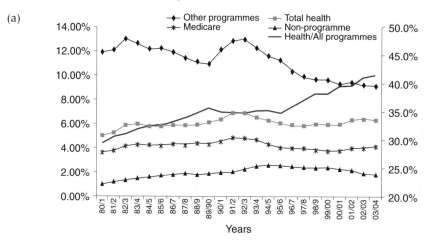

(b)
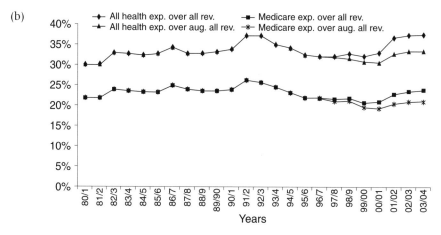

Figure 7.5 (a) Provincial government expenditure as a percentage of GDP, 1980/1 to 2003/04; (b) All provincial government expenditure on Medicare and on all health programmes as a share of total revenue with and without tax cuts, 1980/1 to 2003/04.

The public fisc: still afloat after heavy weather

One explanation might be that for governments, and especially their treasurers, the GDP or its provincial equivalent is something of an abstraction. What is 'real' (subject to the creativity of the public accountants), is the government's own fiscal situation.

GDP patterns certainly affect that situation, insofar as they translate into public sector revenues and expenditures. The 1982 recession ushered in a decade of continuing public sector deficits and growing debt and debt charges; the 1989–91 recession accelerated this fiscal deterioration and raised the spectre of actual bankruptcy for some provincial governments. The harsh public expenditure cuts of the 1992–97 period, combined with subsequent more rapid economic growth, reversed this situation, generating substantial surpluses at the federal level and a falling aggregate public debt. But important as national income trends may be for the fiscal situation of governments, it is the public accounts for which they are accountable.

In those accounts, provincial government expenditures on healthcare programmes have been taking up a rapidly increasing share of total expenditures (Figure 7.5a, right scale).[vii] In the six years between FY1995/6 and FY2001/2, health spending by all provincial (and territorial) governments in Canada rose from 34.8% of total program spending (i.e. net of debt service charges) to 41.1%. This trend appears to provide strong evidence that escalating healthcare costs in the public sector are increasingly crowding out other and important forms of public expenditure – clearly an unsustainable situation. Allegedly, this problem can be addressed only by transferring costs from public to private budgets.

Equally clearly, however, there is something unusual about this particular six-year period. During the seven-year period from FY1988/9 to FY1995/6 there was no change at all in the ratio of aggregate provincial health spending to other programme spending. And in the previous eight years the ratio had risen from 29.6% only to 34.7%.

Moreover, as also shown in Figure 7.5a, aggregate provincial health spending does not show a similar upward trend over this period, relative to national GDP. Both total health spending by provincial governments, and spending on the Medicare programmes alone, took up roughly the same share in 2001/2 as in 1995/6, a share very little different from 20 years earlier. There is a recent uptick in the share absorbed by total provincial health spending, but none at all for hospitals and physicians. (This uptick, which will probably persist in next year's data, raises the question of whether the future will be different from the past, whether the public system has just now become unsustainable. We will try to address this more speculative question below, noting here only that such claims have a long history.)

It follows that provinces must have been cutting back on their non-health spending, and indeed they were. Provincial government spending on other programmes took up a roughly constant share of national income from 1980/1 to 1995/6, between 11% and 12%. It has since fallen steadily, to just over 9% in 2001/2. Yet this quite dramatic reduction was not in fact driven by an 'unsustainable' surge in health spending.

There could still be 'crowding out', if cuts to aggregate spending were being forced by a declining revenue base while political considerations made it difficult or impossible to impose these cuts on health. Other programmes might have had to bear more severe cuts because of the inflexibility of the healthcare as presently structured. But this would imply that health spending was rising as a share of provincial revenues as well as of programme expenditures. This is not so (Figure 7.5b).

Between 1995/6 and 2001/2, when provincial government health spending was rapidly increasing its share of programme expenditures, its share of revenues was virtually flat. Only in the last year do we see the same uptick as in Figure 7.5a. Taking the longer view, health spending now takes up roughly the same share of provincial revenue as it did 20 years earlier.

Moreover, several provincial governments have been taking deliberate steps to reduce that revenue. Starting in 1996/7, they began to introduce a variety of fiscal measures, including, in particular, reductions in their rates of personal and corporate income taxation. By 2003/4, the resulting foregone revenue is estimated at about $23.1 billion annually – $24.9 billion in income tax cuts less $1.8 billion from increases in other tax rates and fees. This reduction represents nearly 15% of aggregate provincial government own-source revenues (excluding federal transfers). Had provincial governments not chosen to use the reviving economy as an opportunity to cut tax rates, the share of provincial revenues devoted to the Medicare programmes would now be lower than it was in 1995/6 (Figure 7.5b, augmented all revenues) – the year in which provincial health spending began to take a rapidly increasing share of total programme spending. In fact, that ratio would have been lower, in the last three years, than in any other year since 1980/1.

Even apart from the impact of these tax cuts, there is no evidence that health spending is placing an increasing strain, over the long term, on the provincial revenue base. The recessions at the beginning and end of the 1980s certainly reduced that base, and each resulted in, among other things, a jump in the proportion of total revenues going to healthcare. Since the economic ground lost in those recessions was never really recovered, that ratio stayed up through the 1980s. In the 1990s, (politically difficult) cuts and rationalisations in the Medicare sector brought the ratio back to its long-term level, consistent with the now lower path of economic growth.

But if health spending has been taking a relatively stable share of revenue while increasing its share of programme spending, then the ratio of revenue to expenditure must have been rising. And it has been, for nearly a decade (Figure 7.6a). Provinces reacted to the recession of the early 1980s by running persistent deficits; the 1989–91 recession exacerbated their weak fiscal positions.[viii] By 1992/3 aggregate revenues were nearly 20% below expenditures (including debt service). This was unsustainable, and serious expenditure cutting began in both the health and non-health sectors. Figure 7.5a shows the corresponding downturn in both spending components, relative to GDP.

But the persistent deficits that were a hangover from the 1980s have now been eliminated (Figure 7.6a). The provincial total is inflated in 2000/1 by a spike in resource revenues, particularly in Alberta; the aggregate ratio drops back to balance in the next year. But Figure 7.6a also shows what provincial revenues would have been, in the absence of the income tax cuts and other fiscal changes that began in 1996/7. Provincial governments would, in aggregate, have reached fiscal balance five years ago, and several would now be rolling up large surpluses.

[And others would not. The unequal distribution of economic development and particularly of resource revenues results in very large disparities between so-called 'have' and 'have-not' provinces. While wealthier provinces have been cutting their taxes and driving the aggregate data, fiscally weaker provinces are still struggling to keep their heads above water. They are also under political pressure to compete in the 'tax cut' game. These disparities generate severe political strains within the federation.]

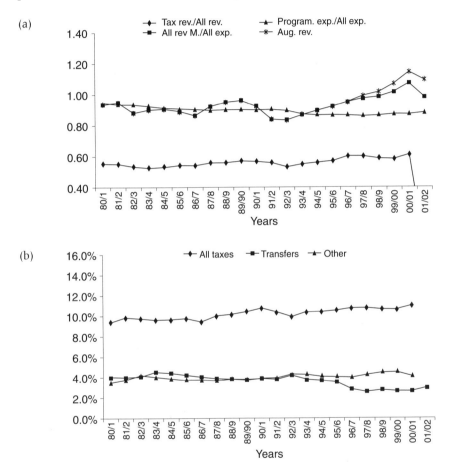

Figure 7.6 (a) Ratios; (b) Provincial government revenue as a percentage of GDP.

Federal–provincial fiscal relations – of course

There is another dimension to the story. The federal government transfers money to the provinces, both as 'tax room' – tax rate reductions to permit provinces to raise their rates – and as block grants of cash, to help provinces support health, education and social welfare programmes. These transfers are a source of continuing friction. Without delving into the fascinating arcana of federal–provincial fiscal relations, the critical point is that after a number of years of chipping away at the cash grants, the federal government introduced a major

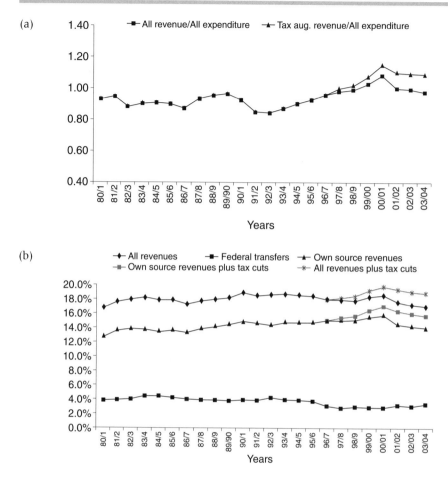

Figure 7.7 (a) Provincial governments, total revenues over total expenditures, 1980/1 to 2003/04; (b) Provincial government revenue, total and components as a percentage of GDP, 1980/1 to 2003/04.

restructuring, effective 1996/7, that consolidated several of them into one item – the Canadian Health and Social Transfer (CHST) – but significantly reduced the overall amount (Figure 7.7b).

Between 1995/6 and 1997/8, federal cash transfers fell by about $5 billion, or nearly 20%, leaving a substantial hole in provincial budgets. Critics argued, with some justification, that the federal government was fighting its own deficit 'on the backs of the provinces'. That federal battle was outstandingly successful: the Government of Canada has been recording surpluses ever since 1997/8 and, barring major recession, seems likely to do so for the indefinite future.

Rather than restoring the cash grants to their pre-CHST rate, the federal government began in 1998/9 to cut its own income tax rates. By 2003/4 the annual federal revenue foregone is estimated to be about equal to the total of the provincial government cuts in that year – $24 billion – and is budgeted to rise to $29.6 billion in 2004/5. The total cumulative revenue foregone through these federal tax cuts is estimated by the Department of Finance to reach $101.5 billion by that year; in comparison, total spending on healthcare in Canada in 2002 is estimated at $112.2 billion, with public sector spending accounting for $79.5 billion.

It is hardly surprising that provincial governments have demanded restoration of the cash transfers unilaterally reduced by the federal CHST.[ix] A substantial amount of new federal money has since begun to flow, but as Figure 7.7b shows, this has not restored the previous relationship of federal transfers to GDP. On the other hand, the federal government seems to have taken the (also understandable) view that there was no benefit to either the healthcare system or its own political fortunes from transferring more revenues to provincial governments whose principal priority was cutting their own income tax rates. The government of Ontario, in particular (ideologically at odds with the federal government during this period), will by 2003/4 have cut a cumulative total of $61.9 billion out of its own revenue base.

Amid the continuing inter-governmental wrangling, one fact is prominent. Between 1996/7 and 2003/4 the federal and provincial governments have between them cut personal and corporate income tax rates so as to remove $170.8 billion from public sector revenues. In 2003/4 the annual public revenue foregone will amount to an estimated $48.9 billion – over 60% of current public sector expenditure on healthcare.

In summary, the Canadian federal and provincial governments have, over the past decade, succeeded in restoring fiscal positions undermined by unfavourable developments in the general economy. But this process has had two distinct phases. Prior to 1996/7, provincial health and non-health expenditures were both being reduced, relative to GDP. In the more recent period there was a resumption of the flow of public funds into healthcare, more or less in proportion to the rise in GDP, while the shrinkage of non-health programmes has continued. Hence the rise, after 1996/7, in the share of health in provincial programme spending.

But the cuts to non-health programmes in the more recent period were no longer being driven by the need to balance provincial budgets. That job, difficult and important, had been done. The tax cuts after 1996/7 were a fiscal choice by right-wing governments in several of the larger provinces, a choice that then necessitated continuing expenditure cuts to maintain the fiscal balance previously achieved. Presumably, finding it politically more difficult to make further cuts in the healthcare sector, these governments made deeper cuts to non-health programmes. One could argue that in this way healthcare was in fact now 'crowding out' other programmes. But the source of the pressure was no longer fiscal exigency generated by poor overall economic performance, rather it was the political decision to take advantage of an improved fiscal situation to cut tax rates rather than to maintain spending on public programmes (or to pay down debt).

Governments are elected to make choices, fiscal and otherwise, and the provincial governments making these choices have been duly and democratically elected. But it would be erroneous, and misleading, to claim that an unsustainably expensive public healthcare system has been the source of the pressure on other public programmes. The argument that the public health programmes are economically 'unsustainable' has no more basis in the public accounts than it has in the national accounts.

What's the real issue? The inegalitarian agenda

So the anomaly remains. These data are perfectly well known in provincial and federal finance ministries; indeed these ministries are their source. They are not known to most of the public; that raises a whole other set of issues as to the role of the media during this period. (The awareness of politicians is always an open question.) So what are the real motives behind the claims of unsustainability?

An important clue lies in the pattern of some of the recent provincial tax changes. Figure 7.8 is calculated from the federal and provincial income tax returns for single residents of Ontario and British Columbia. Between 1997 and 2002, individuals in both provinces with annual taxable incomes of $15 000 and $25 000 (and no other complications) had their tax liabilities reduced by about 4%, with roughly equal reductions in federal and provincial taxes. But the percentage reductions increase steadily with annual income, reaching nearly 9% (Ontario) and 10% (BC) at $100 000. Beyond this point the federal reductions decline as a share of income, but the provincial reductions continue to increase. In Ontario, these increases are quite small, and do not offset the federal decline. But in British Columbia they do, reaching nearly 8% for a taxable income of $1 000 000. At that level, after-tax income would be larger in 2002 by $104 097 ($78 754 from the province, and $25 342 from the federal government). After-tax income at the $15 000 level in British Columbia would rise by $645 ($327 provincial, $317 federal). The comparable provincial amounts for Ontario are $49 293 and $255.

Rate changes immediately introduced by the British Columbia government newly elected in mid-2001 account for most of the increased inequality of after-tax incomes. Later changes in other taxes reinforced this effect.[x] British Columbia, like the neighbouring province of Alberta, levies compulsory health insurance 'premiums' (unrelated to risk status). Public coverage is not, however, conditional upon payment; the 'premiums' are actually a form of poll tax. In May 2002 they were raised by 50%, or $216 for a single individual.[xi] Figure 7.8 shows this premium increase as a proportion of taxable income; it offsets over one-third of

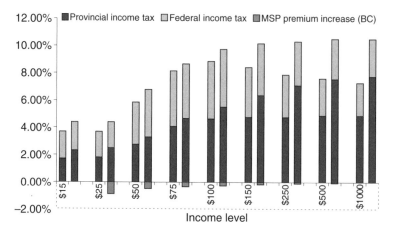

Figure 7.8 Income tax reductions in Ontario and British Columbia, 1997–2002, as a percentage of taxable income, by income level.

the income tax cut at $25 000 per year, 4% at $100 000, and a quarter of a per cent at one million.

The Government of Alberta also increased its healthcare premiums in 2001, by about one-third, but its approach to income taxation was even simpler. On 1 January 2001, Alberta introduced a provincial 'flat tax' of 11% of taxable income above a basic exemption level, substituting for the previous percentage of the (relatively progressive) federal liability. This approach twists the whole tax schedule above the basic exemption level to decrease the relative burden on the wealthy and increase it on middle incomes.

In all three provinces, the higher the income, the greater the percentage gain from income tax reductions. In addition, the cuts to public expenditures imposed in these provinces along with a variety of additional fees for public services were significantly regressive in their impact.

One has to conclude that these provincial governments were pursuing, for whatever motive, an agenda of regressive income redistribution.[xii] Nor are they alone. Historically, Canadian governments have significantly mitigated, through taxes and financial transfers, the degree of income inequality that is generated in the marketplace.[13] Changes since the mid-1990s, however, appear to have reduced this buffering effect, and post-government income inequality is now on the rise.[14,15] And senior politicians at the federal level have recently floated, as a trial balloon, a federal 'health insurance premium' – read poll tax – supposedly to support increased transfers to the provinces.

Taxes and transfers are, however, only part of the process by which governments influence the distribution of economic well-being. Expenditure programmes, such as public education and healthcare, also play a major role in detaching benefits from ability to pay. In all public health insurance systems (at least in the high-income, industrialised countries) people in the upper-income brackets subsidise (on average) the care of those lower down, while at the same time the relatively healthy subsidise the care of the comparatively unhealthy. There is no other way to maintain a modern healthcare system – at least none is known.

But considerable variation occurs among national systems in the nature and extent of this subsidisation. The Canadian Medicare programmes, covering hospital and physicians' services, are almost entirely financed from general taxation and provide care 'on equal terms and conditions' to the whole resident population. In the US, in sharp contrast, people of different incomes receive care on very different 'terms and conditions' depending on their employment status, age and ability to pay. Most European systems make care available on more or less equal terms and conditions to the whole population, but several (unlike Canada) permit providers within the public system to sell, to those willing and able to pay, more timely access to a perceived higher standard of care. Purchasing these advantages for themselves, the better-off are not required to contribute to a similar standard for the rest of the population – that is the whole point of 'two-tier' care.

Moreover, the distribution of the cost of healthcare across the population varies considerably among national systems.[16,17] Financing raised through direct taxation tends to distribute the burden more or less in proportion to income, indirect taxation is more regressive, and social insurance programmes can be either more or less proportional (France) or quite steeply regressive (Germany, the Netherlands) depending on their structure. But private payment, whether through private insurance or directly out of pocket, is by far the most regressive. Low-, middle-, high-, and very high-income people pay the same amounts for the same services, but these payments represent very different shares of their respective incomes.

Since health is correlated with wealth, on average lower-income people would pay an even larger share of their incomes for healthcare through private payment – if they were to get equal service for equal need. But of course they do not. Higher-income people spend more on healthcare through private payments, and get more services, but spend a much smaller *proportion* of their incomes in this way. This pattern is similar for both private insurance and self-payment, because private insurers in a competitive market must set their premiums according to the estimated risk of the insured. For equivalent coverage, healthier people will pay less, regardless of their incomes, and sicker people will pay more.

Thus the 'private/public' debate about financing sources is, in all modern healthcare systems, fundamentally a debate about *Who Pays?* and *Who Gets?* The Canadian universal tax-financed system requires higher-income people to contribute more to supporting the healthcare system, without offering them preferred access or a higher standard of care.[18,19] Any shift towards proportionately more private financing, through user charges with or without private insurance, would reduce the relative burden on people with higher incomes. Insofar as private payments also limit access by people with lower incomes, they also open better access for those willing/able to pay. Relative to universal, fully tax-financed public insurance, an expansion of private payment would thus enable the wealthy to pay less (in charges, private premiums and taxes) and get more (in volume, quality and/or timeliness). The converse would be true for those with lower incomes. This conflict of economic interest is real, unavoidable and permanent in all systems, which is why the 'public–private' debate is never resolved (and why it is typically so occluded with 'econofog').

Cutting across the income spectrum, there is a third and equally deeply entrenched conflict feeding the endless 'public–private' financing debate – *Who Gets Paid?* and how much.

Private insurance systems, for example, incur heavy administrative costs to conduct underwriting and set premiums, to market policies, and to adjudicate and pay individual claims, as well as to reward investors and (sometimes spectacularly) senior executives. These overhead costs absorb between 15 and 20% of the revenues of Canadian private insurers. In addition, there are substantial costs imposed on providers of care and beneficiaries or their representatives, in negotiating with insurers and trying to ensure that claims are in fact paid.

In the US, the only country with significant private coverage, these overheads were recently estimated[20] at 31% of total healthcare expenditure in 1999. In a universal public system, most of these costs vanish; the comparable estimate for Canada was 16.7%, which includes extensive private insurance for dentistry and drugs. The excess administrative costs in the US were estimated at $209 billion or 17.1% of total US health expenditures. But all these billions represent income for insurers, benefits managers, and administrative and financial staff in hospitals and clinics. In a universal public insurance system, most of these jobs would not exist.

Payments to care providers raise exactly the same issue. Insofar as public single-payer systems have been relatively more effective in controlling overall costs of healthcare, they have, to the same extent, controlled the incomes of providers. Hence, the intense opposition to such coverage in North America from economically motivated providers, most notably the for-profit pharmaceutical industry. Again, the conflict of interest is real and fundamental; for a firm whose products have high fixed costs of development but are sold at prices far above variable cost, any reduction in prices comes straight off the bottom line.

Not all providers thrive in a private funding system. Health and wealth are correlated; a high proportion of costs are generated by a relatively small proportion of people with above-average morbidity and below-average incomes. The income base of the provider community as a whole depends on a high proportion of public funding. Even in the 'private' US, about 60% of healthcare expenditure comes directly or indirectly from public funds.[21] But a multi-source financing system, with supplementary private financing and public sources that are indirect and difficult to control, provides the best income opportunities for providers – i.e. higher healthcare expenditures.

Political wolves masquerading as economic sheep

These embedded conflicts of economic interest over *Who Pays?*, *Who Gets?* and *Who Gets Paid?* play roles analogous to the tribal, ethnic or religious divisions in the framework of Figure 7.1. They are always present, but tend to flare up into more intense and self-reinforcing political conflict under economic stress. Such conflicts may pose a real threat to the sustainability of Canada's Medicare. But it is a threat from private interests pursuing a redistributive agenda, rather than from expenditures outrunning public resources.

The relative deterioration of the economic environment in Canada since 1981, with its particularly powerful impact on the public fiscal situation, has resulted (among many other things) in a number of relatively successful efforts to 'do more with less'.[xiii] On the other hand, a number of policy proposals for structural 'reform' represent, in reality, the application of ingenuity to redistribute burdens and benefits – to eat the other fellow's lunch. Efforts to promote – and to expose and combat – such 'reforms' distract from the very real needs for improved system management and adaptation to a less favourable environment.[xiv]

The wealthy in the modern world may be increasingly reluctant to accept a single standard of care for the whole population, with no preference for themselves, while contributing a relatively larger share of the cost. Private financing quite genuinely offers them 'more, for less', while offering the rest of the population 'less, for more'. It may lead to a less efficient and more expensive system overall, through increased overhead costs, weaker control over prices, and reduced potential for managing care patterns, while a diversion of care from those with greatest need to those with greatest resources will result in a less effective distribution of services. But the wealthy still come out ahead.

It also appears that in several countries, including Canada (and for reasons well beyond the scope of this chapter), political systems have become increasingly sensitive to the priorities of the wealthy. Claims that Canada's Medicare is economically or fiscally unsustainable represent part of a broader propaganda campaign to advance those priorities, 'softening up' a generally sceptical and unsympathetic public to accept that the current form of public health insurance (which most Canadians still strongly prefer) is simply impossible to maintain. The agenda is being advanced by right-wing governments in the larger provinces, with sympathetic coverage from the country's dominant newspaper chain. In these circumstances, the political sustainability of the public system is very much an open question. But the claims of economic unsustainability appear from the data to be themselves wholly unsustainable.

That was then, this is now?

Or are they? Unsustainability is a claim about the future, not the past, and that claim is buttressed by current fiscal projections showing public healthcare spending growing much faster than provincial revenues. As noted above, the most recent data available at the time of writing do show a resumption of more rapid rates of cost escalation. Is there now a real economic wolf at the door?

The future is an uncertain place, and all forecasts will be falsified. But why should the future be different from the quite sustainable past? A standard triad of reasons is typically offered – and has been for decades. They are classic examples of 'Zombies' – ideas and arguments that are intellectually dead but will not stay buried,[22,23] and are repeatedly disinterred to advance interests that are very much alive.

The triad consists of interlinked claims about trends in demography, technology and public attitudes, each asserted to be generating increasing needs or demands (the distinction is typically fuzzy) for increasingly expensive healthcare. Ageing populations have greater needs; advancing technology creates ever more expensive possibilities for intervention; and 'public expectations' of the healthcare system are ever increasing. People just want more, and want it now. But (it is further asserted) no government can afford to meet these ever-expanding needs/demands. So we should, indeed must, limit the public liability, and let those who can, buy more for themselves if they wish. There is really no alternative. QED.

When one unpackages these broad generalities, however, and looks at the actual data, a very different picture emerges.

The 'Zombie' of the ageing population, a.k.a. 'apocalyptic demography', has been studied in particular detail. The average age of modern populations is rising, and elderly people generally do have greater health needs requiring more costly care. But it is not true that these patterns will place an unsustainable burden on public healthcare systems.[23–25] Holding age-specific per capita use and cost rates constant, Canadian population forecasts indicate a rise in per capita costs of about 1% per year – well within the range of prevailing rates of economic growth.

Use and cost are primarily driven not by changing age structure, but by changing patterns of care use – what is done to and for patients. These patterns obviously respond to the evolution of scientific knowledge and technical capacity, but the link is neither simple nor direct.[26] New technologies may be inherently either cost enhancing or cost reducing – there are many examples of each – but it is the way in which they are taken up and applied that determines their impact on costs. That process of uptake and application is primarily controlled by clinicians, and the cost-enhancing bias of technology arises, *inter alia*, from the economic incentives that they face.

There is extensive evidence of the provision of questionable or simply inappropriate services, old and new, at unnecessarily high cost. But efforts to evaluate outcomes, eliminate ineffective or questionable practices, and restrain the exuberant proliferation of interventions have typically met indifference from clinicians, if not active resistance. Apart from issues of professional autonomy and pride (and the urge to 'do something'), this reaction has roots in the ineluctable reality that cost containment must always threaten someone's income.[xv]

The potential for transferring a large proportion of inpatient care to ambulatory or day care facilities, for example, has been well documented in Canada since the early 1970s. But large-scale uptake was slow until the rigorous budgetary restraints of the 1990s. The transfer eliminated jobs; widespread claims of 'underfunding' and threats to patient health have not been substantiated.[xvi] If substantial additional funds flow into the healthcare system, the incentives for improved efficiency are likely to be relaxed.

The clearest examples of inappropriate and excessively costly choice of intervention can be found in the pharmaceutical sector. In Canada, the principal driver of rapid cost escalation is the replacement of older, off-patent drugs with new patented ones at prices that may be ten times higher. These are marketed as superior, but the regulatory process does not require new drugs to be tested against those they will replace, only against placebo. In some recent trials, high-profile (and high-cost) new drugs have shown no additional benefits.[27,28] Large additional expenditures, stimulated by intense marketing, are in effect buying nothing.

But what about public demand for the newest and the best, at any cost? Again, the pharmaceutical experience is instructive. Manufacturers have always engaged in intense and highly sophisticated marketing, primarily targeting physicians. More recently the industry lobbied successfully to eliminate American regulatory restrictions on advertising directly to the public, and in 2000 spent $2.5 billion to manipulate public expectations. Such advertising does change physician prescribing behaviour[29] – why else would a for-profit industry spend the money? American pharmaceutical manufacturers – for whom data are available – now spend twice as much on marketing as on research.[30] In this environment, to speak of 'public expectations' as if they represented independent consumer choices is at best dangerously naive, and at worst deliberately deceptive.

Managing patient expectations has always been a significant part of the professional role. The difference between a physician and a for-profit firm is that the former is responsible for the health of patients, the latter for the earnings of shareholders. In both cases expectations management has very significant effects on trends in health expenditures, but those effects depend on the incentives created by the institutional environment in which the process takes place. That environment is determined by public and private policies and is always politically contested – as the pharmaceutical example makes clear.

Such matters as technology assessment, medical practice guidelines and efforts to promote the practice of 'evidence-based medicine' are highly political, interacting with the economic incentives embodied in the different structures for reimbursing physicians and hospitals. Medical and other professional associations and unions take a very active interest in these matters; advancing the economic interests of their members is one of their principal responsibilities. The recent uptick in Canadian healthcare costs includes some very successful physician fee bargaining. To pretend that trends in healthcare use and costs are determined by impersonal forces external to the industry itself is just that, a pretence.[xvii]

Whether or not the recent rise in Canadian Medicare expenditures presages a period of more rapid longer-term escalation is a critical question, but the answer does not depend on external factors. Rather it will, as in the past, depend on the outcome of political and administrative contests between those who pay and those who are paid for delivering or financing care. Projecting cost trends is akin to predicting the outcome of the Stanley Cup, the ice hockey cup final; there is certainly relevant information, but it is not a scientific exercise.

Private morality and public choices – and consequences

In the end, though expenditure trends loom large in the public debate, the question of 'sustainability' may not be about expenditure trends at all. Reinhardt[31] argues that sustainability is actually a moral issue, a debate about what the members of a society owe to each other.

To illustrate, suppose the preceding argument is incorrect, and we are in fact entering a new era in which advancing medical technology really does offer dramatic improvements in health – at dramatically increased expense. Citizens might quite rationally accept this bargain, with healthcare spending rising as a share of GDP – why not? That is exactly what happened in Canada when universal public insurance was introduced; there was consensus (rightly or wrongly) that more spending would produce better health for everyone. At root, the arguments for cost containment have always been about seeking value for money, containing price inflation and paring away waste, not about foregoing effective care.

But who should pay, and who should get the care? Under public insurance, the burden would fall on taxpayers and the benefits would go to patients. Government expenditure on healthcare would rise, as would taxation. The claim that such increases would be 'unsustainable' is tantamount to saying that this pattern of burdens and benefits is morally wrong. People should not get care that they cannot afford. And people who can afford a higher standard of care for themselves should not have to contribute, through taxation, to support a similar standard for others.

This moral position does not appear to be widely shared by the Canadian public. Nor can its advocates credibly claim that governments 'cannot afford' such increased expenditures, while simultaneously advocating and carrying through substantial cuts to income taxes. Considerable ingenuity must therefore be devoted to finding general harms from an expanded public sector.[xviii] This ingenuity might more constructively be directed towards improving the efficiency and effectiveness of the healthcare system. But those who allege unsustainability largely ignore the evidence on waste and inappropriate care, and implicitly or explicitly also allege 'underfunding' – thus coming into alliance with provider interests.

Reinhardt's comment[31] on the US Congress is worth quoting:

> *That no one in the US Congress shows much interest in the glaring inefficiencies that could easily be addressed within the current Medicare program [in the US, covering only those 65 and over] speaks volumes about*

the true, but hidden, agenda that actually drives the quest for privatising . . .
Crisply put, the objective is to shift responsibility for health spending on older
persons from the general taxpayer onto the older people themselves . . . (p. 201)

Canada's universal system has done a much better job of mobilising ingenuity to
deal with these 'glaring inefficiencies', but a much better job than the US still
leaves a lot to be desired. More significant reforms continue to be stalled by the
political struggles over *Who Pays?*, *Who Gets?* and *Who Gets Paid?* Claims that the
Canadian public system is both economically unsustainable and underfunded
seem driven by the same agenda that Reinhardt identifies in the US – containing
public outlays while letting private expenditures go where they will. Such a
mixed system would be more expensive and less efficient overall, as the US
example has shown, escaping the price restraints imposed by the public single
payer and bearing significantly increased administrative overheads. But it would
be better for the wealthy.

Hence Reinhardt's assertion that 'sustainability' is actually a moral issue, of
defining the mutual obligations of the members of a community. Public choices
are private morality writ large. There *is* a wolf at the door of the Canadian
Medicare system. But it is a political wolf dressed in phoney economic clothing to
deceive the sheep.

References

1 Meadows DH, Meadows DI, Randers J, Behrens WW III (1972) *The Limits to Growth.*
London: Earth Island.
2 Homer-Dixon TF (2000) *The Ingenuity Gap.* Toronto: Alfred A Knopf.
3 Homer-Dixon TF, Boutwell JH, Rathjens GW (1993) Environmental change and
violent conflict. *Scientific American.* **268**(2): 38–45.
4 Evans RG (1998) Healthy wealthy and cunning? profit and loss from health care
reform. In: Nemetz PN (ed.) *The Vancouver Institute: An experiment in public education.*
Vancouver: JBA Press, pp. 447–86.
5 Evans RG (1982) Health care in Canada: patterns of funding and regulation. In:
McLachlan G and Maynard A (eds) *The Public–Private Mix for Health: the relevance and
effects of change.* London: Nuffield Provincial Hospitals Trust, pp. 371–424.
6 Evans RG (2002) Financing health care: taxation and the alternatives. In: Mossialos E,
Dixon A, Figueras J, Kutzin J (eds) *Financing Health Care: options for Europe.* Buckingham: Open University Press, pp. 39–58.
7 White J (1995) *Competing Solutions: American health care proposals and international
experience.* Washington, DC: Brookings.
8 Boccuti C and Moon M (2003) Comparing Medicare and private insurers: growth rates
in spending over three decades. *Health Affairs.* **22**(2): 230–7.
9 Evans RG (1990) Tension compression and shear: directions stresses and outcomes of
health care cost control. *Journal of Health Politics, Policy and Law.* **15**(1): 101–28.
10 United States Congressional Budget Office (1992) *Projections of National Health Expenditures.* Washington, DC: Congressional Budget Office.
11 Levit K, Smith C, Cowan C, Lazenby H, Sensenig A, Catlin A (2003) Trends in US
health care spending, 2001. *Health Affairs.* **22**(1): 154–64.
12 Lu J-FR, Hsiao WC (2003) Does universal health insurance make healthcare unaffordable? Lessons from Taiwan. *Health Affairs.* **22**(3): 77–88.
13 Wolfson MC, Murphy BB (1998) New views on inequality trends in Canada and the

United States. *Monthly Labor Review.* United States Bureau of Labor Statistics (April): 3–21.

14 Sharpe A (2003) Linkages between economic growth and inequality: introduction and overview. *Canadian Public Policy.* **29** Supplement (January): S1–S14.

15 Statistics Canada (2003) Family income, 2001. *The Daily Mail.* 25 June.

16 Wagstaff AE, van Doorslaer E, van der Burg H *et al.* (1999) Equity in the finance of healthcare in twelve OECD countries. *Journal of Health Economics.* **18**(3): 291–314.

17 van Doorslaer E, Wagstaff A, van der Burg H *et al.* (1999) The redistributive effect of healthcare: some further international comparisons. *Journal of Health Economics.* **18**(3): 263–90.

18 Mustard CAM, Shanahan S, Derksen S *et al.* (1998) Use of insured health care services in relation to income in a Canadian province. In: Barer ML, Getzen TE, Stoddart GL (eds) *Health, Health Care and Health Economics: perspectives on distribution.* Chichester: John Wiley, pp. 157–78.

19 Mustard CAM, Barer ML, Evans RG, Horne J, Mayer T, Derksen S (1998) Paying taxes and using health care services: the distributional consequences of tax financed universal health insurance in a Canadian province. Presented at the Centre for the Study of Living Standards Conference on the State of Living Standards and the Quality of Life in Canada, Ottawa, October. Available from URL www.csls.ca/oct/must1.pdf

20 Woolhandler S, Campbell T, Himmelstein DU (2003) Costs of health care administration in the United States and Canada. *New England Journal of Medicine.* **349**(8): 768–75.

21 Woolhandler S, Himmelstein DU (2002) Paying for national health insurance – and not getting it. *Health Affairs.* **21**(4): 88–98.

22 Evans RG, Barer ML, Stoddart GL, Bhatia V (1994) *Who are the Zombie Masters and what do they want?* Toronto: The Premier's Council on Health, Well-being and Social Justice.

23 Barer ML, Evans RG, Hertzman C, Johri M (1998) Lies, damned lies and healthcare Zombies: discredited ideas that will not die. HPI Discussion Paper #10. University of Texas-Houston Health Policy Institute, Houston, Texas. Available from URL www.chspr.ubc.ca/hpru/pdf/hpru98-05D.pdf

24 Barer ML, Evans RG, Hertzman C (1995) Avalanche or glacier? Health care and the demographic rhetoric. *Canadian Journal on Aging.* **14**(2): 193–225.

25 Evans RG, McGrail K, Morgan S, Barer ML, Hertzman C (2001) Apocalypse now: population aging and the future of the health care system. *Canadian Journal on Aging.* **20**(Supp. 1): 160–91.

26 Bassett K (1996) Anthropology, clinical pathology and the electronic fetal monitor: lessons from the heart. *Social Science and Medicine.* **42**(2): 281–92.

27 Furberg CD and the ALLHAT Investigators (2002) Major outcomes in high-risk hypertensive patients randomized to angiotensin-converting enzyme inhibitor or calcium channel blocker vs diuretic. *Journal of the American Medical Association.* **288**(23): 2981–97.

28 Rossouw JE and the Women's Health Initiative Trial Investigators (2002) Risks and benefits of estrogen plus progestin in healthy postmenopausal women. *Journal of the American Medical Association.* **288**(3): 321–33.

29 Mintzes B, Barer ML, Kravitz RL, Bassett K, Lexchin J, Kazanjian A, Evans RG, Pan R, Marion SA (2003) How does direct-to-consumer advertising (DTCA) affect prescribing? A survey in primary care environments with and without legal DTCA. *Canadian Medical Association Journal.* **169**(5): 405–12.

30 Families USA (2001) *Off the Charts: pay profits and spending by drug companies.* Washington, DC: Families USA Foundation Publication, pp. 1–104.

31 Reinhardt UE (2001) Commentary: on the apocalypse of the retiring baby boom in northern lights: perspectives on Canadian gerontological research. *Canadian Journal on Aging.* **20**(Suppl. 1): 192–204.

32 Canadian Institute for Health Information (2001) *National Health Expenditure Trends: 1975–2002*. Ottawa: Canadian Institute for Health Information.

33 OECD (2003) *Health Data File 2003*. Paris: Organisation for Economic Cooperation and Development.

34 Barer ML, Evans RG (1986) Riding north on a southbound horse? Expenditures, prices, utilization and incomes in the Canadian health care system. In: Evans RG, Stoddart GL (eds) *Medicare at Maturity: achievements, lessons and challenges*. Calgary: University of Calgary Press, pp. 53–163.

35 Black C (2001) The most boring election in history (editorial). *The National Post*. 1 December.

36 Hurley J (2000) Medical Savings Accounts: approach with caution. *Journal of Health Services Research and Policy*. **5**(2): 30–2.

37 Forget E, Deber R, Roos LL (2002) Medical Savings Accounts: will they reduce costs? *Canadian Medical Association Journal*. **167**(2): 143–7.

38 Pear R (2003) Drug companies increase spending to lobby congress and governments. *New York Times*. 31 May.

Endnotes

i The idea is not entirely new. HG Wells referred to civilisation as a race between education and disaster, and Arnold Toynbee built a theory of history around the success or failure of different civilisations' responses to successive challenges.

ii Advocates of market mechanisms tend to presume on *a priori* grounds that private markets always generate the right or 'optimal' answer – a position typically buttressed against empirical challenge by the implicit assumption that whatever outcome is generated by such markets is by definition optimal.

iii '. . . and presently word would come, that a tribe had been wiped off its ice field, or the lights had gone out in Rome'.

iv The ingenuity requirement to manage an increasingly complex global environment – 'tightly coupled' physically, financially, and even psychologically – does appear to be increasing rapidly, and it is far from clear that our political institutions in particular have the capacity or can even recognise the need to meet that growing demand. But that, O Best Beloved. . . .

v Here and subsequently, calendar year data on GDP and health expenditure back to 1975 are from CIHI (2002).[32] Data back to 1960 can be found in OECD (2003);[33] sources for pre-1960 data are given in Barer and Evans (1986).[34]

vi The pharmaceutical industry and its advocates claim that this increase has made possible the reduction in hospital costs; the claim is spurious. It rests on little more than a correlation of trends, and cannot withstand any serious empirical scrutiny. But that again is another story.

vii Here and subsequently, FY data on provincial and federal public accounts are from the federal Department of Finance, Economic and Fiscal Reference Tables (October 2002) updated and augmented with additional data from Finance Canada staff. FY health expenditures are from CIHI (2002).[32]

viii They may quite reasonably have anticipated a recovery to the long-run growth path, as in previous recessions. That did not happen.

ix It is difficult to know how much of the rhetoric of 'unsustainability' is simply part of the never-ending provincial campaign for larger federal transfers.

x The provincial budget went from a $1.4 billion surplus in 2000/1 to a $1.2 billion deficit in 2001/2. A number of other fiscal changes were made, generally regressive in effect but not so directly linkable to income level.

xi The premium is discounted for those with incomes under $25 000, falling to zero at $15 000.

xii This agenda was spelled out explicitly by Conrad Black (2001)[35] in an editorial bitterly critical of Canadian governments for ' . . . taking money from people who have earned it and redistributing it to people who haven't'. As owner of most of the major newspapers in Canada he had taken the opportunity energetically to promote his personal political views.

xiii The spread of 'managed care' in the US during the 1990s can be similarly interpreted as the application of ingenuity to deal with an increasingly unsatisfactory environment – somewhat less successfully.

xiv Medical Savings Accounts provide a leading example. They would serve no useful purpose in the Canadian context, merely providing a cover for increases in both user charges and health expenditures. But de-bunking the claims of their advocates has taken up a significant amount of research effort (e.g. Hurley, 2000; Forget *et al.*, 2002[36,37]), and diverted public attention from more constructive topics.

xv Accordingly, when technologies emerge that are both therapeutically superior and less costly per patient treated, they are often associated with rapid proliferation – and increased total cost.

xvi A similar pattern was observed in the US when the Prospective Payment System was introduced in 1983. Patterns of care respond to economic incentives.

xvii ' . . . the Pharmaceutical Research and Manufacturers of America, known as PhRMA, will spend at least $150 million in the coming year' on political lobbying activities including ' . . . spend[ing] $1 million for an *"intellectual echo chamber of economists – a standing network of economists and thought leaders to speak against federal price control regulations through articles and testimony, and to serve as a rapid response team"* ' and 'allocates $1 million *"to change the Canadian healthcare system"* ' (Pear, 2003; italics are quotes from industry documents).[38]

xviii Economists have been particularly helpful in this quest, being ingenious in providing rigorous demonstrations – from faulty assumptions – of the general benefit from smaller government and greater inequality. This pays.

Chapter 8

Public–private mix for health in France

Lise Rochaix and L Hartmann

Introduction

The French healthcare system has traditionally been considered inflationary, due to its open-ended financing structure and the large degree of freedom of its participants. Indeed, healthcare expenditure has increased at a rapid rate over the past 20 years (7.8% per year in real terms), representing 9.5% of GDP in 2000, compared to 8.6% in 1990 and 7.8% in 1981.[1] For the early 1980s, this rapid rate of growth can be explained by the extension of public insurance cover, a high rate of investment (both in capital and labour), population ageing and price increases. Two main instruments were used to balance the budget: increases in social insurance contributions and inpatients' cost sharing, particularly for drugs. Contrary to what was happening in most European healthcare systems in the early 1980s, little effort was made to manage the supply side, apart from the setting up of an information system on physicians' activity.[2] The demand side cost containment measures did not succeed in altering the incentives towards over-spending built into the system and expenditure continued its steady rise.

Consequently, structural reforms were called for, both on the finance side and in healthcare provision. The main purpose of the financial reforms was to shift solidarity to a citizen-/resident-based principle rather than a professional one, and to extend coverage and equity of access. Because of the mixed public–private nature of healthcare provision, coupled with the unrestricted freedom of both providers and users, the development of competition (between GPs, between GPs and specialists, and between public and private hospitals) has been fostered. Nevertheless, being mostly based on quality (rather than price), which is difficult to monitor, this competition has not generated the efficiency gains that might have been expected. More importantly, it has been considered unfair in the hospital sector, where different financing rules have long prevailed between competing public and private hospitals, leading to a specialisation of private hospitals in the most lucrative procedures. The failure to generate the expected gains in the ambulatory care sector can be explained by the sole reliance on patients' choice between the different healthcare providers, with no public information on quality, and no effective mechanism to reduce patients' incentives to overuse services.

The reforms of the 1990s attempted to make competition fairer and more effective, while placing a cap on total healthcare expenditure. They have fostered the use of prospective payment schemes in the hospital sector. In ambulatory care, more attention has been paid to the behaviour of providers and incentives created to try and reconcile private and collective preferences. Contracting has developed, either collectively or individually, and with it, the information systems necessary to evaluate quality and performance. The finance side, for its part, has come closer to the Beveridge model by the progressive introduction of tax-based components and the extension of cover to all residents. The focus of this chapter will be on the major changes that have taken place in the financing and provision of healthcare in France in the past 20 years[3–6 i] and how these changes have affected the intricate public–private mix that has long prevailed at all levels of the French healthcare system.

Healthcare financing reforms: the search for universality

Who pays for what?

The French *sécurité sociale*, originally inspired by a Bismarckian philosophy, was set up in 1945 and founded on the principle of professional solidarity. Healthcare financing comes from four sources:

- National Health Insurance (NHI) funds, covering virtually all French residents
- supplementary insurance schemes
- users through out-of-pocket payments
- the State and local authorities.

The largest NHI fund (*Caisse Nationale d'Assurance Maladie des Travailleurs Salariés,* CNAMTS) covers 80% of the population (mainly employees, industrial workers, pensioners, unemployed and their dependants). Until recently, financing came mainly from mandatory employer and employee payroll taxes, with employers contributing, respectively, 12.8% of gross wages and employees 6.9%. The second largest fund is the MSA, *Mutualité Sociale Agricole* (for farmers and agricultural workers) covering 9% of the population, and the third is for self-employed (*Caisse Nationale d'Assurance Maladie des Travailleurs non Salariés des Professions non Agricoles*, CANAM) with 6%. About 16 other small funds cover subgroups of the population (railway workers, civil servants, etc.).

NHI funds provide both cash benefits (for sickness absence) and benefits in kind (partial if not total refunding of healthcare expenditure). They offer one of the most extensive benefit packages (including, for example, homeopathy) in any industrialised country, but with varying reimbursement rates (high for hospital but low for ambulatory care, particularly dental and ophthalmic care). Although benefit packages were harmonised in 2001 between the three main NHI funds, variations remain among the smaller funds, both in variety of services covered and access rules. The insured generally pays the service charge in full (*avance de frais*) for ambulatory care, and is refunded on the basis of a fixed rate. The remaining co-payment, the so-called *'ticket modérateur'* can be partly or totally refunded by privately purchased supplementary insurance schemes (called *assurance complémentaire*). This introduces an additional source of variation. The co-payment varies according to the type of service, with exemptions granted for expenditure relating to long-standing illness. At least 10% of those insured and suffering from a long-term severe and/or chronic illness such as cancer are totally or partially exempt from the co-payment. NHI funds' reimbursements are based on set tariffs negotiated with healthcare professionals. NHI funds act as third-party payers for hospital care, and patients only pay the co-payment for services up to a defined ceiling, to a maximum of 20% of the total bill. In practice, most procedures are above this ceiling and patients' out-of-pocket expenditure for hospital care is very limited. The same applies to diagnostic hospital services, costly drugs or laboratory tests provided on an outpatient basis.

Supplementary insurance schemes covering out-of-pocket payments do not benefit from tax breaks. They comprise mutual aid funds (around 6500 in 2000, covering about 59% of the supplementary scheme beneficiaries), provident societies (about 20, jointly managed by trade unions and employers and covering 16% of beneficiaries) and private for-profit insurance companies (about 80 covering 21% of beneficiaries). Premiums paid into mutual aid funds, can be proportional to income (particularly so in funds enrolling public sector employees), with minor adjustments for age in certain cases. Private for-profit insurance schemes use risk rating within the legal restrictions. Benefits mainly include refunding of co-payments and access to more comfortable care. Supplementary schemes covered a third of the population in 1960, half in 1970, roughly two-thirds in 1980 and up to 86% of the population in 2000. The remaining 14% with no complementary cover are often unemployed or retired. In more than half of the cases (57%), the employer subscribes to the contract for supplementary support on behalf of his employees. These group contracts usually offer more generous coverage than individual contracts.

Between 1990 and 2001, NHI funds have reduced their share of healthcare expenditure (from 76 to 75.4%), while the State and local authorities on the one hand, and patients and their supplementary insurance schemes on the other, have been paying an increasing share (Table 8.1). The slight increase to 1.3% in 2001 paid for by the State and local authorities is mainly related to the financing of the *Couverture Maladie Universelle*, CMU (universal medical cover) which was set up in 1996. Payments for patients and their supplementary schemes accounted for 22.9% of total healthcare expenditure in 1990 and reached 23.3% in 2001, the increase being paid for primarily by mutual aid funds. The supplementary insurance schemes' contribution to healthcare expenditure varies substantially

Table 8.1 Healthcare expenditure* financing in France

	1990	1995	2000	2001
National Health Insurance funds	76	75.5	75.4	75.4
State and local authorities	1.1	1	1.1	1.3
Mutual aid funds	6.1	6.8	7.4	7.5
Private insurance funds		3.1	2.6	2.4
Provident societies	16.8**	1.6	2.2	2.3
Households		12	11.3	11.1
Total	100	100	100	100

Source: DREES (2002).[7]

*This is based on the CSBM indicator (*Consommation de Soins et de Biens Médicaux*, Medical goods and services expenditure).
** Until 1990, the respective shares for households, private insurance schemes and provident societies could not be identified separately.

according to the type of service; it only represents 3.7% for hospital care, but 21.9% for ophthalmic services and prostheses, 18.6% for drugs and 35.9% for dental care.

The steps towards a citizen-based solidarity principle

In the early 1980s, there was a call to move from a professional to a residency-based solidarity principle to extend coverage and regularise NHI funds benefit packages,[8] on the grounds of both efficiency and equity. Indeed, the professional base for enrolment to compulsory insurance schemes has a number of disadvantages, as noted by Bellanger and Mossé.[9] The first is its negative impact on the labour market. When healthcare is mainly financed through employer and employee payroll taxes, it increases labour costs and reduces international competitiveness. Also, resources are sensitive to fluctuations in employment. Nor can competition develop between schemes, since patients are not free to choose. Apart from being inefficient, the professional base for benefit entitlement also fosters inequity. This system caters for the family through the extension of the insured benefits, and for the unemployed and retired workers through special funds, but a small number of residents who do not meet these criteria are excluded. Discrimination also arises between those insured, since supplementary insurance schemes offer packages which vary in terms of coverage. Analysis was undertaken of the distributive effect of healthcare financing in France for 1980 using the ECuity project methodology.[10] Results indicated that the system was marginally regressive, both because of the importance of out-of-pocket payments and of slightly regressive social insurance contributions. Further analyses[11-13] have documented important variations in use (in particular for certain services such as dental care) between individuals registered with different NHI funds and/or enrolled in different supplementary schemes.

Consequently, the 1991 Rocard Government, followed in 1996 by the Juppé administration, initiated a reform process aimed at switching the entitlement rule to citizenship rather than profession and to create a fully universal health insurance system.[14] The implementation of this new principle met with scepticism, since it inevitably brought with it a revision of entitlements and rights for the beneficiaries of the smaller, often most generous, funds. The reform process was slow but the relative importance of social insurance contributions versus earmarked taxes has changed markedly. Between 1992 and 1999, the latter increased fivefold, mainly as a result of the introduction in 1991 of a general levy tax called *Contribution Sociale Généralisée*, CSG. This new tax has a wider base than personal income tax, since it covers all sources of income (patrimonial incomes, shares and bonds, pensions). Originally set at 1.1%, mainly to finance family benefits, the CSG rate was increased to 2.4% in 1993 to include contribution towards financing pensions. The additional 1% increase in 1997 was, for the first time, earmarked to healthcare. In 1998, the global rate reached as high as 7.5% (with a lower rate of 6.2% for pensioners). In 2000, 5.1% of CSG revenues were allocated to healthcare, and this percentage was increased to 5.25 in 2001.[15 ii] At the same time, social insurance contribution rates were reduced by 0.75% and by 2.8% for pensioners. Another tax was created in 1996, originally as a short-term measure, but recently extended until 2014: the *Contribution au Remboursement de la Dette Sociale*, CRDS, meant to cover NHI funds' deficits, with a rate of 0.5% but with a wider taxable base than the CSG. The CSG has now become an important source of finance (estimated in 2000 at about 35% of total NHI funding), while employer and employee contributions now only contribute 51% of the total.[16]

The second major step towards a universal health insurance system was the implementation of a universal medical cover (*Couverture Maladie Universelle* CMU), made law in July 1999 to take effect from 2000. The CMU reform pursued two objectives. The first was to ensure a wider coverage by extending basic insurance provision to the remaining fringe of residents still not covered (estimated at 150 000 individuals). To do so, a residency criterion was added to the traditional employment-related principle (either directly or indirectly through a working member of the household). The second was to offer a basic supplementary cover to those below a certain income threshold (currently set at €6589 per year per person). Although the principles underlying the CMU reform were generally consensual, its implementation raised important questions related, among others, to the desirable level of the threshold and to the possible strengthening of the poverty trap.[17] About 4.5 million residents (7% of the population) benefited from CMU at the end of 2002.[18]

The remaining equity concern with out-of-pocket payments

User charges are of significant proportion, often serving conflicting purposes and creating distortions in access. Governmental reports[19,20] have regularly emphasised the need for a structural reform of user charges but no major change has occurred in the past 20 years, apart from the implementation of CMU.

Net of all insurance refunds, user charges still constitute a substantial share of total expenditure (11.1% on average for 2001). More importantly, they vary significantly according to the nature of the risk (maternity, illness or professional), according to the fund (salaried or not) and to the nature of the service. For instance, in 2001, they represented on average 11.7% for physician services, but they can be as high as 26% for drugs and 28.7% for dental care, while remaining very limited for hospital care (5.2%).

No gatekeeping system exists in France, where patients have direct access at no extra charge to the four following points of entry into the system:

- GPs
- specialists
- outpatient visits in hospitals
- emergency services.

Most GPs and specialists practice outside the hospital (*médecine de ville*) and are paid on a fee-for-service basis. Specialists practising in public hospitals are salaried while fee-for-service is used to reimburse clinicians in private hospitals. Under such systems, where most providers are paid fee-for-service with no gatekeeping, user charges are usually applied to reduce patients' potential overuse of services (or moral hazard[iii]).

In France, two mechanisms are used: the *avance de frais* and the *ticket modérateur*. The first, which implies that the patient pays the full price and is later refunded by his NHI fund, is only used for ambulatory care and is meant to inform the patient of the expenditure incurred. It has always been supported by physicians who strongly object to being paid directly by NHI funds. It is rather unique in Europe (with the exception of Belgium), but has long been criticised both on grounds of efficiency, since its management is labour intensive, and equity, since it tends to create access distortions between hospital and ambulatory care, the lower incomes groups using hospitals more readily, and at a later stage in their illness. The CMU reform, by exempting its beneficiaries from the *avance de frais*, should contribute towards reducing some of these distortions. More importantly, it has led to this seemingly immutable mechanism being questioned. Today, a large number of providers, including pharmacists, accept the new patient's microchip card (*carte Vitale*) which, in effect, waves the *avance de frais*.

The second and main mechanism to reduce moral hazard comes from the *ticket modérateur*. However, there is no legal limit to refund from supplementary insurance schemes, which reduces its expected effectiveness for those benefiting from generous policies. Private insurance companies thrive by offering contracts which, in effect, refund the co-payments that compulsory insurance funds impose in order to reduce users' moral hazard.

User charges also serve the purpose of restricting the range of services to which collective responsibility applies. The exclusion of certain services or drugs from reimbursement and the lowering of reimbursement rates are regularly used by the government. The *Haut Comité de Santé Publique*, HCSP (the national advisory panel on public health) has stressed the importance of a clearer definition of the basket of goods and services (*panier des soins*) to be placed under collective responsibility.[21] Extra billing (called *dépassement*) was introduced in France in 1980 for ambulatory care physicians wishing to join a newly created sector (called *Secteur II*). They were granted the freedom to charge over and above the negotiated fee for all their patients against an increase in their personal social insurance contributions. Those who subsequently moved from *Secteur I* (where fees remained regulated, with some exceptions[7 iv]) to *Secteur II* were mainly specialists practising in already wealthy regions such as Paris and the south of France.[22] Even among specialities, the share of *Secteur II* physicians varies from only 23% for neurosurgeons to 72% for gastroenterology. This use of fee-fixing freedom between physicians according to their sector has affected the utilisation patterns and strengthened the existing access differences. As a result, the right for physicians to opt for *Secteur II* was virtually suspended in 1990, but by then *Secteur II* physicians already represented 26% of fully active physicians in 1991, and the average mark up (*dépassement*) was 25%. In 2002, 25.4% of physicians still had a right to charge over the agreed fee (of which 14.6% were GPs and 37.9% were specialists). Physicians' income from extra billing was doubled between 1990 and 2002 and the percentage of consultations with extra billing has increased rapidly in recent years, going from 8.7% in 2000 to 13.6% in 2002.[7]

Under this system of refundable user charges, some households (usually those for whom private insurance is paid for by companies) may benefit from full cover whereas others still face high user charges, particularly for those services such as dental care, where extra billing is high. The introduction of CMU reduced one of the most blatant sources of inequity in the system, i.e. the fact that any increase in user charges was only paid for by those with no supplementary insurance scheme (the lower income groups). But wide variations still prevail between those who benefit from generous supplementary schemes and those who do not.[23]

Shifting the burden to patients and their supplementary schemes through user charges is likely to be a more widely used strategy in years to come, judging by the nature of the cost control measures discussed by the current government, particularly for drugs (reduction of the number of drugs on the reimbursement list; introduction of a reference price system). Up until recently, supplementary insurance schemes have adopted rather generous refunding strategies for the *ticket modérateur* and the *dépassements*, since competition was mainly in terms of coverage rather than price, but the recent increases in outlay may lead to more restrictive reimbursement conditions in contracts with important equity implications. It has also led to a questioning of the subsidiary role played by supplementary insurers who wish to become more active.

The public–private mix for healthcare provision: towards fairer competition

The provision of healthcare in France is highly mixed for both hospital and ambulatory care. Yet, as will be shown, competition has not always brought the expected efficiency gains and recent reforms have attempted to level the playing field between the public and the private sector in both hospital and ambulatory care to enhance fairer competition.

Hospital care: from market segmentation to DRG-based competition

Due to the strong autonomy of healthcare professionals and the importance of users' freedom of choice, hospital care delivery is characterised by the co-existence of a public and a private sector. Patients can choose freely between these and the refunding by NHI and supplementary insurance schemes makes them financially indifferent between both sectors. Hospitals may be either public, private not-for-profit or private for-profit (the so-called *'cliniques privées'*) but the division is not clear-cut, since public hospitals may house a private sector[v] and private not-for-profit hospitals may choose to carry out a public service, just as public hospitals do (*Mission de Service Public*[vi]).

The relationship between public and private hospitals has traditionally been one of peaceful co-existence, in that both their objectives and financial means were different, the private sector specialising in minor surgical interventions and leaving complex surgery to the capital-intensive hospitals. This division of labour was based on the limited financial resources of the private sector regarding medical equipment, but it has changed substantially in the past 20 years. Developing competition has been impaired by the different financial rules applied to these sectors and recent reforms have sought fairer competition between them through regional planning, performance and quality assessment and the use of DRGs (diagnosis related group) to define budgets.

The mixed provision of hospital care

In 1998, public hospitals in France represented two-thirds of total beds (about 320 000). They enjoy a relative administrative and financial autonomy within the limits of their budget and the State only exerts ex-post accounting control. Three main types of hospitals can be identified according to their size and scope: large teaching hospitals at regional level with heavy technical equipment (called *Centres Hospitaliers Universitaires*, CHU); general hospitals with highly diversified activity; local hospitals with no surgery or maternity services but fulfilling an important access role.

Private hospitals, for their part, are a highly heterogeneous group, some being run on a for-profit basis and others not. Private not-for-profit hospitals often belong to foundations, religious communities or mutual aid funds. They represent about 15% (75 000 beds) of hospital care and most of them carry out a *mission de service public*, providing predominantly postoperative care and rehabilitation (for a third of all beds), with some specialising in certain types of illness, such as cancer.

New, for-profit institutions known as '*cliniques privées*' are much smaller in size than public hospitals (80 beds on average compared to 400 in public hospitals). Ninety-five per cent of these *cliniques privées* have signed a tariff agreement with the third-party payer, and for those that have not (less than 5%), prices are entirely free, with most of the expenses paid out of patients' pockets. They were originally owned by physicians, but the cost-containment measures of the 1990s fostered a strong concentration process. They represent half of all surgical beds and a third of all obstetrics beds. Most of their activity is day care or short-term surgery (they undertake 75% of total day care surgery).

All hospitals, whether public or private, are State-led. They are subject to the same quality controls, with sanctions including closure in the event of inadequate care. They are also placed under capacity and standards controls (both technical and medical). Heavy medical equipment and beds stocks are centrally planned through a *carte sanitaire* and new investments are subject to ministerial approval. One of the objectives of this planning device, set up in 1970, was to affect the spatial distribution of healthcare facilities in order to ensure a fairer regional allocation. Additional planning tools of a more qualitative nature (*Schémas Régionaux d'Organisation des Soins*, SROS) have been developed at regional level as a result of the progressive decentralisation of the system. A tentative evaluation of these planning devices (Cour des Comptes, 2002)[15] indicates that the 1990s' bed oversupply estimate of 60 000 has been halved, with reductions in hospital supply regional variations. Yet, according to the Cour des Comptes, planning tools remain rather crude and the quantitative and qualitative performance indicators poorly combined.[15,24][vii]

Global caps: the unequal treatment of the public and private hospital sector

For public hospitals and some of the not-for-profit institutions, the implementation of a global financial cap (*budget global*) was legally endorsed in 1983 and implemented in 1984–5. It covers most of the hospital resources and replaces the *per diem* system which provided no incentives to reduce length of stay. The *budget global*, originally defined on a historical basis, is modified yearly by a national rate of increase set in accordance with the general economic prospects. The main objective was to curb total hospital care expenditure by increasing hospitals' financial accountability. The marked slowdown of hospital costs which followed is explained by a decrease in the number of hospital beds, a corresponding transfer of activity outside hospitals and a decrease in the average length of stay. Between 1980 and 1990, the rate of growth of hospital budgets amounted to between 2 and 3% for the public sector (respectively 3 to 6% for the *cliniques privées*), compared with an average rate of growth of total healthcare spending of 5% over the same period, and a GDP growth rate of 2.2%. For the year 2000, the occupation rate was 81.8%, the average length of stay 10.9 days and the average density for hospital beds was 10 per 1000 inhabitants, with marked regional variations (the index varies from 84 to 144). However, because the *budget global* was mainly defined by historical costs, rather than expected output, it has proved rather inequitable, some hospitals benefiting from rents and others being under strict financial constraints.

While public hospitals have experienced global caps, *cliniques privées* continue to be paid *per diem*. They are still financed today on a cost-plus basis, with a two-item tariff: fees for specialists' diagnostic and therapeutic services (in line with those agreed for specialists' services outside hospitals) and a *per diem* lump sum payment covering all other costs (patients' accommodation, ancillary services, drugs) multiplied by the number of days. These day tariffs are not harmonised at national level, and vary substantially from one geographical area to another. The resources clearly depend on the volume of specialists' services and the length of stay, which provides a strong incentive to inflate the number of services, thereby increasing the rate of use of medical equipment to pay back expensive investments. The provision by *cliniques privées* of high-tech medicine with little concern for total cost, compared to the strict financial caps imposed on the public sector led to growing concern over the unfair nature of the competition that had developed between the sectors.

A first attempt was made at controlling total costs in the private for-profit sector through the 1991 Hospital Reform which recommended the use of global expenditure caps. Unlike public hospitals, regulation of the private for-profit hospital sector is the joint responsibility of the State, representatives of NHI funds and national trade unions for *cliniques privées*. The implementation of caps, therefore, had to be negotiated between the three partners and led, in 1992, to the definition of a cap called OQN (*Objectif Quantifié National*) with collective sanctions in case of overshooting at the end of the year and tariff increases in case of undershooting.

For the first three years of implementation, undershooting was experienced and tariff increases were subsequently granted. The slowdown was, however, mainly attributable to the powerful concentration of the for-profit sector, a process hastened by the substantial inpatient bed oversupply which *cliniques privées* decided to reduce by converting them into day care facilities and other outpatient activities. The entry, in the 1990s, of private operators (*Générale des Eaux*, for instance) contributed to the merger process, although their share only represents 10% of all *cliniques* beds, as investment has had a lower than expected return.[25] In the following years, overshooting became the rule, but no sanctions were imposed (despite the fact that overshooting reached 2% in 1998), which considerably affected the credibility of the whole mechanism.

DRGs: the drive towards harmonisation

The 1996 Ordinances (known as the 'plan Juppé', after the former prime minister) introduced major reforms in the healthcare system, particularly for hospital care. They led to a regional setting of the *budget global* and fostered the idea of progressive implementation of prospective payment schemes in order to harmonise financial regulations between public and private hospitals and to encourage fairer competition through performance measurement and the development of quality assurance processes. They also opened up the possibility of experimenting with healthcare networks of different types (whether related to a specific illness or not).

Since 1996, the Parliament prospectively sets the global cap (ONDAM, *Objectif National des Dépenses d'Assurance-Maladie*) by annual ballot under the Social Security Law (*Loi de financement de la Sécurité Sociale*, LFSS). This cap is then split between the different sectors: *cliniques privées*, still called OQN; the public hospital sector; ambulatory care (called ODD, *Objectif de Dépenses Déléguées*); and social services.

The allocation of resources to public and private hospitals is undertaken by regional agencies *(Agences Régionales de l'Hospitalisation*, ARH) set up in 1996 to encourage decentralisation. They define contracts with each institution, specifying both objectives and means (*Contrats d'Objectifs et de Moyens*, COM) and are responsible for planning healthcare facilities and heavy medical equipment, through regional schemes (*Schéma Régional d'Organisation des Soins*, SROS). To allocate resources, the different ARH use the PMSI (*Programme de Médicalisation du Système d'Information*) set up in 1985 for public hospitals and in 1996 for *cliniques privées*, which provides information on hospital activity in the form of discharge abstracts, using 512 different DRGs (called GHM, *Groupes homogènes de malades*). The use of resources per GHM is analysed through an implicit price called ISA – *Indicateur Synthétique d'Activité.*[viii]

Both the OQN for *cliniques privées* and the *budget global* for public hospitals have to be decentralised to the regions. The 1996 ruling includes a long-term convergence process according to a formula, similar to the British RAWP (Resource Allocation Working Party) system, and aimed at progressively reducing regional discrepancies. Under this scheme, the financial target for each region is defined with regard to short-term activity and long-term and psychiatric care. The determination of the short-term factor takes into equal account both an indicator of morbidity (namely the population likely to use hospital care) and an indicator of hospital performance (measured by the regional average value of each ISA point). In 1999, two other indicators were added: one accounting for population flows from one region to the other and another based on comparative mortality rates.[15] At the same time, the 17-year horizon initially set for the convergence process was extended to 30 years, up until 2038. Each region is, therefore, endowed with two separate caps: one for the public sector and the other for *cliniques privées* (called OQR, *Objectif Quantifié Régional*). The ARH then allocates resources separately under each cap, but attempts in both cases to encourage performance.

The 1996 Law requires public hospitals to submit a provisional budget to their ARH, which then accepts or modifies the proposal after due consideration of the regional budget and its priorities as defined by the COM, comparing efficiency across hospitals in the region on the basis of performance indicators. For short-term care, the ARH allocates public hospital budgets on a historical basis, with a normative rate of increase (*taux directeur*) but with a correction factor between 1.5 and 3% maximum, given the value of the respective ISA point. The correction is meant to reduce variations in the financial situation of public hospitals in the region by transferring funds progressively from the more affluent hospitals to those less prosperous. Both the aggregate budget constraint for the public hospital sector as a whole and the budget constraint at hospital level imposed by ARH have become more binding over recent years.

In the private for-profit sector, negotiations between the three partners (State, NHI funds and trade unions) take place shortly after the annual budget cap (ONDAM) ballot. As well as setting both OQN and OQR, they also define regional average rates of growth for tariffs and the upper and lower limits for tariff variations within a region. The ARH then negotiates individual tariffs for the coming year with each *clinique privée* under these nationally agreed terms and on the basis of observed performance (value of ISA point of the *clinique privée*). The ARH can revise tariffs according to the rate of growth of expenditure after the first six months, in order to meet the OQR target. Clearly, one of the main difficulties encountered in the definition of this tariff policy is the diversity of the methods used by the different ARHs.

Although budget setting remains separate between the public and private sectors, the introduction of levers at ARH level to reward performance is an important step towards harmonisation. Another is the more systematic use of quality monitoring. In this respect, a national agency for accreditation and health services evaluation (*Agence Nationale d'Accréditation et d'Evaluation des Soins*, ANAES)[ix] has been introduced to encourage the evaluation of healthcare practices in the public and private sector, both for hospital and for ambulatory care. Accreditation carried out by professionals outside the institution has become particularly important to ensure both safety and quality. Indeed, quality adjustments are a likely response to regulation based on performance indicators such as ISA points, which are only quantitative. Although it is compulsory for all hospitals, both public and private, accreditation lags behind for lack of means. A manual for accreditation has been produced, but by the end of 2001, only 131 out of 3000 hospitals had been accredited.

The main milestones (the 1985 global budget for public hospitals, the 1991 introduction of DRG-based information and accounting systems and the 1996 Ordinances for Decentralisation) in public and private hospitals have led to structural reforms in this sector, implementing regional contracting and the progressive use of prospective payment schemes. Today, hospital funding depends, in part, on regional performance which implies a virtual competition in shadow prices.[27] Eventually, performance review based on both efficiency and quality indicators will become an integral part of the prospective financing system for hospitals. Only then can fair and effective competition be developed between both sectors' hospitals.

From user-driven competition to supply-side regulation in ambulatory care

In France, the ambulatory care sector (which covers all non-hospitalised services as well as drugs) is characterised by a large degree of freedom of all parties,

Table 8.2 Recent trends for ambulatory care

	Rates of growth (value)	Rates of growth (volume)
1990–5	4.5	2.7
2000	4.5	4.1
2001	5.1	6.1
2002	7.4	4.2

Source: DREES (2002).[7]

particularly users. Still it is clear that conditions remain unmet for fair competition to develop between providers. Structural reforms, aimed at decreasing incentives to overuse and making competition more effective have been called for since the early 1990s. Indeed, some have been attempted, but they have faced much stronger opposition than in the hospital sector.

Ambulatory care saw a rapid rate of growth (between 7% and 9%) between 1980 and 1990. Over the following decade, there was a notable slowdown in the rate of increase, with an average annual rate of growth of 3.7% (of which 2.5% corresponded to a volume increase). Expenditure for specialists' services increased faster than that for GPs', but expenditure on drugs, which represented 17.8% of total healthcare spending still experienced a rate of 5.7% for the period 1990–2000. In more recent years (2001 and 2002) rapid growth rates have clearly made a come-back (*see* Table 8.2). Drug expenditure is of particular concern today. Its share in total medical care consumption has risen from 18.4% in 1990 to 21% in 2002.

The rate of increase (in volume) of healthcare consumption continues to be twice as fast as that of GDP for the period 1960–2000, and the recently released budget deficit figures for 2003 are alarming. In ambulatory care it is clear that the reforms of the past 20 years have not succeeded in containing costs in an ongoing manner.

From demand to supply-side regulation

In the 1980s, most measures related to cost containment aimed at increasing user charges. In 1983, for instance, the first of a long list of cost-containment programmes (*plan d'économies maladie*), usually named after the health minister of the time, was enacted by Bérégovoy. Its measures mainly froze physician fees and drug prices. Demand-side cost containment entailed the exclusion of certain procedures or drugs from reimbursement, increased co-payments for some pharmaceutical products, physical therapy and laboratory tests, and exempted private practitioners in 'Sector II' from negotiated fee schedules (the patient paying the extra amount). The 1986 *Plan Séguin* instituted a variety of measures mostly designed to exact more co-payments (*tickets modérateurs*) from patients for hospital stays and drug reimbursements. It also introduced distinctions between those illnesses that would be covered fully and those only partially.

Supply-side regulation remained limited to controlling medical density through a *Numerus Clausus* which only affected entries and remained relatively ineffective in improving geographical allocation, since physicians have a right to set up practice regardless of the local medical needs of the population. On the other hand, price regulation through freezing fees has been circumvented by volume increases. The high volume trend in ambulatory care is strengthened by a number of system characteristics:

- absence of a unique third-party payer (due to the *avance de frais*)
- partial if not total refunding of user charges by supplementary insurance schemes, leaving no mechanism for reducing patients' moral hazard
- direct access to secondary care (specialists' consultations, hospital care)
- absence of individual contracting between NHI funds and healthcare providers
- opacity of physicians' activity due to lack of a precise coding system.

The combination of these characteristics has created an environment in which both patients and providers benefit from overspending, in tacit collusion, at the expense of the collective interest of taxpayers.

From the physicians' point of view, there is a strong incentive to induce demand to maintain a certain target income rather than move to frequently less attractive areas with lower physician density. For their part, specialists tend to prescribe excessive return visits and examinations, while generalists are under pressure from both drug companies and patients. The latter try to keep a stable share of the clientele, by gratifying it with, for example, excessive prescribing or signing certificates for interrupted activity, or other healthcare professionals' services. The situation is particularly difficult for generalists in France, because competition with specialists is unfair, patients tending to value specialists' services very highly. These incentives, coupled with the fact that physicians' activity is not adequately monitored, for lack of an appropriate fee schedule and coding procedure, have led to a rapid volume escalation.

'Maîtrise médicalisée' *versus* 'maîtrise comptable': *a false dilemma*

Altering some of the supply-side incentives became the focus of the reform process initiated in December 1990 by the Health Minister, M Durieux. The main objective was to move from an open-ended system to the ex-ante negotiation of a global rate of growth for total healthcare expenditures. The advantage of such a system was to 'trade value for volume', i.e. to enable all parties to move from volume maximisation back to an equilibrium with higher prices, lower volumes and more importantly, better quality.

Global caps were first introduced in December 1991 for private biology laboratories (the rate of growth of total expenditure being fixed at 7% for 1992, compared to 10 to 11% for previous years), for private nurses (set at 9.7% compared to 10 to 14% previously) and for ambulance services (9% compared to 14% previously). Different mechanisms were used to ensure the limits were observed. The sanction on biology laboratories is collective and set in terms of lower increases in tariffs in the following year. Until recently, an annual individual activity ceiling was set for nurses, in terms of a maximum number of services per year. This was in line with the Quebec regulation of GPs, the general philosophy being rooted in public health considerations. In addition, the nurses had to refund the insurer between 70 and up to 90% of the fees received above the quota.

A first attempt at setting a prospective cap for physician services was made in 1993, but was met with fierce opposition from physicians. The principle of caps on physicians' services was only enacted through the 1996 Juppé Ordinances, the target rate of growth for ambulatory care expenditure (ODD, *Objectif des Dépenses Déléguées*) being voted annually by the Parliament, together with the global rate for total healthcare expenditure (ONDAM, *Objectif National des Dépenses d'Assurance Maladie*). The mechanism entailed a comparison between the target rate and the effective expenditure rate. Collective overshooting was sanctioned by lower increases in tariffs in the following year. The 1996 agreement included both physicians' fees and drug expenditure in the cap, with individualised refunding by each healthcare professional in case of overshooting. The individualised sanctions were soon rejected by the State Council (*Conseil d'Etat*) and so never enforced. Subsequently, the LFSS removed physicians' personal financial accountability for drug prescription, leaving collective tariff revisions as the sole mechanism in case of overshooting.

Meanwhile, a number of measures were taken to develop peer review. The precise coding of physicians' activity (procedures, diagnoses and prescriptions) was legally formalised in 1994 (but data are currently collected for laboratory tests and prescriptions only). In order to ensure a more efficient quality audit as well as a check on unnecessary care, physicians were required to submit information on diagnosed illnesses and prescribed drugs to local sickness funds. Peer review also saw the development (beginning in 1993) of utilisation guidelines, termed *Références Médicales Opposables* (RMOs), because a sanction could be imposed on physicians in cases of non-compliance (up to €10 000 per physician per year). Initially, they covered about a third of NHI refundable drugs and the impact was particularly noticeable the following year, but it was maintained for only a small number of drugs. Between 1994 and 1997, the rate of increase of drugs outside the regulated range was 6% compared to only 2.6% for drugs under RMOs. In 1998, 243 RMOs had been defined through consensus conferences, of which 77 focused on pharmaceuticals and 78 on medical practices. From the onset, physicians were strongly opposed to sanctions and few were actually used. In the 1994–7 period, of the 20 983 physicians' practices that were appraised, about half had failed to comply with at least one RMO, 73 had received a reminder, but only 121 had incurred an actual financial sanction. A recent assessment of the impact of RMOs by CREDES (2000) tends to indicate a decrease in the prescription of certain drugs (antibiotics for instance) with a notable effect for a period of up to three years, but results are generally rather mixed.

Over this period (1994–7), a heated debate developed between those who believed that information and activity assessment would successfully curb unnecessary healthcare expenditure and those who supported the view that closed caps were also needed for effective cost containment. Physicians bitterly resented any capping approach (including the vote by Parliament of ONDAM and ODD, effective since 1996) which they called *maîtrise comptable*, as they perceived it mainly in terms of budgetary restrictions. They were more supportive of the so-called *maîtrise médicalisée*, provided it did not impose individual financial sanctions.

By this time, the global cap mechanism had lost some of its credibility, being systematically overshot by €1.72 billion in 1999 and more than €2 billion in 2000, due for the most part to the high rate of increase in ambulatory care. Physicians' growing discontent with the capping approach led to a number of strikes and a general questioning of the capping mechanism. The government responded by setting up a conciliatory body, and a report[26] was submitted in July 2001 to the then health minister M Guigou, arguing in favour of the global cap mechanism provided it was defined over a longer time span than a year, with progressive indexing on the GDP rate of growth. It also emphasised the importance of better connection between the stated objectives of French public health policy (as defined by the HCSP) and Parliament's allocation of prospective financial means (ONDAM) through explicit priority setting.

Other conclusions were drawn from this large consultation process. Among these was the recognition that many regulatory measures had been made law, but were scarcely effective since the incentives necessary to their implementation were for the most part non-existent. Some of the recommendations were, therefore, aimed at providing these incentives to physicians in the form of lump-sum payments for certain services such as collective prevention, active participation in pathology networks or in hospital emergencies, or for physicians practising in less affluent areas. A number of recommendations were included in the 2002 LFSS, including the creation of an observatory for health manpower planning, the development of auditing and reviewing processes for ancillary staff in line with existing practices for the medical profession, and the expansion of further education and medical guidelines. Proposals were put forward to strengthen the role and widen the responsibilities of the existing High Committee for Public Health, *Haut Comité de Santé Publique*, now called the High Health Council. In an effort to promote its independence, this committee is no longer chaired by the Health Minister and it is also expected to help Parliament set priorities through an annual report.

From administered prices to price and volume contracts for drugs

Regulation of expenditure on drugs had a further aim of progressively introducing contracting with drug companies on an individual basis in order to reduce volumes. Since prices are administered by the government and fixed at rather low levels by comparison with European markets, drug consumption has increased rapidly over the past 20 years. The government regularly requested drug companies to contribute a certain percentage of their turnover to reduce healthcare deficits, although no long-term or structural approach to regulation was adopted until the mid-1990s.

A committee for drug regulation, now called *le Comité économique des produits de santé*, was formed in 1996 to negotiate price and volume contracts individually with drug companies willing to enter into such an agreement over a given time period (usually longer than a year), while the government still decides which new drugs are placed on the reimbursement list. To encourage companies to participate, a default clause (*clause de sauvegarde*) was introduced in 1999 which indexed the rate of growth of sales on that of ambulatory care (ODD) for those companies remaining outside the contracting mechanism, with financial sanctions in case of overshooting. This clause was made more stringent in the 2001 LFSS and now stipulates a payment of 50% of the overshoot in the event that the ODD is overshot by less than half a point, 60% if it is between half and one point and 70% for anything higher.

In comparison with other countries, French drug companies were also spending an important percentage of their turnover on advertising, at the expense of research. The industry found itself a hostage to fortune in this respect and in 1994 the government intervened, placing a cap on advertising expenditure, with sanctions (reduction in prices) for non-compliance. A tax was also introduced on advertising and this was raised in 2002. In addition to encouraging individual contracting and the capping of advertising expenditure, the government has long been considering a move towards a reference price system to encourage the development of generic prescribing. The free pricing of truly innovative drugs is also currently under discussion.

Future challenges

The intense reform process of the past decade is in marked contrast to the inertia of the 1980–90 period, with the exception of the introduction of public hospital global budgets in the mid-1980s. A recent econometric analysis, carried out by Caussat *et al.*,[28] of the impact of regulation over the period 1960–2000 shows that the change in total healthcare expenditure in the past decade is due to the accumulation of these regulatory measures. More importantly, structural reforms have been carried out in the hospital sector ensuring fairer competition between public and private hospitals. Many issues still need to be addressed, such as better quality/performance monitoring and rewarding, and harmonisation of information systems between public and private hospital sectors, and between hospital and ambulatory care. Another important achievement is that healthcare financing has effectively moved from an ex-post refunding to the ex-ante vote by Parliament on a global expenditure target rate of growth (ONDAM), subsequently defined in specific targets for hospital and ambulatory care. Although Parliament's ability to vote under adequate information is still debated, this change has made choices more democratic.

The 1990s' experience with supply regulation also helps delineate the obstacles encountered by a regulatory policy based on contracting. There were difficulties with performance monitoring, due to the lack of reliable and precise information systems on costs, volume and outcomes. In this respect, healthcare professionals were clearly reluctant to participate in what is still fundamentally perceived as a control over their activity. More importantly, major political obstacles were met when sanctions had to be enforced on healthcare professionals.[29] Political considerations were also invoked against any structural reform of users' financial participation and access rules, however inefficient. In fact, one of the major limitations of the 1990s' regulation is that it only focused on healthcare professionals, leaving the demand side untouched. Providers were still able to use patients' moral hazard to justify increasing healthcare expenditure, particularly for drug prescription. These unresolved issues constitute serious challenges for the future.

The difficult relationship between NHI funds (in particular, the salaried workers' fund CNAMTS) and the State is still to be overcome. The CNAMTS is jointly managed by employers and employees' unions and is a quasi-public organisation: on the one hand, it has its own management and finances but on the other, it is under the close scrutiny of the State, which sets the level of insurance premiums and benefits and takes part in the negotiation process with healthcare professionals. Many attempts have been made to clarify respective roles and responsibilities (in 1991 and also in the Juppé Ordinances of 1996) but little progress has been made. In July 2001, the employers unions' resentment of government interference was such that they withdrew from the CNAMTS board of directors. A recent Government report[30] addressed these issues more explicitly, legitimising the State's intervention, but to date no proposal has been made.

The relationship between NHI funds and representatives of the healthcare professions is also a matter for concern. The *Mission de concertation* recommended a three-tier contract, the first two levels to signed collectively and the last based on the professionals' willingness to undertake certain activities (disease prevention) and conform to standards of good practice. As a result of these recommendations, a law passed on 6 March, 2002 defines conditions for a structural change in the negotiation process between private healthcare professionals and insurance funds. However, implementation of this law has been considerably delayed by the June 2002 presidential election and subsequent change in government.

Above all, what is needed now is to convince healthcare professionals, and the French population at large, that there is a need to prioritise among competing uses of resources to improve the health of the population. There is still a general consensus in France that healthcare is a priority and that the rate of growth of ONDAM, albeit set annually at a level comparable to that of the GDP, would be too low, if one takes into account the growth determinants of the healthcare sector. To most, therefore, caps are at best acceptable as long as they are not closed and adequately reflect the trends in healthcare demand (driven by ageing, increased insurance coverage and technological progress). In effect, what remains unacceptable to most parties in the French healthcare system is the concept that as well as reducing overspending, there is a need to set priorities. The temptation to seek additional sources of revenue to avoid such choices, either through user charges or by private for-profit schemes, is stronger than ever.

The change in government should not, however, alter the spirit of the supply-side regulatory policies adopted in the 1990s. Nor should it soften constraints on healthcare spending, considering the expected 2003 deficit[31] x and the European Union's additional demand for public deficit reduction. The new government may be tempted to balance the accounts by reverting to the device which prevailed exclusively before 1980, i.e. increases in social insurance contributions and user charges. While some mechanism is required to reduce patients' moral hazard (if only to weaken their tacit collusion with physicians who are paid on a fee-for-service basis), it should not necessarily take the route of increased user charges. Other instruments have been advocated, such as the introduction of gatekeeping on a voluntary basis, giving patients incentives to enter long-term relationships with their GPs,[31] a recommendation based on the limitations of patient-driven competition in the French ambulatory care market, where quality cannot be monitored. The 1996 Juppé Ordinances introduced this option under the name of *médecin référent*, freely chosen by the patient who would then benefit from *tiers payant* (i.e. no *avance de frais*), but it met with little success, for political reasons. Clearly, if such a gatekeeping system were to be reconsidered, it would imply more substantial changes in GPs' payment schemes than previously envisaged, with a move towards mixed payment schemes, including both fee-for-service items and lump-sum payments.[32,33] Such changes would take time, however, for they call into question both the dominant payment mode for physicians (fee-for-service) and patients' right to choose between providers.

Another method for reducing the public deficit in healthcare would be to follow a proposal backed, for nearly a decade, by some private for-profit insurance companies such as AXA. They are willing to play a more substantial role by offering full rather than the current supplementary coverage. Private operators argue that they would be better purchasers of care than NHI funds and the government sees in this proposal a chance to reduce its current healthcare deficit at a time when the EU is compelling France to reduce public spending. Again, the main concern is patient selection, since the present market shares of not-for-profit and for-profit insurers is already unbalanced, the latter benefiting from a younger and healthier insured population. This solution, which is currently under serious consideration, needs a regulatory approach, with community rating and basic benefit package definition as prerequisites. A recent report[34] has examined this proposal thoroughly, but it met with such hostility that the government decided to postpone the discussion of this rather structural reform of NHI until 2004.

Over the past 20 years, major reforms have been made law, but few have led to the desired change. Evaluation, quality assessment and performance review have become more acceptable to most players in the field, but it clearly takes time to change daily practices and the evidence base is still very poor. What remains hotly debated is the macroeconomic constraint imposed on the healthcare sector. The argument between *maîtrise comptable* and *maîtrise médicalisée* is strategically used by physicians to avoid addressing the painful issue of priority setting and the government, for its part, is strongly tempted to circumvent it by shifting some of its responsibilities to the private insurance sector.

References

1 DREES (Direction de la Recherche, des Etudes, de l'Evaluation et des Statistiques) (2001) Données sur la situation sanitaire et sociale en France en 2000. Collection Etudes et Statistiques, la Documentation Française.

2 Lacronique J-F (1982) The public private mix in France. In: McLachlan G and Maynard A (eds) *The Public–Private Mix for Health: the relevance and effects of change.* London: Nuffield Provincial Hospitals Trust, pp. 471–511.

3 Hartmann L, Rochaix L, de Kervasdoué J (2000) L'économie de la santé en 1999 (Health economics in 1999). In: de Kervasdoué J (ed.) *Le Carnet de Santé (The Health Notebook).* Paris: Edition Syros.

4 Lancry PJ, Sandier S (1999) Twenty years of cures for the French Health System. In: Mossialos E and Le Grand J (eds) *Health Care and Cost Containment in the European Union.* Aldershot: Ashgate, pp. 443–70.

5 Rodwin V, Sandier S (1993) Health care under French National Health Insurance. *Health Affairs.* 3: 111–32.

6 Sandier S, Polton D, Paris V (2003) *Health Care Systems in Transition: France* (Thomson S and Mossialos E, eds). Copenhagen: European Observatory on Health Care Systems.

7 DREES (Direction de la Recherche, des Etudes, de l'Evaluation et des Statistiques) (2003) Comptes Nationaux de la Santé 2002. Document de Travail, Série Statistiques, no. 55.

8 Rodwin V (1982) Management without objectives: the French health policy gamble. In: McLachlan G, Maynard A (eds) *The Public–Private Mix for Health: the relevance and effects of change.* London: Nuffield Provincial Hospitals Trust, pp. 289–325.

9 Bellanger MM, Mossé Ph-R (2000) Contracting within a centralised health care system: the ongoing French experience. Paper presented at the first meeting of the European Health Care System Discussion Group (EHCSDG), London, 14–15 September.

10 Lachaud C, Rochaix L (1993) The case of France. In: van Doorslaer E, Wagstaff A, Rutten F (eds) *Equity in The Finance and Delivery of Health Care: an international perspective.* Oxford: Oxford Medical Publications, Commission of the European Communities, Health Services Research series no. 8.

11 CREDES (Centre de Recherches et de Documentation en Economie de la Santé) (1999) Santé et protection sociale en 1998. Rapport, Paris.

12 CREDES (Centre de Recherches et de Documentation en Economie de la Santé) (2001) Santé, soins et protection sociale en 2000, Questions d'économie de la santé, no. 46.

13 HCSP (Haut Comité de Santé Publique) (2002) La santé en France. Rapport général, La documentation française, Janvier.

14 Bouget D (1998) The Juppé Plan and the future of the French social welfare system *Journal of European Social Policy.* **8**(2): 155–72.

15 Commission des Comptes de la Sécurité Sociale (2002) Les comptes de la Sécurité Sociale. Rapport, Paris.

16 Les comptes de la Nation en 2000. Institut National de la Statistique et des Etudes Economique, no. 773, April 2001.

17 Couffinhal A, Henriet D, Rochet JC (2001) Impact de l'assurance maladie publique sur l'accès aux soins et la participation au marché du travail. Une analyse théorique. *Economie Publique.* **9**(3).

18 CREDES (Centre de Recherches et de Documentation en Economie de la Santé) (2003) Santé, soins et protection sociale en 2002, Questions d'économie de la santé, no. 1509.

19 Commissariat Général du Plan (CGP) (1994) *Livre Blanc sur le Système de santé et d'Assurance Maladie* (*White paper on the healthcare and health insurance system*). Rapport au Premier Ministre, Coll. des Rapports officiels, la Documentation Française, Paris.

20 Commissariat Général du Plan (1993) *Santé 2010: equité et efficacité du système de santé* (*Equity and efficiency of the healthcare system*). (Soubie R, ed.) Edition: la Documentation Française, Paris.

21 HCSP (Haut Comité de Santé Publique) (2001) Le panier de biens et services: du concept aux modalités de gestion. Document de travail, Février.

22 Carrere MO (1991) The reaction of private physicians to price deregulation in France. *Social Science in Medicine.* **33**(11): 1221–8.

23 Grignon M, Polton D (2000) Inégalités d'accès et de recours aux soins. In: Ministère de l'emploi et de la solidarité (ed.) *Mesurer les inégalités.* DREES, pp. 188–200.

24 Polton D (2001) Quel système de santé à l'horizon 2020. Rapport préparatoire au schéma de services collectifs sanitaires, Ministère de l'emploi et de la solidarité, DATAR, CREDES, la Documentation Française.

25 Hartmann L (2000) Tarification, régulation et incitations dans le secteur hospitalier privé. Thèse pour le Doctorat de Sciences économiques, Université de Droit, d'Economie et des Sciences d'Aix-Marseille.

26 Mougeot M (1999) Régulation du Système de Santé. Rapport no. 13, Conseil d'Analyse Economique, la Documentation Française, Paris.

27 Bruhnes B, Glorion B, Paul S, Rochaix L (2001) Bilan de la Mission de Concertation pour la Rénovation des Soins de Ville (Report from the taskforce on reforming ambulatory care). Ministère du Travail, des affaires Sociales et de la Santé, Paris.

28 Caussat L, Femina A, Geffroy Y (2003) Les comptes de la santé de 1960 à 2001 (Health Accounts from 1960 to 2001). DREES, Document de travail, Série Statistiques, no. 54.

29 Rochaix L, Wilsford D (2005) State autonomy, policy paralysis: paradoxes of institutions and culture in the French healthcare system. *Journal of Health Politics, Policy and Law.* **30**(1).

30 Ruellan R (2002) Rapport sur les relations entre l'Etat et l'Assurance maladie. Rapport de la Commission des Comptes de la Sécurité Sociale, Décembre.

31 Rochaix L, Khélifa A (1993) Rémunération des producteurs et incitations financières des usagers (Providers payment systems and user charges). In: Commissariat Général du Plan (eds) *Santé 2010: equité et efficacité du système de santé (Health 2010: equity and efficiency of the health care system)*. Edition: la Documentation Française.

32 Rochaix L (1998) Performance-tied payment systems for physicians: evidence from selected countries. In: Saltman R, Figueras J, Sakellarides C (eds) *Critical Challenges for Health Care Reform in Europe*. Edition: Open University Press, pp. 196–217.

33 Robinson JC (2001) The end of managed care. *JAMA*. **285**: 2622–8.

34 Chadelat JF (2003) La répartition des interventions entre les assurances maladie obligatoires et complémentaires en matière de santé. Rapport de la Commission des Comptes de la Sécurité Sociale, Avril.

Endnotes

i The interested reader can usefully refer to more exhaustive presentations of the French healthcare system (*see* Hartmann *et al.* 2000; Lancry and Sandier, 1999; Rodwin and Sandier, 1993; Sandier *et al.* 2003).[3–6]

ii The remainder finances other sectors of social protection (1.1% for family benefits, 0.1% for dependency and 1.05% for pensions (Rapport de la Commission des Comptes, 2002).[15]

iii The notion of moral hazard refers to the change in behaviour from the part of the insured, due to the presence of insurance (such as overuse of service).

iv In some limited cases, Secteur I physicians also have a right to extra bill. This practice, which had remained very limited, is increasing (from 2% of all consultations in 2000 to 13.1% in 2002; DREES, 2003[7]).

v Restricted to 8% of the beds of a public hospital medical ward and no more than a day a week workload for doctors. This right had been removed but was placed back partly to curb public hospital doctors' drift towards private hospitals where remuneration is higher.

vi Following the 1958 hospital reform, all public hospitals must fulfil the requirements for a public (or universal) service: continuity of care, equal access and fight against social exclusion, 24-hour access to emergency wards, prevention, screening.

vii See Polton 2001 on long-term planning of healthcare facilities.[24]

viii Public and private information systems are still disconnected, which makes performance comparisons somewhat tentative. While information is based on average costs per DRG for public hospitals, it is based on average prices for the private sector, prices being negotiated between the profession and the regulator who ignores true costs.

ix Formerly called ANDEM, *Agence Nationale pour le développement de l'Evaluation Médicale* (set up in the 90s), its missions were extended to accreditation and therefore renamed in 1996.

x The latest report by the Commission des Comptes de la Sécurité Sociale (15/05/2003) estimated the 2003 deficit of the healthcare branch of social security at €9.7 billion. In fact, healthcare expenditure for the 1999–2003 period has grown at a rate of 26.6% compared to a GDP growth of 15.5%.

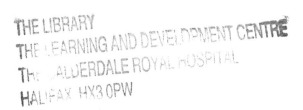

Chapter 9

The public–private mix in Scandinavia

Kjeld Møller Pedersen

Introduction

Despite the obvious interpretation of the term 'public–private mix', it never-theless requires clarification. Often an overly simple concept of private and public is used, i.e. either something is public *or* private. But is it 'public' if the government owns and finances a hospital that the same government has decided to let a private company operate (so-called facility management), which is the situation in at least one Swedish hospital and envisaged in England for some of the zero-star hospitals? Is it 'public' if a government-owned and operated hospital allows a private firm to invest in and operate a MRI-scanner, located within the hospital and integrated in the day-to-day running of the hospital, and further-more, allows the private company to use it for private patients? The company also receives a fee-for-service whenever the hospital uses the scanner, as is the case for at least one Danish hospital. There are many examples of such mixed arrange-ments, and there are also many contracting-out arrangements in areas like cleaning, catering and building maintenance.

Over the past 10–20 years, Scandinavia has witnessed a gradual softening of the once-clear distinction between private and public in healthcare. Undoubtedly, the sharp distinction was due to the fact that in the post-war years the universal free and equal access to healthcare became almost synonymous not only with collective financing, e.g. taxes, but also with government provision of services, i.e. government-owned and operated healthcare facilities, in particular hospitals.

But the integration of public financing and public production of healthcare has increasingly come into question. For instance, a recent Danish white paper on healthcare states: 'it is not a condition for free and equal access that the production of healthcare services takes place at publicly owned and managed hospitals. Services can be financed collectively, but at the same time produced based on different forms of ownership and management, for instance self-governing hospitals, hospitals owned by patient associations or privately owned and managed hospitals'.[1] This goes hand in hand with a more general tendency towards 'modernisation' of the (Scandinavian) welfare state. The idea is to maintain solidarity, somehow defined, and at the same time increase efficiency with diversity in the provision of health and social care.

The rhetorical level of the popular, professional and political debate about more private involvement in the essentially public Scandinavian healthcare systems is in marked contrast to the actual modifications in the mix which have taken place over the past one to two decades. Relatively small changes have occurred, towards more private involvement in terms of financing or provision, e.g. contracting out, private hospitals or private management of hospitals. They are in no way akin to a shift in general policy, to say nothing of revolutionary transformations.[i] Not revolution, but evolution, according to the needs of the period, has characterised development. The *really* important change has been the 'zeitgeist', the spirit of the age, introducing concepts and management of the production and provision of care, while retaining much of the 'publicness' of healthcare, in particular tax financing. However, this has led to important changes in institutional framework, such that the public healthcare systems are not what they used to be. Internal markets have been introduced, hospitals have been corporatised, contracting out has been implemented and free choice of provider has been developed.

Terms and definitions

Often, the general understanding of ideas like 'free and equal access' and 'solidarity' is based on a confusion of financing and production of services. At the general level, one has to distinguish between the financing and the provision of healthcare, Figure 9.1, but in view of development, this must be supplemented with updated management and allocation practices. The term 'market orientation' is used, despite the fact that it is a far cry from anything vaguely resembling real and unregulated private markets. Also, much of this development takes place within a public framework, e.g. internal markets and corporatisation of (public) hospitals. Entrepreneurship or entrepreneurialism,[8] is a more apt term, which better captures the spirit of current practices and avoids some of the (ideological) notions associated with 'market' and 'market orientation'.

In a Scandinavian context, financing can be subdivided into three categories: tax financing, co-payment and supplementary voluntary health insurance. Clearly, the first is public, while the two latter categories are examples of private financing. The empirical question is whether the balance between these three has changed over the past decade – and why. If it has, then it makes sense to speak of increased private financing.

Purely public provision consists of publicly owned and managed institutions, e.g. hospitals or general practices. So a change in the public–private mix denotes a shift from public to private ownership and management (e.g. general practice in Norway) or a combination of publicly owned facilities, privately managed and with services paid for by a public third party. The term 'privatisation' is often used in this context. Strictly speaking, privatisation refers to turning a public asset over to private ownership, as has happened with many public utilities. Much of the change in the public–private mix is not privatisation in this well-defined sense. The public – and for that matter scientific debate – would benefit from using clearly defined terms to avoid the resulting ideological and political heat, with little substantive light.

Figure 9.1 also shows the difficulty in using descriptive terms like 'Beveridge System' and 'Bismarck System' to characterise healthcare structures. Generally, the Beveridge system is thought to cover the upper right-hand quadrant, i.e. a universal, totally payer–provider integrated system. The Bismarck system would be found in the upper left-hand quadrant, with almost universal coverage but (many) private (not-for-profit or for-profit) institutions. The reality is far too complex for the differences to be described in terms of funding and ownership/

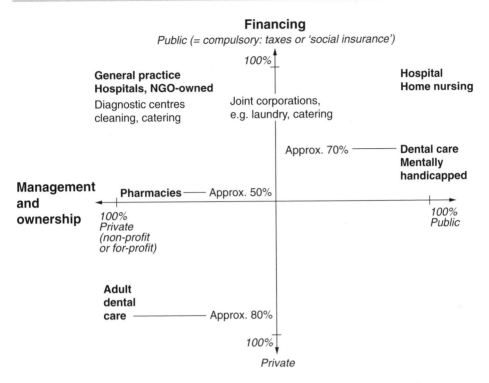

Figure 9.1 Public–private financing and provision: illustrations from Denmark.

management. Much of the public–private mix discussion has roots in somewhat stereotyped images of different healthcare systems.

As noted above, there is more to the public–private mix than just financing and provision. Management and resource allocation practices can alter without affecting the public nature of financing or provision, but logic may shift a 'traditional' public set of principles and values to a more private sector-oriented form.[ii] For instance, the 'corporatisation' of hospitals[14] is an attempt to mimic private sector practices while retaining public ownership and management, but with important adjustments to the latter. In introducing internal markets, allocation methods were altered to simulate certain features of the private market, but as the term indicates, this is a market that is largely internal to the public sector. Free choice of hospital is yet another example. Indeed, much of what is classified as 'privatisation' actually refers to such phenomena.

Overview of the Scandinavian healthcare sectors with focus on ownership and financing

To understand public–private changes, it is necessary to grasp a few elements of the healthcare systems in Denmark, Finland, Norway and Sweden. Essential features are: universal access; tax financing; publicly owned hospitals; and either publicly employed GPs or heavily regulated independent GPs financed almost 100% from taxes.

The Scandinavian healthcare systems can be characterised as a decentralised NHS. None of them are state run, but managed, planned and largely financed either by the counties (Denmark, Sweden), the municipalities (Finland and to a certain extent Norway) or 'corporatised' (the hospitals in Norway, where the state is the sole owner/shareholder of the regional corporations that run the hospitals), Table 9.1.

It is difficult, in the face of a decentralised system such as this, to make sweeping national generalisations. Considerable local autonomy has led to different solutions, e.g. the rather radical development in Stockholm County towards more private involvement cannot be generalised to the other Swedish counties. However, in all countries, national legislation establishes a set of rules and a regulatory framework for financing and provision, e.g. the Danish Hospital Law requires the counties to provide health services free of charge, but does not prevent the counties from contracting with private parties for the provision of services. Among other things, decentralisation means that taxes are levied locally by the relevant political bodies to cover most of the costs of running the local healthcare system supplemented by unconditional block grants from central government.

The healthcare sector can be defined by the types of services provided. Many think of it primarily in terms of hospital care and that provided by GPs and practising specialists. But for the purpose of studying the public–private mix, areas more sensitive to public–private change must be included, i.e. adult dental care, ambulance services and pharmacies. For this reason, Table 9.2 lists present ownership and financing of the major parts of the various sub-sectors of the healthcare system.

Changes in financing

About 75–85% of total health expenditures in Scandinavia are tax financed (Table 9.1). Table 9.1 also shows that co-payment has been increasing over the past 10 years, except in Norway.[iii] However, if the period covered included up to 1980, marked changes would be observed in all countries, for instance a private share of 7–8% for both Denmark and Sweden. In addition, supplementary health insurance has gradually been accepted, particularly in Denmark.

Private health insurance

With the exception of Denmark, at present, voluntary supplementary health insurance (VHI)[iv] is not widespread in Scandinavia, although it is beginning to gain a foothold in the other countries.

Today almost 34% of all Danes (1.8 million)[v] are members of 'denmark', a non-profit mutual health insurance that grew out of the sickness fund system abolished in 1973. At that time, membership was about 270 000, but by 1990 the number had reached about 1 million.

Until 1990, the insurance was, in essence, a 'co-payment insurance',[vi] in the sense that it covered part, but never all, of the co-payment for adult dental services, drugs, physiotherapy, etc. There is no doubt that the growth in membership is parallel with and largely driven by increased co-payment in Denmark.

Table 9.1 Overview of essential features of the healthcare systems of Scandinavia

	Hospitals	GPs	Main political body	Financing	Health expenditures	1990	1995	2000
Denmark	Financed, owned and operated by 14 counties and the Copenhagen Hospital Trust	Privately owned, but financed and regulated by the counties	Directly elected county councils	Income and property taxes levied by the county councils plus unconditional block grants from central government	% GDP	8.3	8.0	8.1
					$ PPP per capita	1453	1880	2398
					% private expenditure	17.3	17.5	17.5
Finland	Financed, owned, and operated by about 20 districts based on associations of municipalities	Municipal employees, usually located in municipal health centres	Directly elected municipal councils	Local taxes levied by the 470+ municipalities plus block grants from central government	% GDP	7.5	7.3	6.5
					$ PPP per capita	1295	1414	1698
					% private expenditure	19.1	24.4	24.9
Norway	Owned by the state, managed by five regions with independent boards. Financed by approbations from national parliament to the regions	Largely privately owned, but financed and regulated by the 435 municipalities	Parliament (hospitals) and directly elected municipal councils	State taxes for hospitals, municipal and social security financing ('folketrygden') for general practice	% GDP	7.3	7.5	7.2
					$ PPP per capita	1363	1865	2787
					% private expenditure	17.2	15.8	15.0
Sweden	Financed, owned and operated by 18 counties and three regions	Most are county employees, usually working in centers ('vårdcentraler')	Directly elected county councils	County taxes	% GDP	7.6	7.8	8.0
					$ PPP per capita	1492	1680	2195
					% private expenditure	10.1	13.3	15.0

Note: Data on health expenditures taken from OECD Health Data 2003.

Table 9.2 Ownership and financing in the Scandinavian countries 2003 (several possible modifying details omitted to provide a general overview)

		Denmark	*Finland*	*Norway*	*Sweden*
Hospitals	Ownership	Public	Public	Public	Public
	Financing	Public	Public	Public	Public
General practice	Ownership	Private	Public	Private	Public
	Financing	Public	Public	Public	Public
Specialist practice	Ownership	Private	Private	Private	Public
	Financing	Public	Public	Public	Public
Dental care	Ownership	Adult: private Child: public	Adult: Public (and P) Child: public	Adult: private Child: public	Adult: public (and P) Child: public (and P)
	Financing	Adult: P & P Child: public	Adult: private Child: public	Adult: private Child: public	Adult: P & P Child: public
Pharmacies	Ownership	Private	Private	Private	Public
	Financing	P & P	P & P	P & P	P & P
Ambulance services	Ownership	Private	Private (and P)	Private (and P)	Public (and P)
	Financing	Public	Public	Public	Public

Note: 'P & P': Public and private (co-payment makes up a substantial part of total expenditures, usually > 15%). The section on co-payment elaborates/modifies the 'public' financing for hospitals, GPs and specialist practice – 'Public (and P) or Private (and P)' means that public (private) ownership (financing) dominates, but with a substantial private (public) component, e.g. ambulance services in Sweden where half of the counties have their own ambulance service, but where one-third also contract with private ambulance companies; or dental care in Sweden where 57% of all dentists are public employees.

When the first for-profit private hospital was established in 1989/90, 'denmark' extended coverage to elective surgery for two of the membership groups, comprising about 450 000 in 2003. In addition, a third group can join for a modest increase in premium, about £40 a year. About 75 000 have chosen this option, so that more than 500 000 Danes (about 10% of the population) can choose elective surgery at private hospitals or clinics for a fairly modest co-payment (about 15% of the price of, for instance, a hip replacement).

The pay-out to members of 'denmark' amounts to about 2% (1.6 billion Dkr) of total Danish health expenditure. But as a percentage of expenditure for adult dental care and drugs, a more relevant comparison, it is much higher. For dental care, the pay-out is equal to about 50% (600 million Dkr[vii]) of public expenditure in this sector, and about 14% (about 600 million Dkr) of public expenditure for prescription drugs. In other words, 'denmark' provides substantial financing for these two items.

Commercially based health insurance has gained a stronger position in Denmark over the past 5 years. It is estimated that around 250 000 Danes now hold an insurance for (essentially only) elective surgery. However, in contrast to 'denmark', this type of insurance is usually paid by the employer and stops when the insured leaves the workforce.

Discounting double membership, a total in excess of 2 million Danes, almost

40% of the population, carry a voluntary supplementary health insurance, and about 20% have an insurance that allows them to 'jump' waiting lists for elective surgery at public hospitals.

It should be noted that no health insurance – commercial or non-profit – is offered for acute care, so the type of health insurance discussed here covers only 15–20% of hospital-based treatment.

When the present right-right government came into power, its declared intention was to change the tax rules for commercial health insurance. In accordance with normal tax policy for fringe benefits, company premiums had been tax deductible, reducing company taxation, but the premium was taxable income for the insurance holder (the employee). The change meant that, provided all employees in a company were covered by health insurance, the premium would be tax-free for the insurance holder. This is an indirect tax subsidy worth about 80–100 million Dkr (£8–10 million). It is a clear example of political support for a move to more supplementary coverage.[viii] The idea is not to substitute tax-financed healthcare, but to supplement and to provide more free choice.

One might think that with this number of voluntary supplementary health insurances there should by now be a solid base for private hospitals and clinics offering elective surgery. As will become clear in the section on provision, this is hardly the case, one reason being that the prevalence/incidence of, for instance, cataract or needed hip replacement is heavily skewed towards the elderly, i.e. 60+ years old. However, at that age they leave the labour market – and most of the commercial insurances only cover working life, so the paradox is that people do not have insurance when they most need it.

Turning to the other Scandinavian countries it should be noted that there is no 'old' tradition like the non-profit mutual 'denmark'. Hence, all supplementary health insurance is offered by commercial companies.

Only within the past 2–4 years has supplementary health insurance grown in Norway and Sweden. Prior to the late 1990s, it was largely non-existent. Compared to Denmark the numbers are, therefore, small.[ix]. It is estimated that about 120 000 Swedes in 2003 now carry supplementary health insurance,[18] largely allowing them to jump the waiting list for elective surgery. As a percentage of the population it is a miniscule 1.3%. In about 90% of cases – compared to almost 100% in Denmark for commercial insurance – the employer pays the fees. It is usually justified, as in Denmark, by the idea that it will reduce long-term sickness absence because of the possibility of jumping the waiting list.

In Norway it is estimated that about 30–40 000 have supplementary health insurance,[19,20] allowing them, as in Sweden, to jump the waiting list by obtaining treatment from a private provider paid by the insurance. As a percentage of the population it is only 0.6%. However, the Norwegian government in 2003 introduced the same tax rules as in Denmark, hence providing a tax subsidy. The two references used here are 10 months apart, and allowing for uncertainty, it seems that this legislative change – along with other things – has increased demand, increasing the number of persons by 10 000 from October 2002 to July 2003.

In Finland the only data are from a 1996 national survey which showed that 12% of the population have some type of health insurance. Most of this, however, is insurance cover for child healthcare and often taken out by citizens of the larger cities where there are many private physicians.[17] In terms of coverage (percentage in group covered) the numbers are: children aged < 7: 34.8%; children aged 7–17: 25.7%; and adults: 6.7%,[16] Table 5. Other data show that health insurance is 2% of total healthcare financing in 1997.

Thus, voluntary health insurance plays only a minor role in Scandinavia, even in Denmark. As long as publicly owned and managed hospitals are not allowed to take in private and paying patients (like the private wing concept in England), the importance of VHI lies in (potentially) providing a patient base for a private sector, independent of the public sector. It also allows for citizens to partially opt out, at least as regards elective surgery, but still be taxpayers and hence contributing to the public healthcare system.

Critics of this development fear that – in the long run – a two-tiered healthcare system will emerge: a largely VHI-financed private sector and a public sector for the rest. In view of the extent of VHI, this debate and fear seem to be overblown, and it is premature to 'cry wolf'. In many respects this development is unlikely unless supplementary health insurance gradually turns into a substitute for tax financing. At present this is not a probable scenario. However, there is no doubt that catering to individual wishes and relying on their willingness to pay not only their taxes but also supplementary insurance will create a more individualised and diverse healthcare sector.

Co-payment

Co-payment has increased steadily over the past 20 years in all the Scandinavian countries. However, often a ceiling model is used. This means that after a certain cumulative level of user payment has been reached, either there is no or only symbolic co-payment. In this way it is believed that the most harmful effects on social equity are avoided. Increased co-payment can then be achieved by increasing the value of the ceiling.

Some care must be taken, however, in interpreting this trend. Take pharmaceuticals as the best example. The percentage of total health expenditure going to pharmaceuticals has increased from a one-digit number in the mid- and late 1980s to a two-digit number in 2003, e.g. around 15% in Sweden. Depending on the exact co-payment structure this will at the same time tend to drive up the share of total health expenditures paid for through user payment.

Co-payment in Sweden varies by county. Within established national maximum limits the counties are free to vary co-payment, for instance by income or age. Typically children are exempt.

Table 9.3 shows examples of current co-payment. In both Norway and Sweden it is combined with ceilings, which are also used in Denmark for pharmaceuticals. The general impression is one of rather widespread co-payment in Scandinavia, contrary to the picture of 'free' access. Table 9.3 does not show the increase that has been witnessed in most areas. For instance there was no co-payment for GP visits in Finland prior to 1993. Overall there was a dramatic increase in co-payments in the early 1990s. In 1990, it made up about 13% of total healthcare expenditures, but by 1994 it had increased to 20.4%.

In Sweden and Norway there has been, in effect, privatisation of adult dental care for many adults above a certain income. In Denmark, co-payment now makes up about 80% of expenditure for adult dental care.

Table 9.3 Current co-payment situation

	Denmark	Finland	Norway	Sweden
GP (per visit)	Free	80–160 Dkr	110 Dkr	100–150 Dkr
Practising specialist	Free	80–160 Dkr	185 Dkr	150–250 Dkr
Outpatient visits	Free	160–560 Dkr	185 Dkr	150–250 Dkr
Hospital (per day)	Free	200–560 Dkr	Free	80 Dkr
Adult dental care*	75–80%	40% (for a limited set of services)	Normally 100%	Considerable
Prescription pharmaceuticals*	Percentage** varies with total annual expenditures	After the first cumulatative amount of €10 there is 50% co-payment up to a ceiling	36%, maximum 400 Nkr per prescription	Percentage** varies with total annual expenditures

Source: Reference 1, Table 4.2, plus information from NOMESCO.[21] This source gives details in English.
* only a very rough picture. For details see reference 21.
** General idea: 100% co-payment for the first 700–900 Dkr, then 50% for the next expenditure interval followed by 25% etc., and after a certain maximum expenditure limit has been reached there is no co-payment.

Even though co-payment for pharmaceuticals has also increased somewhat, it should be noted that the increasing use of drugs has increased the absolute and relative amounts that individuals pay for drugs.

It is natural to ask whether the increased co-payment is a conscientious move towards more individualised financing – a move away from solidaric financing. In general the answer is no. First of all, the changes have taken place both during social democratic and right-right governments, usually thought of as, respectively, opponents and supporters of co-payment. In fairness, the speed of change has been slower during social democratic governments. Second, the move is basically a way of trying to cope with the difficulties of tax financing the increasing expenditures for healthcare without straining the total level of taxation too much. The level of taxation in the Scandinavian countries is the highest in the world. Third, in at least one country, Finland, some of the changes were simply necessary in the early 1990s in view of the almost total melt-down of the economy following the collapse of the Soviet Union with almost 25% unemployment. As noted, attempts have been made to protect either low-income groups through ceilings or high-usage groups with a specially designed reimbursement system like that for drugs.

Changes in provision

Even though some small moves towards more individual ('privatised') financing can be observed, greater changes are to be found on the production side. Across the Scandinavian countries there has been a general move towards contracting out via tendering, in particular for non-clinical hospital services. A few – but much-talked-about – private hospitals have been established in all the countries. There have been important changes for GPs in one country. There has been some liberalisation of the pharmacy system in two countries. Furthermore, in Sweden two private 'health corporations' have appeared, Capio (described in a later footnote) and Praktikertjänsten; and ISS in Denmark is also interested in the market.

All in all then, greater diversity can be observed on the production side while retaining the basic solidaric tax-financed system. However, as with financing, the change in relative terms has been modest. It is not a landslide but a gradual adaptation to a new environment focusing on increased efficiency by using different providers in order to infuse a degree of competition.

The greatest changes can be observed for primary care. Despite the much publicised changes in Sweden, the change in the public–private mix is modest here. From 1993 to 2000 the number of employees in for-profit healthcare companies increased by 5000,[22] out of a total health sector workforce of around 300 000 persons. Within institutional healthcare, i.e. hospitals, the proportion of private contractors is slightly below 3% in terms of number of employees, and increased by one percentage point from 1992 to 2000. One single hospital, the St Göran in Stockholm, accounts for much of the change. In Denmark, the first private for-profit hospital was established in 1989. There are several small private hospitals providing elective surgery. However, in terms of hospital beds the number of private beds is about 1% of the public beds. The same holds for Norway, and in Finland about 3–4% of all inpatient care is private.

Figure 9.2 shows the interaction between funding and provision. There are two main points. First, it is very difficult to create a sustainable private supply side, in particular for hospitals, without either a very strong base of private insurance (VHI) or public funding. It is telling that in Denmark, with substantial supplementary insurance, the take-off point has hardly been reached yet. Hence, to a considerable extent the growth of privately based provision depends on the rules/laws/norms governing tax funding of privately produced services. Second, the growth of VHI depends on availability of services covered by the insurance, e.g. elective surgery. However, if public hospitals are prohibited from taking insurance-paid patients – for instance by law, as in Denmark – the growth of VHI depends on the growth of (for-profit) private hospitals.

A better understanding of changes in the public–private mix of the financing and production side assumes an understanding of the forces driving what is depicted in Figure 9.2. Laws and/or politically-based behaviour to a large extent determine changes in the flow in the figure. If, for instance, private wings were allowed as part of public hospitals in Scandinavia[x] it would create competition vis-à-vis private for-profit hospitals. However, politically many would fear that this would open up 'first- and second-class' patients in public hospitals creating an inequality that would be politically unacceptable, even for some right-right parties.

General practice

Primary healthcare is a very important component of the overall healthcare system in Scandinavia. It is embodied in the GPs who in all the countries but

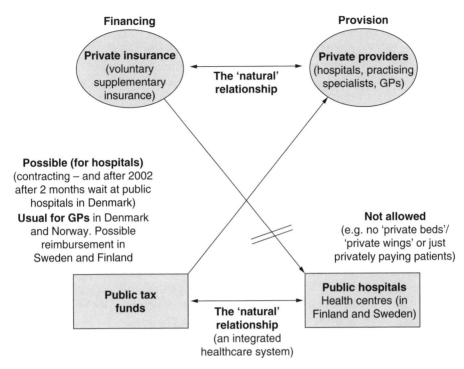

Figure 9.2 The mutual dependency between funding and provision.

Sweden act as gatekeepers, i.e. a referral from a GP is usually needed to get access to more specialised healthcare. Apart from Denmark, the past decade has witnessed changes.

The most sweeping change over the past decade is the privatisation of Norwegian GPs. Prior to 2001 most GPs in Norway were municipal employees. A reform in 2001 introduced a list system combined with the possibility for GPs to become independent entrepreneurs contracting with the public funding authority. Today about 90% of GPs have chosen this mode of operation. However, as in Denmark, they are heavily regulated and derive close to 95–100% of their income from contracts with a tax-financed public agency. The remuneration system was changed from basically a salary system to 30% capitation and 70% fee-for-service (much the same as in Denmark).

In the early and mid-1990s Sweden experimented with changing the employment status of GPs from public employment to that of independent entrepreneur. However, it is telling that much depends on the party in power, i.e. Social Democrats after 1994 versus the right-right government from 1991 to 1994.

With the Family Doctor Act of 1994, along with the Act on Freedom to Establish Private Practice, the road was paved for a move from GPs as public employees to GPs as independent entrepreneurs. However, these two laws enacted by the right-right Government in 1994 were withdrawn by the Social Democratic Government mid-year 1995 before they were fully implemented. However, due to the decentralised nature of Swedish healthcare, several county councils had already implemented part of the laws, and those changes were retained meaning that the two acts and the preceding decision process, e.g. the recommendations from 1992 by the Association of County Councils,[23] overall led to an increased privatisation of primary care in some counties with partial free choice of GP, namely those GPs working on contract with the county councils.[23,24] In the Skåne Region (southern Sweden) about 40% of primary care is private, compared with 20% in the rest of Sweden,[25] and according to the Swedish Association of counties, about 25% of all physician visits in primary care (outside hospitals) were handled by private practising doctors,[26] but the number of doctors involved has decreased from around 1400 in 1998 to 1211 in 2001.

In Finland the employment status of GPs has not been changed, i.e. they are still public employees, but the idea of a list system was introduced in the early 1990s. Initially it was called the 'personal doctor system', later 'population responsibility'. Today about 50% of the population has been assigned to a personal doctor. The system was accompanied by a change in the remuneration system, from salary to a four-component system: fee-for-service (15%), capitation (20%), basic salary (60%) and 5% local allowance.

It seems that the number of visits to private practising doctors, but reimbursed by the relevant public authority, has decreased by about 20% from 1990 to 2000 (private communication). About 8% of Finnish doctors work full time in private practice,[27] but about one-third of all physicians working full time in public employment have some kind of part-time private practice.

Hospitals

In Scandinavia there have always been a modest number of non-profit hospitals run by charities, church organisations or patients' associations. The new feature of the past 10–15 years is the entry of for-profit hospitals in all four countries. The important thing to note is their very existence and their modest size. None of them are acute hospitals,[xi] and most of them have carved out niches in elective surgery. With one exception they are small, with fewer than 75 beds. Typically they have 20–40 beds, but much of their activity is same-day surgery. As noted earlier, their share of the market is very small, at most 3–5% in some areas of surgery. There are relatively few full-time employed doctors in the private hospitals. Most of their doctors work on a part-time basis, for instance five hours a week, often nights and Saturdays, and have full-time employment in public hospitals.

The private hospitals are careful to point out that they consider themselves as a supplement or a free-choice alternative, but they rarely or never position themselves as fully-fledged alternatives to public hospitals.

If for-profit hospitals are to survive financially there must either be a good base of voluntary health insurance, or the hospitals must contract with the responsible public authorities, e.g. the counties in Denmark (*see also* Figure 9.2). Apart from in Denmark, voluntary health insurance is not widespread, and even there the base is not big enough to create a sustainable financial base for the present number of private hospitals or large clinics. Hence, the decisive factor is either public contracts or outright 'automatic' public funding. The usual pattern has been contracts where counties, after a tendering process, typically for waiting-list surgery like cataract or hip replacement, contract with a private hospital. In Denmark a more automatic mechanism was created in mid-2002 with a new national law about expanded free choice. This means that after two months' waiting time for elective surgery at a public hospital citizens have the right to treatment either at a private hospital or to go abroad, also with public payment. The private Danish or foreign hospitals are usually paid on a diagnosis related group (DRG) basis – with DRG rates equal to what public hospitals would receive. It remains to be seen whether this will create a sustainable financial base for private hospitals. It is obvious that they are vulnerable to a decrease in waiting time for elective surgery at public hospitals.

The establishment of private hospitals has required 'patient' investor money before profits began to emerge. Very few of the private hospitals make a profit. In Denmark the net result across all the private hospitals has been negative. In total, over the past 10 years investors have lost around 150 million Dkr (£15 million). However, a number of small clinics, for instance specialising in cataract or other same-day surgery, have made a profit, but many of them exist on a hit-and-run basis due to the rather modest level of the entry investment.

The entry of private hospitals has, of course, been surrounded by heated public debate, whereas changes in primary healthcare, e.g. GP organisation, go largely unnoticed. In Sweden the sale of the St Göran hospital in Stockholm to the Capio Corporation[xii] in 2000 led the Social Democratic Government to introduce a law temporarily preventing the counties from selling (or managing) public acute hospitals to private for-profit parties.[29] The law has recently been extended to 2004 while awaiting a more permanent set of rules surrounding the involvement of private for-profit companies in the healthcare sector (see below for details). Similarly, the Danish Social Democratic Government in 1993/4 changed the hospital law to prevent public hospitals from taking in insurance or privately paid patients. However, the law clearly allows the counties to use private hospitals for providing whatever services the county council approves for funding. Also, the counties are not allowed to enter into commercial joint activities with private for-profit hospitals. In other words, national legislation to a considerable extent governs the boundaries of public–private cooperation. This legislation obviously mirrors the political stand of the government in power.

Pharmacies

Norway liberalised the heavily regulated pharmacy system in 2001. Before the reform a pharmacy had to be owned and operated by a licensed pharmacist. This was repealed, opening the way for non-pharmacist investors. However, a pharmacy must still employ at least one trained pharmacist. The result has been that three chains now dominate the market compared to the many pre-reform independent pharmacies, and the number of pharmacies has increased without a concomitant increase in the number of employees. The average number of opening hours also has increased.[30]

Denmark has witnessed a small liberalisation in that the pharmacy monopoly on distribution of both prescription and over-the-counter (OTC) drugs was changed in 2001. A rather small, but gradually increasing, number of OTC drugs can now be sold by, for instance, supermarkets fulfilling certain conditions. This is the first change in the pharmacy monopoly on distributing drugs since 1972. Norway is following Denmark along this path in 2004 – and the Norwegian monopoly goes as far back as the Danish.

Changes in management and allocation principles: 'market orientation'

As noted several times, actual changes in ownership and financing have been modest in relative terms. However, the trend is clear despite small changes. Real, almost dramatic, changes have occurred in the way management and resource allocation takes place. In many respects – and expressed in a variety of ways – there has been a basic change in the approach to running public institutions. Many of the ideas resemble or outright mimic private sector methods. Hence, the imprecise term 'market orientation' has often been used as a cover-all term, both with positive and negative connotations.

The changes can be split into production- and patient-side changes. On the production side:

- principle-based discussion of diversity of providers
- increased use of contracting out
- 'corporatisation' of hospitals
- modern management methods in general
- provider-purchaser split
- incentive systems
- pay systems for personnel
- reimbursement, in particular hospitals.

On the patient side:

- free choice of hospital
- various waiting list/time guarantees
- strengthening of patient rights in general.

Sweden has led the way in embracing these changes, but they have to varying degrees, except for the purchaser–provider split, been introduced in all the Scandinavian countries since the early 1990s.

There is no doubt that these changes together have had a greater impact on how the healthcare sector is run in Scandinavia than 'privatisation', in the sense discussed in the previous sections.

Discussion of principles for provider diversity

Until recently there has only been heated public debate surrounding 'privatisation', mainly driven by reflexes dictated by ideological stances, not analysis.[xiii] However, the Swedish government, in the wake of the law following the Stockholm County sale of a public hospital (see above), decided to develop a White Paper to look more systematically into the ownership forms in healthcare. This has resulted in two rather lengthy and wordy reports, and a short English summary of the first of these reports.[22,31,32]

A Social Democratic member of parliament acted as chairman for the work , i.e. the reports are not based on work by independent experts. Hence, most of the recommendations naturally mirror thinking by the current Swedish government. The focus has been on the question of how to, at one and the same time, safeguard (publicly spirited) priorities, basic principles and values as the Swedish healthcare system gradually opens up for a greater diversity of providers. The recommendations basically call for diversity of providers, in particular non-profit providers, but also recommends that a sale like the St Göran case should not be allowed. All in all, the recommendations argue to a considerable extent for the status quo. How this will translate into legislation is not yet clear.

Hence, it is not the recommendations that are important. The importance of this work lies in the nascent recognition that many laws and regulations have been developed which implicitly and almost unknowingly mirror a totally integrated public healthcare system, and that much needs to be changed if one wants to open up for a more diverse set of producers, i.e. rules for setting up contracts and the like along with a changed legislation, while retaining public financing. The same basically holds in the other countries. For instance, the Danish 2003 report also calls for a non-dogmatic use of diversity of providers.[1] Reports like these help focus on what constitute 'true public values' as regards production, for instance democratic insight into the running of enterprises that provide (100%) publicly provided services. Much clarification and myth debunking undoubtedly is needed here.

In a recent Finnish government report,[33] there is another principle-based discussion, namely of the extent and nature of work undertaken by full-time publicly employed physicians in private hospitals or private practice. In Finland and the other Scandinavian countries this is quite common. Ideas like those of the Finnish government have also been discussed in Denmark.[xiv] The important point is how to avoid conflict of interest. The Finnish Medical Association, Health Care Sector Service Organisations and hospital district management have compiled recommendations to prevent such problems arising. Some rather obvious examples are that publicly employed physicians must not refer patients to their private clinics in a manner that conflicts with their official duties. Admission of a patient to a hospital or polyclinic must be arranged according to equitable principles based on the need for treatment. A physician may not participate in person in the decision making about admission of a patient that the same physician has referred for treatment, unless there are compelling reasons for so doing. Also, physicians participating in decision making or the preparation thereof pertaining to outsourced services may not serve as members of the board of directors, supervisory board or comparable organs, or as managing director of enterprises engaged in the provision of outsourced services for a hospital or health centre.

Contracting out

Contracting out of non-clinical services is common, but not required by law or regulation in any of the Scandinavian countries. However, contracting out of clinical services is more rare, e.g. of an X-ray department, a laboratory or management of a suite of operating theatres. It has been impossible to identify the extent and the change over, for instance, the past decade. It is mentioned in a Swedish report that the proportion of private contractors increased from just below 6% in 1993 to approximately 12% in 2000. Although often met with hostility by public hospital employees, contracting out has gradually been accepted, in particular because rules have been set up for transfer of employment status for persons working in the areas contracted out to private contractors.

There have been instances where counties in Denmark have set up jointly owned companies with a private party, for instance in laundering or catering. Typically the public party owns 49% of the company in question. However, this practice is in no way widespread, but shows how public–private partnership evolves in interesting ways based on a softening of attitudes and prejudices.

Corporatisation of hospitals and modern management practices

In Norway and Sweden 'corporatisation' of hospitals has become quite common. This means that a hospital becomes a public corporation, with the county (or state in Norway) holding 100% of the shares. Sometimes it approaches the status of an independent legal entity, i.e. outside the traditional public sector bureaucracy.[xv]

In Norway the whole hospital sector was reorganised on 1 January 2002.[35][xvi] Ownership of hospitals was transferred from the counties to the state, and hospitals essentially became independent legal entities (with considerable similarity to private companies) with the state as sole shareholder. There is considerable freedom in operational matters, while there is still central control with larger investment projects. Furthermore, the country was divided into five regions. Each region has a government-appointed board (without politicians) that is given considerable responsibility. The hospitals in a region are, in essence, daughters of the region, i.e. mirroring a private sector corporate structure. Each hospital has its own board, again without appointed politicians, and as in a corporation is usually chaired by a director from the 'mother' company.

Several Swedish hospitals, in particular in the Stockholm County and the Skåne region, have been corporatised – and 'de-corporatised': two hospitals in the southern-most Swedish county, Skåne, were corporatised in 2000 following an election victory by the Conservatives, but the next election was won by the Social Democrats and they turned these two hospitals into traditional public governance structures.[25,38] This example shows – in contrast to the Norwegian reform – how contentious the change to 'private-like' governance forms can be. In essence corporatised hospitals are still publicly owned (100% shareholder) and financing is still 100% public.

Similarly, the recent Danish expert report to the government,[1,25,38] recommended increased autonomy to the hospitals without going as far as in Norway and Sweden. The keywords were 'arm's length' to the political level. In practice this means a clarification of what constitutes genuine political decisions and what is acceptable political interference, and hence, what is the responsibility of hospital management. In general, operational decisions – for instance labour force composition, ongoing capacity adjustment and contracting out – should be the autonomous decision of hospital management. The report also discusses the possible added value of introducing a model similar to Norway, but sees no added value if the principle of arm's length is followed.

In these ways hospital management is allowed greater freedom to run hospitals along more business- and professional-oriented lines. Basically it allows the establishment of a solid arm's length principle to the political overseers and paymasters and lets professional judgement be of decisive importance. It is believed that this will increase productivity, quality and responsiveness to patient wishes. However, the empirical evidence in a traditional scientific sense is scant.[35][xvii] On the other hand, 'causal empiricism and observation' does suggest that freer reins and associated increased responsibility have a positive effect on how hospitals are run. In addition, it should be noted that these changes have gone hand in hand with, and in essence been reinforced by, increased used of explicit contracts between county politicians and the individual hospitals setting down production and quality targets to be reached within the (capped) budget and/or increased use of activity-based financing, i.e. DRG-based reimbursement. The latter, almost by assumption, requires increased operational responsibility by the hospital management.

Purchaser–provider split

This idea has only been adapted in some Swedish counties, as usual led by Stockholm County, and appears to be firmly entrenched, but it has not been adopted by the political decision makers in the three other Scandinavian countries.

In Finland the possibility of its adoption actually exists, in that there is a natural administrative split, namely with the municipalities as purchasers and the 20 hospital districts as providers. However, the idea has never been pursued vigorously. The Danish 2003 report[1] devoted a whole chapter to a discussion of the model, but concludes that the empirical evidence from England, New Zealand and Sweden in terms of productivity and quality does not show clear advantages compared to the current Danish practice. There is contracting between the 'purchasers' (county politicians) and providers (county-owned hospitals with increased operational autonomy). This concept was introduced from 1993 onwards, and today embraces all counties. In a sense it was the Danish response to the internal markets movement in the UK.

As illustrated by the Swedish experience,[39,40,41] the issue is whether it is the purchaser–provider split and the ensuing (potential) competition that can explain possible efficiency increases or the concomitant and often necessary DRG-based reimbursement of hospitals that make a difference. Something indicates that it is the latter. Norway and Denmark have gradually introduced DRG, most systematically in Norway, where between 50 and 60% of hospital reimbursement is through DRG. Some (weak) productivity increases seem to have been demonstrated in Norway.[42]

Incentive systems

DRGs are used to some extent in all the Scandinavian countries apart from Finland.[xviii] Earlier capped budgets were the standard way of 'reimbursing' hospitals. Line-item budgets were scrapped in the 1980s, and unconditional block budgets were introduced, leaving considerable discretion to hospital management. However, the idea of a more automatic funding mechanism that to a certain extent could mirror actual activity, and hence demand, gradually gained prominence.[43][xix] At the same time, it was believed that this would be more conducive to productivity than the unconditional system with block budgets. However, the main problem with activity-based funding is that budget control –

and hence taxes needed – become far more difficult. This was clearly illustrated in the early years in Stockholm County. Therefore the introduction of DRG-based reimbursement has been followed by a variety of measures to ensure 'budget adherence', i.e. staying within stipulated annual overall expenditure frames, but at the same time blunting some of the postulated efficiency effects.

The salary system for public employees – based on seniority-based increases – has been modified to provide better performance-oriented incentives for individual employees. In Denmark, a system called 'new wage system' has been introduced in the whole public sector opening up the possibility of individual pay contracts. It is unclear what the effects of such changes will be. The importance of the new system is that it mirrors the quest for improved performance in the public sector, including hospitals, and that means a change in the age-old system of fixed salary, seniority-based pay systems for public employees.

Free choice of provider

In 1993 Denmark introduced a national law giving citizens free choice of (public) hospitals, except for highly specialised university hospitals. It was extended in 2002 to include private hospitals or hospitals abroad, provided that the patient had waited for treatment for more than two months at a public hospital.

The idea of free choice of provider has gained general prominence in Scandinavia. The last country to join is Finland. However, it is official government policy to implement free hospital choice in Finland by 2005.[33]

Free choice has almost become an independent value attracting political support from right and left. The reasons given for free choice vary, however. Some stress the possibility for (reputation) competition among hospitals or the possibility of evening out waiting times by letting patients choose hospitals with low waiting times, while others consider free value a natural development of the advanced welfare society so that it is possible to cater for different needs and wishes, including freeing citizens from the psychological straitjacket of a monopoly supplier.

It should be noted that, at least in Denmark, there has always been free choice of GP. The same is now the case in Norway, but not as a general rule in Sweden and Finland.

Waiting time initiatives

All the Scandinavian countries are struggling with waiting lists, mainly for elective surgery. It is undoubtedly a consequence of inadequate tax financing and probable hospital inefficiencies. It obviously creates dissatisfaction with the healthcare system and raises questions about the causes and possible alternatives. There is no doubt that the existence of private hospitals is to a large extent due to waiting lists.

Waiting time problems have been at the centre of much political debate and have gained an importance that is out of proportion to the extent of the problem. However, they are a visible sign of some of the inadequacies of the healthcare system, and attempts to do something are equally politically visible, and success is fairly easy to measure. The analysis of the underlying waiting time/list dynamics, however, is never debated. The political response has been to give waiting-time guarantees. Fulfilment of the guarantees has varied considerably, and the various strategies chosen have succeeded unevenly, none of them close to perfectly.[43–50]

The most radical approach has been taken in Denmark, where, in effect, a (maximum) two-month waiting-time guarantee was introduced mid-2002. It was decided to include Danish and foreign private hospitals in the free-choice scheme once patients had waited two months or more for treatment at a public hospital, and to let the counties pay for this. In this way (excess) private capacity was being put to use, while the county payment requirement put pressure on the public county hospitals because the marginal costs for surgery at the public hospitals are usually lower than the average DRG rates the counties pay for patients opting for the private sector. This seems to be working, not only for the reason indicated, but also because additional central government funding was paid on a per case basis (DRG rate) – not a general block grant as in the past. Hence, the public hospitals also got a chance to honour the two-month limit through very targeted funding, but if unsuccessful, private hospitals stepped in.

The Norwegian government also has taken drastic measures. In 2001, separate funds, a little less than £100 million, were approved to treat waiting-list patients abroad, hence using (excess) private hospital capacity in other countries.[51] More than 3000 patients have been treated abroad, in particular in Denmark, Germany and Sweden.

To many doctors and hospital administrators it seems somewhat of a paradox that the same politicians who are responsible for the financing and running of public hospitals, and hence in essence are also 'responsible' for the waiting lists, are willing to finance treatment of waiting list patients at private hospitals. They have argued for increased funding to public hospitals as an alternative. However, it seems that public hospitals that have received additional funds have found it difficult to combat the waiting lists. In a sense then, the use of private hospitals in the waiting list battle has infused some degree of competition and made public hospitals acutely aware that alternatives for elective surgery are available.

Patient rights

The patient rights legislation in all the countries, along with the free-choice movement, has firmly shifted more power to the demand/patient side. Thus the picture of a supply-driven health system has changed considerably. Some of the elements in various laws are fairly obvious, but important. In the Danish legislation the right to decide is clearly spelled out and clearly moves away from a paternalistic supply-side attitude. A patient should decide (consent to) whether an offered examination or treatment is to be carried out – also in cases when only one type of treatment is possible. If a doctor changes the treatment, the patient has a right to receive new information and again should choose. The patient can withdraw consent at any time, and if they do so, the relevant staff members should propose other treatment possibilities.

Effects of changes in the public–private mix: efficiency and equity

The question of the effects of changes in the private–public mix has been touched on only superficially, and only for (technical/production) efficiency ('productivity'). Generally, from an economist's point of view there are two effect issues: is it possible to observe changes in efficiency and in equity due to a changed public–private mix?

It is well known that a trade-off exists between efficiency and equity when organising and regulating market and non-market activities. Usually it is assumed that increasing equity has a cost in terms of stagnating or decreased efficiency. Orthodox economics furthermore assumes – almost by construction – that efficiency[xx] is highest in market situations, providing a somewhat unconvincing argument for further private involvement in the healthcare sector. There is no doubt that the interest in changing the public–private mix in the direction of more private involvement has been motivated by the quest for increased efficiency without changing equity markedly.

In this section the focus will be on equity. In terms of efficiency in Sweden, the results are somewhat inconclusive.[39,40] In a 1997 study using data from 1974 to 1989 for the hospital sector,[54] it was shown that Denmark was the only country out of 19 showing any significant productivity growth. In summary then, there is very little evidence for increased technical efficiency due to changes in the public–private mix.

Equity has always been an important concern in Scandinavia. In a sense it has been the raison d'être for the Scandinavian welfare states. Whenever changes are contemplated, in particular for co-payment, there is an outcry about (expected) decreasing equity. In the healthcare area there are four separate equity issues: equity in health, in healthcare consumption, in healthcare financing and in geographical equity. Is it possible to observe changes in one or more of these dimensions of equity?

The analytical issue is whether equity is influenced positively or negatively by changes in the public–private mix. Many observers would posit a one-sided hypothesis, namely that an increasing private component increases inequity in the case of changes in ownership and financing. On reflection, however, there need not be changes in equity in a situation with larger private involvement in healthcare provision if financing is unchanged, while increased private financing might influence (economic) equity negatively. It is somewhat unclear whether to expect a negative influence from market-oriented changes.

It is clear, however, that in view of the relatively few changes in financing and ownership, one should not expect big changes in equity. To this should be added the empirical question of how much time must elapse before changes can reasonably be observed – probably 5–10 years for use of service and financing, and longer for changes in health. In addition there are only a few studies addressing the core question directly,[55–58] and these studies do not link changes in equity – however defined – to changes in the public–private mix in any causal sense, but at best in a correlation fashion, and not always using time series. In short then, no convincing evidence exists about changes in equity caused by or correlated with changes in the public–private mix. However, for the sake of completeness, a few of the available studies are summarised briefly below. Only in Finland and Sweden has this issue been addressed and mainly in terms of utilisation of services.

For Finland, Keskimäki,[57] in a cross-section based analysis for 1987–8, i.e. before any dramatic changes, asked whether private surgical procedures contributed to socioeconomic differences. Noting considerable difficulties in ascertaining this, he nevertheless claims that his data support the view that the private sector has at least contributed to the socioeconomic differences in rates for hysterectomy, prostatectomy and cataract operations. A (not very) critical reading of the article and evidence presented, i.e. graphical displays, lead to questioning this conclusion.

In 2003, Keskimäki published a study covering the years 1988–96 on the effects of the Finnish economic recession in the early 1990s and consequent changes in the healthcare sector.[58] A slight shift towards a pro-rich distribution could be observed – mainly due to a larger increase in surgical care among the high-income groups. The article proposes – but does not provide any data-based evidence – that the increasing inequities were due to the high profile of the private sector in specialised ambulatory care and in the supply of some elective procedures, and semi-private public hospitals requiring supplementary payment from patients. It is noted that in 1988, 2.5% of surgical procedures were performed in private hospitals compared to 4.5% in 1995, but a substantial part of surgical operations in private hospitals are purchased by the public sector, however, and can hardly distort equity. Furthermore, 43% of all private hospital procedures in 1996 were carried out by two private non-profit hospitals, i.e. 'private' in the sense of not being publicly owned, but not private for-profit hospitals.

Bruström asks whether one could observe increasing inequalities in healthcare utilisation across income groups in Sweden in the 1990s.[55] The analysis is based on representative surveys from 1988/9 and 1996/7. Based on a stratified analysis it was concluded that 'the overall proportion who had visited a doctor, who had sought emergency services and who had needed but not sought care was very similar in the two periods'.[55] A multivariate analysis modifies this conclusion somewhat. It is noted that the pro-poor bias for hospitalisation, which could be observed in 1988/9, was not evident in 1996/7. The author speculates, but in no way makes it probable by outlining possible causal mechanisms, that the reduction in hospital beds during the first half of the 1990s caused this. Similarly there are speculations about the effect of (slightly) increased co-payments, but there is no link to the data analysis. As in the case of Finland, the question of changes due to various reforms is not an integrated part of the data analysis, and must fairly be categorised as 'speculations', usually based on popular beliefs about the direction of change in equity, not a scientifically rigorous discussion.

There are other articles besides the ones presented above,[59–61] but the important point to note is that the available data, integration of data and reforms, and research methodology at present are insufficient to demonstrate clearly changes in equity, apart from the fact that changes in the public–private mix have been minor, meaning that at best only small changes in equity can be expected. These changes then have to be detected by rather imperfect data and imperfect methodology.

Summary and what has shaped changes in the mix?

The essence of the above is summarised in Table 9.4. It does not do full justice to all countries, but nevertheless captures important trends in the public–private mix.

Three forces shaped this development:

- the macroeconomic situation
  - unable to sustain the public sector growth rate of the past
  - need for increased efficiency
- increased 'consumer orientation' in healthcare
- political swings and a trend towards a clearer understanding of, at one and the same time, the need to have solidarity in tax financing and (some) private production.

These three factors are to some extent interdependent, but there is no doubt that in publicly funded healthcare systems the driving force behind changes is the macroeconomic situation of a country. The direction of changes then are influenced by which political coalition is in power,[xxi] combined with general trends in society, i.e. the somewhat paradoxical move towards increased individualism while at the same time maintaining a (still) mainly supply-driven healthcare sector based on solidarity.

In all the Scandinavian countries but Norway, where oil money flows, macro-economic policy for a variety of reasons has been very tight, in particular from the

Table 9.4 Summary of changes in Scandinavia over the past 20 years

	Production	*Management principles (hospitals)*	*Consumption/ demand*	*Financing*
Up to mid- and late 1980s	Only public production	Public bureaucracy, line-item budgets	No choice – take it or leave it	Tax financing and relatively modest co-payment
1990s–2003	Some diversity. Still mainly public production but small private hospitals/clinics and private contractors entered the sector. More contracting out and innovative public–private cooperation	Modern, 'private sector-like principles'. Contracts and/or activity based reimbursement. Purchaser–provider split (Sweden). Corporatisation of hospitals In total: greater market orientation	1 Choice of provider 2 Waiting list guarantees 3 Patient rights All in all creating some demand-side pressure, to some extent placing the patient in the driver's seat	Overwhelming tax financing, but increased co-payment plus some voluntary health insurance

mid-1980s to the mid-1990s. The growth of the (tax-financed) public sector had to be curbed along with at least a levelling out of the taxation of personal income, but without sacrificing too much of the Scandinavian welfare model.

For instance, overall expenditure on healthcare in Finland fell by over 10% in real terms in the early years of the 1990s, but began to rise again in 1995. This was caused by the economic crisis following the breakdown of the Soviet Union. The Soviet Union was Finland's largest trading partner. The Danish economy was 'reconstructed' from the mid-1980s to the early 1990s. This meant, among other things, that hospital expenditure in the late 1980s decreased in real terms for three years in a row. This obviously created pressure for rationalisation and introduction of new management techniques. However, compared to Sweden, Denmark and Finland did not introduce very many 'market-oriented initiatives'.

As seen from Table 9.1 three of the four Scandinavian countries have actually experienced a decrease in the share of GDP going to health. This is exceptional in the Western world. There are several explanations. First of all it should be noted that $ PPP per capita increased by between 31% and 102% in the last decade of the twentieth century; it was lowest in Finland, the economically hardest hit country, and highest in Norway with the 'oil' economy. This means that the percentage of GDP reflects differences in the overall growth rate of the economy and that of the healthcare sector.

Changed attitudes to the public–private mix and hence private involvement in the provision of public services also characterised the mid-1980s and the 1990s. These trends in the Western world in general were reinforced/weakened by government coalitions nationally and locally (centre-right versus left-left (with social democratic participation)), and the economic situation of the respective countries. As a rule – but certainly not without important exceptions – there has been a push towards more private involvement during right-right governments and retrenchment of public involvement under left-left governments. This is most clearly demonstrated in the case of Sweden. However, fiscal pressure has created unusual alliances.

Although there have been changes towards more private involvement, the Scandinavian welfare model for healthcare is basically intact, provided one does not see 'market' orientation within an essentially publicly funded healthcare system and a largely publicly owned and managed supply side as something negative. As the debate about provider diversity shows, evolution of ideas of how to cope with, on the one hand (reasonable) free and equal access, and hence collective financing, and on the other hand efficient production of the needed services continually challenge the supply side. The existence of waiting times for elective surgery has introduced novel ways of reducing the queues. There is no doubt that politicians realise that the population's belief in the capabilities of the current healthcare system in general and the supply-side organisation in particular depends to a considerable extent on how well it is able to cope with waiting times.

There is, of course, no direct causal link between the public's satisfaction with their healthcare systems and the public–private mix, although it is one among several possible explanatory elements. Table 9.5 shows that the two countries that have 'experimented' the least with their healthcare systems experience the highest degree of satisfaction.

Table 9.5 Public's satisfaction with healthcare systems, in four EU countries 1996 and 1999

	Very and fairly satisfied		Neither satisfied nor dissatisfied		Very and fairly dissatisfied	
	1996	*1999*	*1996*	*1999*	*1996*	*1999*
Denmark	90	75.8	3.8	Not used	5.7	23.9
Finland	86.4	74.3	7.0	Not used	6.0	24.7
Sweden	67.3	48.7	16.7	Not used	14.2	38.9
United Kingdom	48.1	13.0	10.0	Not used	40.9	42.3

Source: Reference 62 and Eurobarometer 52.1, 1999. Norway is not an EU member and has not been included in the surveys. Note the difference in wording of the satisfaction question in 1996 and 1999. It obviously influences the response pattern.

Unless the degree of 'publicness' or 'privateness' is considered as an ultimate end (ideology/value: more private or public is ultimately what is desired, what is 'good') the public–private mix should be considered in a means context. In other words, do differences in the mix result in a better healthcare sector? 'Better' should be measured on several dimensions: responsiveness/satisfaction, health outcome productivity, quality and innovation to mention some key dimensions. Unfortunately it is impossible to find reliable evidence on this crucial issue.

Declaration of interest: the author is a board member of for-profit, non-profit and public hospitals. He has been a member of government commissions under both left-left and right-right governments.

References

1 Sundhedsministerens RU (2003) *Sygehusvæsenets organisaton. Sygehuse, incitamenter, amter og alternativer* (The organizaion of the healthcare sector. Hospitals, incentives, counties and alternatives). Sundhedsministeriet: Copenhagen.
2 Diderichsen F (1993) Market reforms in Swedish healthcare: a threat to or salvation for the universalistic welfare state? *International Journal of Health Services*. **23**: 185–8.
3 Ham C, Calltorp J, Rosenthal M (1992) Future directions. *Health Policy*. **21**: 181–6.
4 Saltman RB, von Otter C (1992) *Planned Markets and Public Competition. Strategic Reform in Northern European Health Systems*. Buckingham: Open University Press.
5 Saltman RB, von Otter C (1990) Implementing public competition in Swedish county councils: a case study. *International Journal of Health Planning and Management*. **5**: 105–116.
6 Saltman RB, von Otter C (1992) Reforming Swedish healthcare in the 1990s: the emerging role of 'Public Firms'. *Health Policy*. **21**: 143–54.
7 Saltman RB, von Otter C (1989) Public competition versus mixed markets: an analytic comparison. *Health Policy*. **19**: 43–55.
8 Saltman RB, Busse R, Mossialos E (eds) (2002) *Regulating Entrepreneurial Behaviour in European Health Care Systems*. Buckingham: Open University Press.
9 Le Grand J (2001) *The Provision of Healthcare: is the public sector ethically superior to the private sector?* London: London School of Economics Health and Social Care, Discussion Paper Number 1.

10 Jørgensen TB, Bozeman B (2002) Public values lost? Comparing cases on contracting out from Denmark and the United States. *Public Management Review.* 4: 63–81.

11 Williamson OE (1985) *The Economic Institutions of Capitalism. Firms, Markets, Relational Contracting.* New York: The Free Press.

12 Williamson OE (1996) *The Mechanisms of Governance.* Oxford: Oxford University Press.

13 Williamson OE (2000) The New Institutional Economics: taking stock, looking ahead. *The Journal of Economic Literature.* 38: 595–613.

14 Preker AS, Harding A (eds) (2003) *Innovations in Health Service Delivery. The Corporatization of Public Hospitals.* Washington, DC: The World Bank.

15 Mossialos E, Thomson S (2002) Voluntary health insurance in the European Union. Report prepared for the Directorate General for Employment and Social Affairs of the European Commission, 27 February 2002. Available from URL http://europa.eu.int/comm/employment_social/soc-prot/social/vhi.pdf 2002

16 Øvretveit J (2002) *The Changing Public–Private Mix in Nordic Healthcare. An Analysis.* Gothenburg: The Nordic School of Public Health.

17 Nilson M (2003) 120,000 betaler sig förbi vårdkön (120,000 pay to jump the waiting lists). *Aftonbladet.*

18 Methi LN (2003) Flere tegner privat helseforsikring (More carry private health insurance). *Aftonbladet.* 3 July.

19 Olsen IA (2003) Helseforsikrede havner på privat sykehus (Health insured end up in private hospitals). *Aftonbladet.* 7 October.

20 NOMESCO (2001) *Health Statistics in the Nordic Countries.* Copenhagen: The National Board of Health.

21 Can for-profit benefit Swedish healthcare? (English summary of white paper SOU 2002–3). Stockholm, 2002.

22 Landstingförbundet (1992) Framtidens Primärvård. Delrapport om familjeläkare/husläkare (The future of primary healthcare. Report on the family physicians). Stockholm: Landstingsförbundet.

23 European Observatory on Health Care Systems (2000) *Health Care Systems in Transition: Sweden.* Copenhagen: WHO.

24 Aidemark L-G, Lindkvist L, Rydberg L (2003) Mångfald i vården. Att skapa alternative driftsformer (Diversity in healthcare. Creating alternative governance, ownership, and management organizations). Stockholm: Landstingsförbundet (Association of Counties).

25 Landstingförbundet (2002) Privata läkare och sjukgymnaster i öppen vård med ersättning enligt nationell taxa 2001 (Private practising physicians and physiotherapists with remuneration according to the national rate scale). Stockholm: Landstingsförbundet.

26 European Observatory on Health Care Systems (2000) *Health Care Systems in Transition: Finland.* Copenhagen: WHO.

27 'Better services for the same money' – interview with Capio's president and CEO. *Health Europe* (published by McKinsey Health Care Practice) 2002; 1: 62–5.

28 Regeringen (2000 and 2002) Sjukhus med vinstsyfte prop 2000/01:36 and prop 2002/03:9 (Government proposal about for-profit hospitals). Stockholm: Riksdagen (Swedish Parliament).

29 Dalen MB (2003) Lekemiddelmarketdet etter apotekerreform. Oslo: HERO, University of Oslo, report: 11.

30 SOU and Commission on For-profit or Not-for-profit in Swedish Health Care (2002) Vinst for vården (Can for-profit benefit Swedish Healthcare). Stockholm: SOU 2002: 31.

31 SOU (2002) Vårda Vården (Take care of healthcare: cooperation, diversity and fairness). SOU 2002: 23.

32 Ministry of Social Affairs and Health (2003) Memorandum of the national project on

safeguarding the future of healthcare services. Helsinki: Working Group Memorandum 2002:3 eng. Ministry of Social Affairs. Available from URL www.vn.fi/stm/english/publicat/publications_fset.htm

33 Amtsrådsforeningen (2003) Undersøgelse af lægers bibeskæftigelse (Survey of doctors' sideline occupation/activities). Copenhagen: Amtsrådsforeningen (Association of Counties).

34 Pedersen KM (2003) Reforming decentralized integrated healthcare systems: theory and the case of the Norwegian reform. Working paper 2002:7, University of Oslo: Health Economics Research Programme.

35 Norges Offentlige Utredninger (1996) Hvem skal eii sykehusene? Oslo: NOU 5.

36 Norges Offentlige Utredninger (1999) Hvor nært skal det være? Tilknytningsformer for offentlige sykehus. Oslo: NOU 15.

37 Aidemark L-G, Lindkvist L (2004) The vision gives wings. A study of two hospitals run as limited companies. *Management Accounting Research*. (In press.)

38 Gerdtham U-G, Rehnberg C, Tambour M (1999) The impact of internal markets on healthcare efficiency: evidence from healthcare reforms in Sweden. *Applied Economics*. **31**: 935–45.

39 Gerdtham U-G, Löthgren M, Tambour M, Rehnberg C (1999) Internal markets and healthcare efficiency: a multiple-output stochastic frontier analysis. *Health Economics*. **8**: 151–64.

40 Tambour M (1997) The impact of health care policy initiatives on productivity. *Health Economics*. **6**: 57–70.

41 Biørn E, Hagen T, Iversen T, Magnussen J (2002) The effect of activity-based financing on hospital efficiency: a panel data analysis of DEA efficiency scores 1992–2000. Oslo: HERO, University of Oslo, Working Paper 8.

42 Mikkola H, Keskimaki I, Hakkinen U (2002) DRG-related prices applied in a public healthcare system – can Finland learn from Norway and Sweden. *Health Policy*. **59**: 37–51.

43 Hanning M, Spångberg UW (2000) Maximum waiting time – a threat to clinical freedom? Implementation of a policy to reduce waiting times. *Health Policy*. **52**: 15–32.

44 Hanning M, Lundstrom M (1998) Assessment of the maximum waiting time guarantee for cataract surgery. The case of a Swedish policy. *International Journal of Technology Assessment in Health Care*. **14**: 180–93.

45 Hanning M, Spangberg UW (2000) Maximum waiting time – a threat to clinical freedom? Implementation of a policy to reduce waiting times. *Health Policy*. **52**: 15–32.

46 Iversen T (1997) The effect of the private sector on the waiting time in national health service. *Journal of Health Economics*. **16(4)**: 381–96.

47 Kristoffersen M, Piene H (1997) Criteria for waiting list guarantee. An attempt at precision (in Norwegian). *Tidsskr Nor Laegeforenin*. **117**: 358–61.

48 Lian OS, Kristiansen IS (1998) Waiting list guarantee between medicine and bureaucracy (in Norwegian). *Tidsskr Nor Laegeforenin*. **118**: 3921–6.

49 Piene H, Hauge HK, Nye KG (1997) Waiting lists guarantee in healthcare. Some theoretical reflections. *Tidsskr Nor Laegeforenin*. **117**: 370–4.

50 Piene H, Loeb M, Hem KG (2000) Hospital capacity and waiting time for treatment – is there a connection (in Norwegian). *Tidsskr Nor Laegeforenin*. **120**: 2988–92.

51 Botten G, Grepperud S, Nerland SM (2003) Pasientbehandling innenlands eller utenlands? An analyse ave ressoursbruk i Pasientbroen (Domestic or foreign treatment? An analysis of resource usage in running the 'patient bridge'). Oslo: HERO, University of Oslo, report 2003:2.

52 Rice T (1997) Can markets give us the health system we want. *Journal of Health Politics, Policy and Law*. **22**: 383–426.

53 Rice T (1998) *The Economics of Health Reconsidered*. Chicago: Health Administration Press.

54 Fare R, Grosskopf S, Lindgren B, Poullier JP (1997) Productivity growth in health-care delivery. *Medical Care.* **1935:** 354–66.

55 Brüström B (2002) Increasing inequalities in healthcare utilisation across income groups in Sweden during the 1990s? *Health Policy.* **62:** 117–29.

56 Gissler M, Keskimäki I, Teperi J, Järvelin M-R, Hemminki E (2000) Regional equity in childhood health – register-based follow-up of the Finnish 1987 birth cohort. *Health and Place.* **6:** 329–36.

57 Keskimäki I, Salinto M, Aro S (1996) Private medicine and socioeconomic difference in the rates of common surgical procedures in Finland. *Health Policy.* **36:** 245–59.

58 Keskimäki I (2003) How did Finland's economic recession in the early 1990s affect socioeconomic equity in the use of hospital care? *Social Science and Medicine.* **56:** 1517–30.

59 Gerdtham U-G, Trivedi PK (2001) Equity in Swedish healthcare reconsidered: new results based on the finite mixture model. *Health Economics.* **10:** 565–72.

60 Grytten J, Rongen G, Sørensen R (1995) Can a public healthcare system achieve equity? The Norwegian experience. *Medical Care.* **33:** 938–51.

61 Lindholm L, Rosén M (1998) On the measurement of the nation's's equity adjusted health. *Health Economics.* **7:** 621–8.

62 Mossialos E (2003) Citizens' views on healthcare systems in the 15 member states of the European Union. *Health Economics.* **6:** 109–16.

Endnotes

i   Much English language literature has been written about the changes in Sweden, but to a considerable extent based on examples drawn from one or two counties, e.g. Stockholm County, or a few, rather isolated changes, for instance the St Göran Hospital in Stockholm.[2–7] Often changes are to be found more in principles of management and allocation than in changes in financing (hardly any changes) or ownership (very few changes). Some of these changes may appear 'revolutionary' to some participants set in their established ways of approaching production of health-care, but looked at in a larger perspective they are natural and must be expected in view of the development that will take place over a period of 10–20 years in response to changed economic conditions, e.g. the meltdown of the Finnish economy after the collapse of the Soviet Union, and new challenges, e.g. waiting lists, free choice, and patients' rights.

ii *See* Le Grand[9] for a clear-headed discussion of, on the one hand, the public ethos, the presumed altruism associated with the public institutions etc., and, on the other hand, the selfishness and greed of privately owned companies. In Jørgensen and Bozeman[10] there is a fairly comprehensive statement of 'public values' – values that according to the political debate may be threatened by increased entrepreneurialism. They list the following: political accountability, 'rechtsstaat' (rule of law, legality, impartiality, etc.), equal treatment, regime stability, balancing of interests, transparency, professional standards, personnel altruism and engagement, employee safety, social cohesion, local self-governance, involvement of citizens, user orientation. It is debatable whether they are all 'values' in the basic sense of the word. There is no doubt regarding accountability and rechtsstaat, while others more probably are established practices, norms or ideals, for instance altruism or employment security. Where does one find it, and how is it distinguished from individual or collective selfishness? Is employment security not an example of private and collective selfishness? Vis-à-vis new manage-ment forms, e.g. contracting out, the question is whether these values are threatened. However, a necessary prior discussion should focus on two issues: are these values widely accepted, e.g. why should a publicly employed nurse have greater employment security compared to her private-sector counterpart and is it really a value, and is there any reason to believe that they are threatened if, for instance, services are contracted out? Most of them can be handled within a contract setting – not necessarily a complete contract but incomplete contracts with ex-post negotiation based on trust, i.e. the spirit of the contract thinking of Williamson.[11,12,13]

iii The Danish percentage of 17.5% in reality is higher – and has been increasing. The explanation is that the Danish definition of healthcare expenditure was changed around 1998 to include part of nursing home expenditures and home help, areas where co-payment is non-existent.

iv See Mossialos[15] for a clarification of terminology and a good overview for the EU. However, Norway, not being a member of the EU, is not included.

v However, children up to the age of 16 are automatically covered if their parents are members. Hence, the percentage in reality is higher. The principles behind membership and premium payment in 'denmark' resemble some of the thinking behind sickness funds, i.e. considerable solidarity. Joining 'denmark' presupposes absence of chronic diseases and being below 60 years of age, i.e. standard health and age requirements. However, having joined, members can stay on for an unchanged premium even if they get a chronic disease, and they retain membership as long as they pay their premiums, i.e. no 'dumping' of older members or when reaching pension age like in most of the commercial insurances. Members decide on which one of three groups they want to join. The premium in each group is the same for everybody. The groups differ only according to services reimbursed. The annual premium of the two most expensive groups is around 2500 Dkr (about £250). Having joined one of the groups, members are free to change group at any time.

vi In a sense contradicting normal insurance thinking: not large, unexpected expenditures, but predictable and rather small amounts.

vii For easy conversion: £1 = 10 Dkr.

viii Interestingly enough, the government did not reintroduce the tax deduction of premiums for privately paid health insurance. This existed prior to 1987 and thus was a tax subsidy for members of 'denmark'.

ix Reliable numbers are hard to obtain because the commercial insurers hesitate to publish, in part for business reasons, in part to be able to let out hot air about the market.[16,17]

x It is a proposal put forward early in 2003 in Denmark by the Advisory Committee to the minister of health.[1]

xi The exception is the St Göran hospital in Stockholm, owned by Swedish Capio. It is by far the largest privately owned and operated hospital in Scandinavia. From 1994 to 1999 this hospital was a public corporation with the county of Stockholm holding all the shares. In 1999 the shares were sold to Capio, and a seven-year contract with guaranteed number of patients, etc., paid for by the county of Stockholm was written. However, whenever private ownership is introduced complicated deals are made. In reality the Stockholm county retained ownership of the hospital building and collected rent through the county owned property management firm Locum AB (www.locum.se). Apparently then, Capio (at the time called Bure) only bought goodwill and possibly some equipment. The purchase price was net 225 million Skr. The annual value of the contract initially was around £70 million (www.sll.se) – St Göran has a substantial annual turnover, about £100 million in 2002, and made a profit of £2 million. In addition it should be noted that the X-ray and lab functions have been spun off as independent companies. In order to compare turnover with a public hospital the turnover from these two units should be added. It is claimed – but not shown in a scientific manner – that productivity at St Göran is substantially higher than at public hospitals.

xii In reality the first healthcare company operating throughout Europe with locations in eight countries, including England and all the Scandinavian countries. For background and perspectives see reference 28. See also www.capio.com. Capio was spun off from the Swedish equity fund Bure in 2000. Bure to a certain extent is based on now closed wage-earners funds, and about 16% of the shares are owned by the state-run supplementary pension fund ATP. However, Capio is owned wholly by private shareholders.

xiii See, however, Saltman and von Otter[4–7] for an early analysis of the trends and a proposal for public competition in planned markets.

xiv Many physicians working full time in public hospitals have considerable spare time due to working rules. It is estimated[34] that more than 13% of senior doctors have sideline activities, in particular surgeons working for private for-profit hospitals or running their own private clinics. This percentage, however, has been stable over the past five years.

xv It is quite clear that the autonomy for these units is greater than for the English trust hospitals or the upcoming Foundation trust hospitals.

xvi In the Scandinavian tradition preceded by government reports[36,37] setting the scene for possible changes. The reform, however, was far more radical than suggested in the latest of the reports.

xvii However, in a report published by the Swedish Association of Counties[25] the experience from two cases of corporatisation is recounted. In both cases waiting time was reduced dramatically, volume increased considerably, and in one case an economic turnaround took place. There was no report on changes in productivity. From the available source it is not possible to decide whether the budget ceiling that exists for traditional public hospitals was removed or eased. If it was the case, changes in waiting time and volume may simply be due to this – employee satisfaction was good – and one of the hospitals became corporatised on the urging of the employees.

xviii Researchers, however, argue for the advantages, but the most recent Finnish government report does not touch on the issue.[42,43,33]

xix There seems to be a tendency to associate such a reimbursement scheme with the market, as witnessed in several paragraphs in a 1994 Danish white paper. It is hard to understand why – in particular because per diem reimbursement is still in use in some areas and was widespread in the 1960s, and because funding is tax financed and tightly politically controlled. It more probably mirrors how tied down most people are by what has been an established norm for 10–20 years, and where almost any change is termed 'market'.

xx On both the consumer and producer side – relying on the results from welfare economics/general equilibrium theory, i.e. the marginal conditions for consumption and production are usually identified with (pareto optimal) efficiency. See, among others, Rice for a rather polemical approach.[52,53] This issue is, however, too general to be pursued here.

xxi The rule in Scandinavia is minority governments. Hence the incumbent government must rely on either 'support parties', i.e. parties that recommended the formation of a particular government or go for compromises that can generate a majority, ideally almost consensus. Major changes in policy usually rely on a large majority because it is realised that sustainable solutions require stability.

Chapter 10

Public–private mix for healthcare in Germany

Martin Pfaff and Axel Olaf Kern

Introduction

The German healthcare system, in its organisation, financing and service provision, is based on the 'Bismarck Model' of social or public insurance. Sizeable private elements exist within the system, in the form of co-payments required for utilisation of the benefits or services granted by the Social Health Insurance (SHI) services; private health insurance coverage for the more affluent, purchased either in lieu of social health insurance or as a supplement; private purchase of health goods and services and private provision of health services through office-based physicians and pharmacists; and privately owned hospitals.

The public–private mix for healthcare in Germany is dominated by the SHI, but the role of the private sector in finance and provision are considerable.

Objectives and principles of the German Social Health Insurance (SHI) system

The German social insurance system in general, and the social health insurance system in particular, were set up by Chancellor Bismarck in 1883 to meet the demands of the labour movement. By providing social protection to the industrial workforce against the multiple perils of ill health, accidents, old age and unemployment, the 'Iron Chancellor' hoped to neutralise the political impact of labour unrest.

Subsequently, the 'Bismarck Model' has become deeply entrenched in German society, not so much as an institution geared to the needs of the poor but as a generalised 'institution of the middle class', and has been replicated in a large number of countries worldwide.

The basic principles of this system are simple:

- utilisation of health services dependent solely on the basis of need
- financing in the form of individual wage-related contributions to particular health insurance funds; those with higher incomes pay a higher absolute amount for the same insurance coverage. Dependent family members do not pay any contributions. There is no risk-related supplement.

The financing system *appears* highly egalitarian, but is not so in practice. The introduction of income-related upper limits to compulsory membership ('Versicherungspflichtgrenze') allows upper-income individuals to opt out of the social health insurance system altogether. Application of a similar upper limit to the amount of contribution ('Beitragsbemessungsgrenze') limits the extent of upper-income individuals' solidarity. The incidence of the contributions paid by those better-off individuals who are still within the limit, and those who opt for voluntary membership, is essentially regressive in nature. They pay a lower share of their earnings than lower-income individuals. Non-wage income which, as a rule, is more likely to be accrued by wealthier or higher-income individuals, is not included in the financing base.

Even on the utilisation side, a range of cultural, social and (indirectly) economic factors contribute to patterns which favour the more affluent. Social stratification still exists in healthcare use in Germany, although it may not be evident at first sight.

Clinical success was rarely measured in the past, but more recent laws require all sectors of healthcare provision to implement quality control. Individual health insurance funds are made responsible for supporting their members' claims in case of medical errors. The quality of health services is now a policy issue, and consumer rights relating to health services have been strengthened.

Physician autonomy remains largely unchallenged and available evidence shows considerable variations in medical practice and outcomes. There are now calls for clinical practice guidelines and for hospitals to be benchmarked.

Finally, the pharmaceutical industry is affected in the main by government's attempts to control costs and regulate prices, although in most other aspects, it remains largely unchallenged because of its effect on employment. The health versus wealth trade-off favours industry rather than patients in Germany.

Nonetheless, there is public agreement that the German system, on the whole, performs adequately. There are almost no queues in the doctor's office or waiting lists in hospitals.[1] The technical and physical infrastructure is of a very high standard and satisfaction with the healthcare system is generally high, even though lately dissatisfaction has been mounting as a result of large deficits of SHI funds and rising contribution rates.

The financing and utilisation sides taken together (budget incidence), show a pattern of redistribution which conforms to overall social policy aims.[2] A system of transfers results, which many consider to be the very heart of solidarity or even the socially oriented state: between the healthy and the sick, and thereby generally; between the young and the old; between men and women; between the childless and those with children; between the working and the non-working population; between the more affluent members who are within the system and the worse off.

Political debates generally rage about the magnitude of these transfers. 'Conservatives' and 'Liberals' wish to reduce them, 'Progressives' wish to stabilise them or even to enhance them. Relatively few wish to abolish the compulsory SHI system in favour of an 'obligation to be insured'. Usually, such advocates of 'market-radical' reforms come from the better-off segments of society, in particular from those individuals who finance egalitarian transfers.

A large number of health insurance funds have been set up over time, at the local level, for particular groups of employees and workers, for craftsmen, for particular firms, for miners, for farmers and for seamen/sailors. These largely self-administered funds provide an attractive role model to countries with differential rates of economic development. They may be more adaptable to the peculiarities of the current situation than a fully integrated national scheme. Furthermore, countries that distrust centralised governments and fully privatised alternatives may prefer a social health insurance system. This is evident in the choice of healthcare system expressed by many post-Soviet Union states.

Most Germans cling to the concept of multiple health insurance funds rather than the concept of a unified insurance system ('Einheitsversicherung'), perhaps influenced by the experience of the notoriously underfunded healthcare system of the now defunct German Democratic Republic (GDR). Neither is any German likely to voice serious objection to the highly unified system of old-age insurance also introduced by Bismarck. Societal styles and political preferences are often the product of historic developments and traditions rather than of rational analysis.

Main transactions within the German healthcare system

The German healthcare system is complex, with the public and private systems overlapping.

Figure 10.1 illustrates the main transactions between the insured, the patient, the sickness fund, the hospital and providers, and the government. These transactions consist of financial and real flows of various types. It shows that the SHI system itself is a 'mixed system', financed with contributions from employees and employers, co-payments of the insured in case of illness, and with general taxation.

Contributions account for about 56% of financial resources and are channelled by the sickness funds directly to the associations of accredited providers.

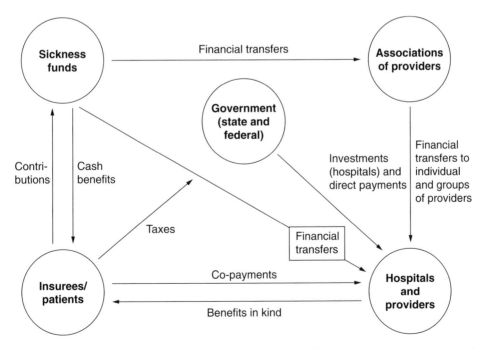

Figure 10.1 Main transactions within the German healthcare system. *Source*: Original presentation based on Pfaff and Nagel (1994).[13]

Physicians, dentists and pharmacists are remunerated indirectly via their intermediary associations. The latter allocate shares of the financial flows to the individual providers in line with the latter's' claims for benefits in kind provided.

There is a 'dual financing mechanism' in place for hospitals. The state governments finance, from their revenues, both the purely public health institutions who are responsible for health promotion and disease control, and the fixed costs of hospitals, primarily for investment in buildings and expensive medical equipment (e.g. computer tomograph, lithotriptor, cyclotron). Health insurance funds finance the variable costs of running the hospitals.

Hospitals have to be recognised within the official hospital plan, which is the responsibility of state governments; only with inclusion in the plan can the hospital be allocated public resources. The variable hospital costs, being related to services provided to the insured in case of illness, are paid by sickness funds (currently on a mostly per diem basis, but soon on the basis of diagnosis related groups, DRGs), from contributions paid by their members. In addition, the state government supervises regional and local sickness funds.

Health benefits, goods and services are provided in the form of real and also cash benefits. Except for co-payments, there is no direct financial relationship between service providers and patients in SHI. The latter, and also the remuneration of hospitals, are negotiated and contracted for between sickness funds and each of the 2200 hospitals declared by the state as essential to inpatient services in Germany. Similar contracts are formulated for ambulatory care with the 16 Associations of Accredited Physicians (Kassenärztliche Vereinigungen) and the 16 Associations of Accredited Dentists (Kassenzahnärztliche Vereinigungen), respectively.

Public elements

Organisation of the SHI

Given the traditions of the German social market economy ('Soziale Marktwirtschaft'), the organisation and financing of healthcare is to a large extent transferred from the government to the self-administering organisations of the sickness funds and of provider associations.

Sickness funds are separate from service providers. This split established the principle of negotiation between purchaser and provider. The Federal Government sets the framework for about 90% of the population and also the overall budget constraints within which the parties operate. Physicians, hospitals, dentists, state governments responsible for investments in hospitals, the pharmaceutical industry, pharmacists, professional bodies, hospital associations, statutory health insurance funds and the like are involved, through negotiations and contracts, in the provision of healthcare services for the population with the federal budget constraint.

According to the Social Code, the provision of health benefits has to heed the principles of economy, so may not exceed what is considered to be 'necessary treatment'. The terms of economy and necessity, however, are not specified explicitly, leaving room for considerable discretion.

Negotiations to establish the budget for ambulatory and hospital care as well as for all other services take place annually, but vary from fund to fund or by groups of funds. A ceiling is negotiated for pharmaceuticals prescribed by office-based physicians. Within this framework, the organisations or associations of service providers and of sickness funds play a significant role. The government seeks to achieve a balance of power among the competing actors, but when in doubt, it has often sided with the sickness funds, which are considered less well organised and hence the weaker party.

In practice, health policy making is a politically hazardous enterprise, particularly for ministers of health or those in other responsible positions. A former Minister for Health Policy compared the network of competing interests and organisations to a 'pool full of sharks'.

Association of Accredited Service Providers

Physicians and dentists accredited to provide ambulatory and dental care within SHI become affiliates, receiving remuneration from their own association. Their associations submit the claims of individual physicians to the sickness funds for reimbursement.

Since 1989, the number of physicians in private practices has been restricted to the number of practices which existed in 1987 and relative to the population. Consequently, not every physician who is registered as a medical doctor has the right to take part in healthcare provision for SHI. But every physician remains free to open a practice treating people on a private basis.

Individual physicians receive remuneration through the respective Association of Accredited Physicians. There are general contracts at federal and state levels for the delivery and monitoring of medical services, regulating provision of medical devices, principles of reimbursement, fees for services, processing of claims, and monitoring of effective and efficient provision of services. This general framework and individual regulations within it are formulated without the direct involvement of the government. General guidelines are set by the Association of Sickness Funds and the Association of Accredited Physicians at federal and state levels.

The Associations of Physicians distribute among their members the total payments that have been negotiated individually and paid for by the SHI funds. This is done according to the importance of specialised physicians and family physicians and their subgroups, e.g. radiologists, ophthalmologists, orthopaedists (Remuneration Distribution Scale – Honorarverteilungsmaßstab) and then according to the Uniform Value Scale (UVC). Every medical procedure and service is listed explicitly in the UVC and assigned a certain value, expressed in points. At the end of each quarter, the office-based physicians provide an invoice of the total amount of points rendered for the services provided by their Association. Due to the negotiated fixed budget and the differing volume of points submitted, the euro-value of each point is variable and dependent on activity levels.

Sickness funds

Membership of sickness funds is compulsory for all employees whose gross income per year does not exceed a set level. The level moves according to the growth of wages, and in the year 2003 amounted to €46 350 per year (and to €3863 per month for persons paid on a 12-month basis). Unemployed and retired persons and certain others, like farmers, artists and students, are included in SHI as mandatory members. The self-employed and employees with an income above the threshold may be voluntary members if they have been a member previously or if they opt for SHI at the beginning of their freelance career. Currently about 90% of the population is covered by SHI, i.e. 51 million members plus 21 million dependents. Of these, 75% are mandatory members, and 14% are voluntary members, including dependants. Ten per cent of the German population is fully covered by private health insurance contracts or by free healthcare (police and soldiers). Public assistance ('Sozialhilfe') covers expenses for health services for people without any income or means.

The law requires that all dependent working persons, and to a certain extent the self-employed, such as artists and farmers, have to obtain statutory health insurance based on a contributory income (this being the part of an employee's income which is assessed for the purpose of calculating his contribution liability to social health insurance and so to 'his' sickness fund).

As a result of mergers, the number of sickness funds decreased from about 11 000 around the year 1900, to 1815 funds in 1970, to 1209 funds in 1991 and to 554 funds in 1997. By 2002, there were about 355 different sickness funds operating at regional or federal levels in Germany. Since 1996, all persons in the statutory health insurance system are free to choose their sickness fund and to change from one to another once a year. As all relevant parameters for competitive comparison (e.g. premium calculation and provided services) are regulated, the number of people changing funds is limited.

Insurance contributions are calculated from the employee's gross wage per month and the rates of contribution are set by each of the sickness funds individually. The calculation of rates is determined by the monthly gross income of the working insured and the total expenses for medical goods and services (including expenses for spouses and children who are insured without having to pay an additional insurance premium).

The law determines 95% of the services for which sickness funds have to pay and supply in cooperation with service providers. Details of service provision and reimbursement are negotiated within the framework of the self-government of SHI. In consideration of the reimbursement for ambulatory care, the Associations of Physicians are responsible for providing necessary medical diagnosis and treatment to the public at a level considered to be sufficient and economical. About 5% of total expenses for services is determined by the funds themselves, so they contract with physicians for certain special services, e.g. acupuncture.

Financing of the healthcare system

The SHI provides both cash and kind benefits, with the healthcare system funded from public (SHI) and private sources (private insurance and co-payments).

Figure 10.2 also shows the distribution of funds covered by SHI, other social insurance institutions, employers, private households and private non-profit organisations in the year 2000. SHI has the dominant role, but a large number of other institutions and actors are involved in healthcare in Germany.

Every citizen not compulsorily insured in SHI is free to contract for private health insurance with one of the 52 private health insurance companies that are

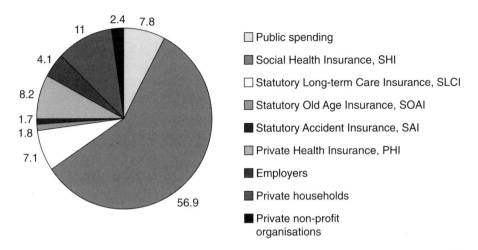

Figure 10.2 Health spending in 2000 by type of institution or source, as a percentage of the total (€218.4 billion). *Source*: Federal Bureau of Statistics (2002).[15]

for-profit companies as well as private mutual health insurance funds. Given the current limit of contributory income of €3863 per month for dependent workers, it is primarily the more affluent who hold a private insurance contract. For a premium which is risk rated according to sex, age and health status, the insured chooses a preferred package of services, including different co-insurance plans. Additionally, members of the SHI funds are free to contract with private health insurance funds for benefits not provided for by their SHI fund (e.g. for single rooms in hospitals).

Health spending and types of benefits granted

Until recently, the health expenditure's share of the GDP and also health spending per capita remained below the level expected, simply on the grounds of Germany's relative overall economic performance.[3] But in the course of German reunification, health spending in Eastern Germany increased much faster than economic growth, with a consequent rise in health spending as a proportion of the GDP (Table 10.1). Overall health expenditure (for benefits in cash and in kind) rose from €160.3 billion in 1992 to €218.4 billion in 2000.

SHI alone, however, has been remarkably stable. For example, between 1975 and 2000, SHI health expenditure remained within 6 to 7% of the GDP,[4] which many observers saw as the result of mechanisms introduced to contain costs in order to meet the requirements of 'payroll tax stability' (control of labour costs). These mechanisms ranged from budgeting to price controls and also included increases in co-payment and some reductions in the types of benefit financed by SHI funds. Although the main aim of attaining a stable payroll tax rate was not achieved for any length of time, these measures nonetheless served to curb expenditure growth to some extent.

Relative shares of particular categories of services may be seen from Figure 10.3 for the year 2000. Hospital care (28.8%) and ambulatory medical care (13.4%)

Table 10.1 Development of total health spending until 1995 in billion DM, since then in billion euro

Year	1970	1975	1980	1985	1990	1995	1996	1997	1998	1999	2000
GDP (billion DM/euro)	672.3	1023.9	1476.1	1817.1	2434.4	3522.2	1833.7	1874.7	1934.9	1982.4	2032.9
Health spending (billion DM/euro)	42.3	90.1	129.9	168.9	211.8	359.2	203.0	203.9	208.4	214.3	218.4
Health spending as a % of GDP	6.3	8.8	8.8	9.3	8.7	10.8	11.1	10.9	10.8	10.8	10.7

Source: OECD Health Data 2001, Federal Bureau of Statistics 2002.[7]

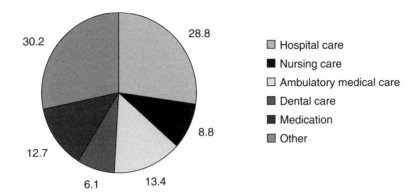

Figure 10.3 Healthcare expenditure by category of services/goods, percentage of total expenditures, 2000. *Source*: Own presentation based on data from the Federal Bureau of Statistics (2002).[15]

account for the majority of expenditure, followed by medication with 12.7%. Labour costs are almost three-quarters of hospital expenditure.

Ambulatory care, dental care, hospital care and pharmaceuticals are described in Appendix 1.

Private sector

In theory, if not in practice, the private sector is based on the model of market exchange. Co-payments are supposed to provide incentives to users to eliminate excess demand. Private insurance payments (premiums) are risk related. In reality, however, there are significant deviations from these idealised market characteristics.

Co-payments

The law for the Modernisation of the Social Health Insurance System, passed in 2003, provides several changes in payment rules. Those on low incomes, the chronically ill and children are exempt from co-payments. Benefits that are considered to be atypical of health insurance are excluded from the SHI package, e.g. death benefits or sterilisation. Maternal benefits, contraceptives for women under 18 years of age, legitimate abortions and sickness benefits in case of the illness of a child are financed with taxes levied on the consumption of tobacco products.

Figure 10.4 compares the co-payments before the Act with those likely to result once the Act is implemented in 2004, with and without exemptions (limiting co-payments to 2% of gross annual income for all, and to 1% of gross annual income for the chronically ill) and differentiating between non-pensioners and pensioners. It is apparent that the Act will lead to a sizeable increase in co-payments.

Generally, for each benefit used there is a 10% co-payment, minimum €5 and maximum €10, except for medical devices and home care services where the duration of co-payments is restricted to 28 days during one year (*see* Appendix 2).

In Table 10.2, the total sum of co-payments for goods and services under SHI is

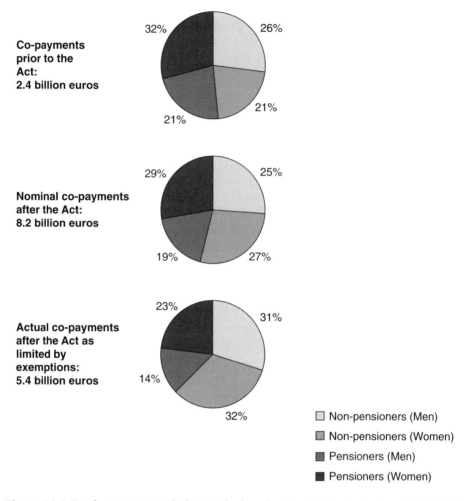

Co-payments prior to the Act: 2.4 billion euros

Nominal co-payments after the Act: 8.2 billion euros

Actual co-payments after the Act as limited by exemptions: 5.4 billion euros

- ☐ Non-pensioners (Men)
- ▨ Non-pensioners (Women)
- ▨ Pensioners (Men)
- ■ Pensioners (Women)

Figure 10.4 Total co-payments before and after the Health Modernisation Act 2003/4, with and without exemptions and their distribution by sex and status (non-pensioner, pensioner). *Source*: Pfaff *et al.* (2003).[16]

Table 10.2 Co-payments per type of benefit, 1992–2001 (selected years), in billion euro

Benefit	1992	1995	1998	2000	2001
Dentures	2.4	2.5	2.2	2.2	2.3
Pharmaceuticals	0.6	1.5	2.8	1.9	1.9
Hospital care	0.4	0.4	0.6	0.6	0.6
Transportation	0.1	0.1	0.1	0.1	0.1
Rehabilitation	0.0	0.1	0.1	0.1	0.1
Total	3.6	5.1	6.5	5.3	5.7

Source: Federal Bureau of Statistics (2003).[17]

shown in billion euros for selected years between 1992 and 2001. With the exception of 1998, the highest totals accrue from dentures, followed by pharmaceuticals and hospital care.

Private health insurance (PHI)

Ideally, in private health insurance the premium should reflect the price of the risks covered. Some major elements present in the German system of private insurance do approximate this ideal. Separate premiums are charged for each insured person (i.e. also for non-working dependents) and there are surcharges in cases of special health risks.

On the other hand, premiums are calculated for a whole cohort of the insured. Insurance rates for the young are often considered to be artificially low to encourage the eligible young people to opt for private rather than public insurance. Furthermore, if premiums for the young are too low, not enough reserves are being built up to subsidise the person's premiums in old age. As a result, there have been dramatic increases in premiums for the elderly, leading to a legal intervention. Finally, the reserves built up in earlier years are not earmarked specifically for each individual but for a cohort of similar individuals. Beyond a certain age, change-overs from one private health insurance fund to another are virtually unknown, as individuals are not allowed to carry their share of the reserves to the new private health insurance fund. Should a person choose to change funds in any event, they have to pay very high insurance rates, thereby reducing incentives for change among competing private health insurance funds. Consequently, there is more competition present between social health insurance funds in Germany than between private health insurance funds. Table 10.3 illustrates the growth in the number of insured persons with full and partial (supplementary) coverage for the period 1991 to 2002, and Table 10.4 shows the number of persons changing between full coverage and SHI for the same period.

With the passing of the law introducing long-term care as a separate branch of the SHI system, private health insurers are obliged to provide also for nursing home care for the elderly. For children as well as for non-working dependants, separate contributions have to be paid towards their long-term care. The latter poses the question of horizontal equity of persons with children and those without, so the Federal Constitutional Court has ruled that households with children should be treated more favourably regarding their contributions while their children are in education.

Private purchases of health goods and services

There are oligopolistic or even monopolistic elements in the markets for health goods. European unification is likely to enhance competition in these markets. The Treaty of Maastricht (1992) and the Treaty of Amsterdam (1999) contributed to making health for the European Union a Community responsibility and hence an element relevant to the European integration process. But there was no reduction in the member states' responsibilities for organising their own health systems and the supply of healthcare. The decisions of the European Supreme Court affect national healthcare systems in so far as ambulatory services and

Table 10.3 Private health insurance: number of fully insured persons and number of persons with supplementary insurance, 1991–2002

Year	Number of fully insured persons (in millions)	Number of persons with supplementary insurance 1991–2000 (in millions)*	Total number of persons (in millions)
1991	6.333""	5.3	11.7
1992	6.686	5.6	12.3
1993	6.829	5.7	12.6
1994	6.934	5.9	12.9
1995	6.945	6.0	13.0
1996	6.977***	6.0	13.0
1997	7.065	7.0	14.1
1998	7.205	7.6	14.8
1999	7.356	7.5	14.9
2000	7.494	7.5	15.0
2001	7.710	7.6	15.3
2002	7.924	7.7	15.6

* Microcensus data or extrapolation thereof.
** Elimination of duplicate counting; net increase in 1991: 262 000 persons.
*** Change in counting methods; 6 945 800 according to old method.
Source: Association of Private Health Insurance Funds, 2002/2003, p. 12.[8]

Table 10.4 Persons switching between private comprehensive medical insurance and social health insurance, 1991–2002

Year	Switches to the private health insurance	Losses to compulsory insurance	Difference
1991	356 000	125 000	+231 000
1992	483 000	154 000	+329 000
1993	307 000	175 000	+132 000
1994	195 000	103 000	+ 92 000
1995	271 000	186 000	+ 85 000
1996	247 000	181 000	+ 66 000
1997	315 000	144 400	+171 300
1998	327 800	154 800	+173 000
1999	324 800	149 200	+175 600
2000	325 000	148 600	+176 400
2001	360 700	147 500	+213 000
2002	362 000	129 800	+232 200

Source: Association of Private Health Insurance Funds, 2002/2003, p. 14.[8]

goods can be used by patients in every member state without prior permission of the health insurer. Incurred costs are refunded to the patient according to reimbursement rules of national SHI.

Healthcare reforms

Since the mid-1970s, healthcare reforms have been mainly motivated by the goal of cost containment. The first Health Insurance Cost Containment Act took effect in 1976, followed in succession by several other similar pieces of legislation (e.g. the Hospital Cost Containment Act of 1981). They all were designed with the primary goal of controlling prices and volumes, or, as was already the case with the 1976 law, shifting costs from the budgets of the health insurance funds to those of the insured, more specifically of the sick, in the form of exclusion of certain benefits or of cost sharing. These early laws already tried to bring about structural changes in the healthcare system. As exemplified in the Health Reform Act of 1989, some of the earlier legislation sought structural reform based on recommendations which were to be developed with the participation of the major actors, i.e. by wider consensus.

These reforms included an effort to control spending within limits laid down by revenues received; the use of prospective budgets to contain spending; measures aimed at enhancing the transparency of benefits provided by the healthcare system (better use of information and more standardisation), although these measures were rarely evidence-based or effective; the use of co-payments, with the stated aim of influencing the utilisation of services; and rules affecting the contracts to be entered into by health insurance funds and providers, largely with the aim of improving efficiency. On balance, the success of these measures of cost containment and more far-reaching reform was limited, at least in comparison with the original policy aims of controlling contribution rates to the SHI system.

This failure was due to measures of conflict resolution often being inadequate in reconciling the claims of different interest groups, concerning the respective shares of the 'economic pie'. Often the political will was absent when decisions, once made, were to be implemented in the face of strong opposition by affected groups. Also, there was a lack of explicitly stated policy goals or of specific indicators which were to be applied for judging the effectiveness of policies.

Ultimately, the affected interest groups opposed the implementation of measures and this was responsible for the limited success of the reforms. Decisions were made collectively within the Concerted Action in the Health Field (representing all major societal actors related to healthcare). But in the end, such 'decisions' were treated as 'recommendations', as no immediate sanctions could, or would, be applied to those interest groups which did not conform to the guidelines.

Experience was similar in the processes leading to the formulation and enactment of the Health Reform Act of 1989. The opposition of affected groups, including that of powerful states (as with the process affecting hospital cost-containment provisions), led to a 'softening' of measures aimed at structural reform.

Furthermore, responsibility was placed on the health insurance funds on the one hand, and on providers' associations, on the other, for implementing the structural reforms required to assure stability of contribution rates. It was hoped that 'self-management' on the part of these actors would influence volumes and prices of health services by providing information aimed at increasing the transparency of this process and introducing new procedures for testing and controlling its efficiency. Clearly, the capacity for resolving conflicts among and between 'self-managing' representatives of health insurance funds and providers was significantly overestimated. A consensual implementation of collectively agreed measures proved impossible to achieve. At the same time, measures aimed solely at particular healthcare sectors were inadequate for the task of influencing the global indicators of health spending and related contribution rates.

With the failure of measures aimed at the 'supply side', the only instruments left for stabilising costs were those directed at the 'utilisation or demand side'. In particular, exclusion of benefits formerly paid for by health insurance funds, increased co-payments, payment of a 'bonus' by the health insurance funds to individual members for non-utilisation of services (e.g. when using preventive measures of dentists) and reimbursement in part of contributions paid where benefits were not used, or only up to a certain limit.

Other interventions were no more successful in changing organisational structure or limiting resource use effectively, so structural reforms were not enacted and the aim of cost containment was not achieved, largely because the instruments aimed at influencing providers' behaviour proved too weak.

In the face of vested interest groups' concern to expand their share of the economic pie, it is clear that use of an information policy alone (taking the form of economic or financial indicators of resource use) was insufficient to curb expenditure growth and to stabilise contribution rates since 1976.

Similarly, processes of 'self-management' of health insurance funds and providers' representations were inadequate in the face of conflicts over distributional shares. In this regard, the Health Reform Act of 1989 proved as ineffective as the earlier cost containment acts. This institutional structure remained almost unchanged until the Health Care Structure Act ('Gesundheitstruktur Gesetz', GSG) of 1993. (*See* Table 10.5 for the main acts and regulations since 1977.)

Since 1977, purchasers and providers of healthcare have been required to pursue the goal of stability of SHI contributions. The Fifth Book of Social Law (§71 SGB V) prohibits the level of contributions from rising faster than the rate of increase in income of all employees covered under social health insurance. To achieve this aim, or at least to pursue cost containment, a variety of policies were adopted: budgets for sectors and individual providers; restriction of expensive medical equipment; restriction of the number of single practices of physicians and dentists; co-payments for pharmaceuticals (depending on size of package), stay in hospital per day, medical and technical aids; limited reimbursement for dental services. Budgets were variable in both form and effect. Table 10.6 lists budgeting for healthcare sectors in Germany in the 1990s.

While the German healthcare system is neither a 'state system' nor a 'market system', it combines the use of 'market-style' incentives with indirect (regulations) and direct (financial) government involvement. Debate over the amount of competition required on the one hand, and government involvement on the other hand, is also reflected in the legislative measures of the past two decades.

Specific measures of various health reform acts are shown in Appendix 3 for the period 1993 to 2003.

Table 10.5 Acts and regulations affecting social health insurance, 1977–2002

Specific Act	Year
Health Insurance Cost Containment Act (KVKG)	1977
Retirement Pension Adjustment Act (RAG)	1981
Cost Containment Amendment Act (KVEG)	1981
Hospital Cost Containment Act (KHKG)	1981
Regulation of Medical and Technical Aids (H&HMRl)	1982
Budget Support Act (HBG)	1983
Hospital Financing Act (KHNG)	1984
Hospital Reimbursement Regulation (BPflV)	1986
Improvement for Planning Accreditation of Physicians Act (GVKBP)	1986
Health Care Reform Act (GRG)	1989
Health Care Structure Act (GSG)	1993
First and Second Health Insurance Restructuring Act (1. & 2. GKV-NOG)	1997
Improvement of Solidarity Act (GKV-SolG)	1998
Harmonisation of Health Insurance Act (RAnglG)	1999
Health Care Reform Act 2000 (GKV Reform 2000)	2000
Diagnosis Related Groups Financing in Hospitals Act (DRG-Einführungsgesetz)	2001
Risk-Structure Compensation Amendment Act (RSA-ReformG)	2002
Health System Modernisation Act (GMG)	2004

Source: Schneider (1994) and own presentation.[9]

Table 10.6 Budgeting in social health insurance in the 1990s

Sector	Budget constraints
Total system	No budget but goal of stability of contributions
Ambulatory and dental care	Fixed budget (negotiated in 1992, 1996, 1997, growth rate set by law for 1993–5, 1998–2001).
Hospital	Individual budgets (until 1992 and from 1997–2001, growth rate for budget set by law for 1993–5).
Pharmaceuticals	Spending caps for physicians working under ambulatory budgets and at fixed prices (since 1994 negotiated between sickness funds and associations of physicians in 23 regions).
Other	No budgets

Source: Busse and Howorth (1999), p. 306.[10]

Frequently, new measures were enacted before the previous law could be put into effect. At times, measures agreed upon in consensus across party lines and made law were simply ignored or openly disregarded by the executive branch (as was the case, for example, with the 'positive list' of pharmaceuticals, openly derided and shredded with the full knowledge of the Minister of Health). And changes in government at times led to the cancellation of previous legal measures, only to be reinstated later.

The political economy of cost control has been less than transparent in Germany. The classical dichotomy between 'right-wing solutions' (entailing co-payments and shifting the funding base from contributions to private insurance) and 'left-wing solutions' – mainly via budgeting of health spending – has not always applied to political parties. Parliament has not seen a single-party majority for many years. Coalitions are usual, and in addition, the second chamber (Council of States or 'Bundesrat') generally has a different majority than the Parliament ('Bundestag'). Consequently, negotiation and bargaining is common, with most major pieces of legislation assuming the character of a 'smorgasbord', containing elements that please either the governing coalition or the opposition.

This situation sustains an ultra-stable political system, with little chance of a major change in health policy. Indeed, one may conclude that in Germany all health reforms are possible if they promise to change very little!

The left and right wing near consensus about the need to improve efficiency has not culminated in agreement on the regulatory structures needed to shift financial and quality risks from payers to providers. Some experts call for risk-related premiums in the SHI system, but such proposals stand little chance of realisation because in the eyes of many policy makers this would be tantamount to a conversion from SHI to private health insurance. By relating financial transfers among SHI funds to the degree of morbidity, the current, individualised risk-related premiums become less attractive to some. More recent SPD Party Convention resolutions (November 2003) call for a risk-equalisation or transfer scheme between private and social health insurance systems – a step towards equalisation of financial risks across public and private insurers.

The interplay between public and private elements over time

Time patterns

As may be seen in Table 10.7, while in absolute terms both public and private sources of financing healthcare have grown over time, the actual shares of various types of public or private resources has not conformed to a simple pattern. Social health insurance started with 58.3% of total spending in 1970, increasing (with some fluctuations) to 68.0% in 1995. Particularly in the wake of the reunification of Germany, and as a result of policy decisions to finance the unification process mainly via contributions rather than taxes, the share of SHI funding rose steadily from 65.4% (1990), to 65.9% (1993), to 69.5% (1994), to 68.0% (1995). The tax share in health finances declined steadily from 14.5% (1970) to 10.1% (1995), a pattern unaffected by the reunification process. The share of co-payments fluctuated. From a high of 13.9 (in 1970) and a low of 9.6%

Table 10.7 Sources of funding 1970 to 2000, selected years (as a percentage of total health spending)

Source of funds	1970	1975	1980	1985	1990	1993	1994	1995	1996	1997	1998	2000
Public												
– SHI	58.3	66.6	67.0	66.1	65.4	65.9	66.8	68.0	68.9	69.5	69.4	69.0
– Taxes	14.5	12.4	11.7	11.2	10.8	11.6	10.6	10.1	9.4	7.1	6.4	6.0
Private												
– Co-payments	13.9	9.6	10.3	11.2	11.1	11.4	11.4	10.9	11.0	12.2	12.8	11.0
– Private health insurance	7.5	5.8	5.9	6.5	7.2	6.7	6.8	6.4	6.5	6.9	7.1	13.0
– Others	5.8	5.6	5.1	4.9	5.4	4.4	4.3	4.4	4.2	4.3	4.3	n/a

Note: Data up to 1990 refer to Western Germany, and from 1991 to total Germany (East and West).

Source: OECD Health Data 1999 and OECD Indicators 2003, p. 128.[11,12]

(in 1975), it varied over time, reaching 11.0% (in 2000). The share of private insurance varied only slightly, from 7.5% (1970) to 6.4% (1995), but it increased to 13.0% by 2000. 'Other' sources of private spending stayed roughly within a general band (5.8 to 4.3%).

Likely effects of competition on the public–private mix

Ironically, in present-day Germany more competition exists between social health insurance funds than among the private health insurers. Furthermore, competition is very real between social health insurance funds as a whole and private health insurance funds, particularly for younger and higher-income individuals. Critics point out that the latter is ultimately an unfair type of competition, since the current rules favour private health insurance funds.

Social health insurance funds competing for members was the consequence of the broadening of choice resulting from the Health Structure Reform Act 1993. Prior to that date, only about half of the insured (mainly white-collar workers) could choose among funds as individuals or as members of a group (i.e. as employees of a firm). The Act extended this right to choose to practically all members of the social health insurance system, and at the same time, funds were (and still are) liable to accept every applicant regardless of individual risks.

A system of risk-structure-related transfers was also instituted in 1993, in order to neutralise those factors in the competitive process which the individual fund could not change by its own efforts, e.g. age and sex of the insured, number of dependants, health status (disability) and basic wage. For the majority of those insured, this system led to a substantial reduction in the range of contribution rates payable.

However, recently, some skilled entrepreneurs have used the provision of legislation allowing the institution of corporate health insurance funds and craftsmen's health insurance funds. By organising the flow of information (e.g. via the Internet) they ensured that, as far as possible, the young and the healthy would join the new fund, enabling it to charge substantially lower contribution rates. So the 'better risks' moved from the larger local and special health insurance funds to those newly formed. Since the transfer formula of the risk adjustment system allocates to each age and sex group (etc.) a transfer computed on the basis of average costs of all members, the difference between the lower actual costs of funds with a healthier-than-average membership and the imputed average costs acts as a further subsidy allowing the newer funds to lower rates even further. In this way, a dynamic process of desolidarisation was initiated which has not been corrected by the recent amendment of the act.

Such a process has an indirect bearing on the public–private mix. When 'better risk' individuals leave a larger fund with a mixed risk membership, their surplus of income over costs is lost and the fund must raise general contribution rates for all of its members. Those now motivated to change to a fund with more favourable contribution rates may choose to go directly to a private health insurance fund if they are entitled to do so. Among these, in particular, there are higher-income individuals who preferred membership of a social health insurance fund because they have a large number of dependants for whom they would have had to pay separate contributions to the private fund, or with health problems for which they would have had to pay a surcharge to the private fund.

Of greater importance are the unequal starting positions between private and public funds in competing for younger members. Some argue that private funds entice them with contribution rates which are too low, so that insufficient reserves accrue to help subsidise their contribution rates during old age. In fact, a recent law obliges private funds to make a 10% surcharge on the initial contribution rates of the young, to be used to build up reserves for the future.

Private funds are advantaged, not only by the right of the well-to-do to opt out of the SHI system. All else being equal, private funds can ask for lower rates from wealthier individuals to finance a given level of spending. So indirectly it is the privileges granted by law to private funds which give them an advantage in the competitive race. Also, private funds can eliminate *de facto* competition among themselves by the very fact that an individual member wishing to choose another private fund cannot transfer funds accrued in his name. There is evidently ample scope for reform to create efficiently fair and functional competition.

Given these institutional arrangements, it is surprising that private insurance has not seen greater growth. Evidently, socioeconomic factors (e.g. the number of individuals with higher income eligible to opt for private insurance) place greater constraints on the growth of private insurance than other factors. Similarly, limits determined by public policy on the rise of co-insurance act as a further curb to the expansion of the private element in the overall mix.

Outlook: whither the public–private mix in Germany?

Unless major legal measures are enacted, significant change is unlikely. Much depends on the ongoing policy debate about necessary reforms in the healthcare sector. Ultimately, it is a question of the appropriate ideological reference model for the future role and development of the public versus the private subsystems of the healthcare system. Will the two converge and become very similar in mode and operation or diverge in reference model and operation? If the path of convergence is chosen, there are still two polar extremes which may serve as ideal types to inform the process.

Convergence type 1: partial 'privatisation' of the SHI system

A far-reaching form of privatisation moulds SHI into a system increasingly similar to the private health insurance system existing today. Advocates of radical market-liberal reforms implicitly hold such a view. Future forms of government coalition will decide whether such a 'liberalisation' of the system continues to take place beyond the shift to a greater private role brought about by the Health System Modernization Act of 2003/2004, though it is unlikely that the concept of a total privatisation of the SHI will command much support in the political domain.

Major stepping stones on the path of liberalisation of the SHI system may be further increases in co-insurance, leading to the introduction of regular and optional benefits (together with differing contribution rates geared to differing benefit packages) and partial reimbursement of contributions in the event that use of benefits is avoided over a certain period of time.

Convergence type 2: partial 'socialisation' of the private health insurance system

If private health insurance institutions are permitted to establish separate departments offering insurance packages according to SHI principles (utilisation on the basis of need; financing on the basis of ability to pay), another type of process of convergence will be initiated, the prototype of which can be found in Germany's long-term care insurance system. Private insurers are obliged to offer a 'standard package' of benefits – in addition to the different packages based on classical private insurance principles, turning them, in effect, into 'partial SHI institutions'.

Even if such measures are not put into practice on the benefits side, there are measures on the financing side creating solidarity between the privately and publicly insured. In particular, the risk-adjustment concept could be applied to private health insurance. Differences in the basic wage could lead to a pooling of finances which would lead to sizeable transfers in favour of the SHI system.[5]

Convergence type 3: 'equivalence' departments for SHI funds

In addition to the two polar types, there may be a convergence towards an 'in-between' type 3, where SHI funds would be entitled to offer optional additional packages of benefits in consideration of extra premiums. This would have to be financed on the basis of the equivalence principle, i.e. the 'price' would have to correspond to the benefit granted or the risk covered.

In the German context, where private health insurance funds already exist which offer individual add-on benefit packages to members of SHI funds, it is hard to justify such measures on the grounds of enhancement of the freedom of choice. In effect, such proposals only make political sense if the standard package of benefits available equally to all members in case of need is reduced significantly, leaving room for various packages of benefits to be chosen individually by the members of SHI funds. However, such a 'solution' is really a strategy to reduce solidarity in the SHI system, financing a lower-level package of benefits and leaving individuals to insure against more far-reaching risks or for more generous benefits. There is a widespread conviction in Germany that such a system would lead to a 'two-tier' system of provision of health goods, wherein the weight of an individual's wallet would determine their quality of healthcare – an evident violation of SHI principles.

An example of convergence may be found in the Netherlands. Under the 'Dekker Plan', the rules for raising contributions and for awarding benefits were to be equal for all insurance organisations, thus causing the differences between public and private health insurance funds to disappear. All health insurance funds, public or private, would be open to all-comers. The same rules would apply for the competition between private and SHI funds and they would all be included in a risk-adjustment mechanism aimed at neutralising the effects on competition of different age and sex structures, etc.

Alternatively, future development may proceed along the lines of what may be termed a *'divergence model'*, where both the SHI and the private health insurance system would be reduced to their essential features, and remain separate from each other to an even greater extent than they are today.

A more *moderate type of a divergence model* would reaffirm the basic principles of SHI systems by progressively reducing or even excluding private elements: co-payments, partial refunds of contributions in the event of non-use of benefits and the (few) optional benefits already present in today's SHI system.

As a corollary, the restrictions present in today's private health insurance (premiums or benefits) would have to be reduced or eliminated entirely. In order to conform more closely to the ideal type of market exchange, elements restricting competition today would have to be abolished, in particular the non-transferability of accumulated reserves when moving from one private fund to another; the transfer elements present in the rate structure; the 'social' elements present in the form of 'standard benefits package'; and other rules restricting the freedom of choice of fund.

Furthermore, a radical variant of a divergence model would make all resident citizens compulsory members of the SHI system, and raise contributions on all types of income over and beyond wage income, restricting the private health insurance to the provision of supplementary benefits, as is currently the case in some countries. Alternatively, a more complete convergence along the following lines is also being discussed (in 2004). Both SHI and PHI funds would offer identical social health insurance packages financed on the basis of ability to pay (measured not only on the basis of wage income but of total income). Additionally, both SHI and PHI funds would offer supplementary insurance on an individualised basis, i.e. on the basis of risk-related premiums. Both of these measures should provide the grounds for further forms of competition between all health insurance funds. In fact, the notion of a 'citizens' insurance' ('Bürgerversicherung') gained a sizeable majority in the November 2003 Party Convention of the Social Democratic Party (SPD), against the wishes of the party leadership. The Green Party has called for a similar long-term reform of the financing system.

Conclusions

The German healthcare system may be reformed in many different ways. The country's fiscal crisis, with high unemployment and low levels of economic growth, is creating pressures for the radical reform of the public sector, in part to reduce budgetary deficits. However, the choice of reform is not so much a question of imagination, but of political preferences and the distribution of power between groups striving to assert their interests in the competitive societal and political struggle. Given the dominance of coalition governments, reform may be slow and it will always be difficult electorally.

Appendix 1: Particular categories of services

Ambulatory care

Physicians in private practice provide ambulatory medical services. In most practices, 80 to 90% of revenue results from the treatment of members of SHI funds, with additional revenue accruing from treating patients with private health insurance. Private rates for all services are about three times higher than those from SHI.

Until recently, there were no co-payments. The current legislation provides for a co-payment of €10 for doctors' visits each quarter (except for referrals by other doctors and for control visits related to preventive measures). Physicians are allowed to offer SHI clients, on the basis of a private contract, additional services that are not covered by SHI.

In 2001, of the 297 893 medical doctors in practice, 129 986 were working in their own practices and 142 310 in hospitals.

Dental care

Traditionally, members of statutory health insurance received dental care according to statutory healthcare standards free of charge. Over time, coverage for crowns and dentures was reduced, leaving room for the emergence of private dental insurance. Co-payment for these public services has risen from 20% in 1980 up to about 50% in 2003.

Thus far, dentures are offered mostly under private treatment and patients are billed. Quality assurance is handled directly via the Association of Accredited Dentists. The dentist's bill is based on a fee-for-service schedule similar to the one in ambulatory care, with the Associations of Dentists settling accounts with the sickness funds every three months.

The Health Care Modernisation Law of 2003 brought about far-reaching changes to the dental care sector. With effect from 1 January 2004, a co-payment of €10 covers dental appointments per quarter, not payable in the case of a referral by other dentists. More importantly, with effect from 2005, dentures will no longer be covered by SHI without additional contributions. Individuals will be under obligation to insure themselves by membership of either a SHI fund or a PHI fund. Under the former, a member's monthly contribution earmarked for dentures will amount to €6 per month. His or her family members will be covered without additional contribution.

Hospital care

Since the Hospital Law of 1972, hospitals and sickness funds have fixed the daily rate per patient at the beginning of each year. They have to cover the expected operating expenses of the hospital, including doctors' pay and the salaries of medical and non-medical staff.

The 2200 hospitals are required to have cost and service records, which provide an outline of their cost structure. Additionally, a uniform compensation scheme exists for a number of treatments and procedures and the states develop hospital planning for the overall number and allocation of hospitals and beds. Most hospitals are publicly owned; only 15% (and less than 7% of all hospital beds) are in the private for-profit sector. Long-term investments in hospitals are subsidised up to 100% from the public funds of the federal states.

The reimbursement scheme and centralised planning have produced an average length of stay of 9.8 days in acute hospital care. This is still higher than in other EU countries (Denmark averages 6.1 days and Sweden 6.8). But with the implementation of diagnosis related groups (DRGs), the length of stay is expected to decline.

There is widespread dissatisfaction with the planning process associated with hospitals: it often reflects political interests, and is cumbersome and inefficient.

Since the mid-1990s, hospitals do provide a limited outpatient treatment service in the form of day surgery, though hospitals rarely run outpatient clinics. Hospitals are used for inpatient care and with the exception of emergencies, hospital care depends on referral by an ambulatory care physician.

As hospitals are financed in a 'dual fashion', conflicts can and do arise. The responsibility for financing the renewal of buildings and equipment is a case in point. Should this rest with the individual states (Länder) or the sickness funds? Also, hospital planning is the responsibility (and the right!) of the state governments. Associations of health insurance funds have only to be heard in the planning process, not necessarily listened to!

Finally, hospitals are organised rather loosely. There are no regional hospital associations responsible for negotiations and contracts. The state hospital associations and the German Hospital Association represent the interests of individual hospitals, but only hold the status of private associations ('Vereine'). They cannot regulate an individual hospital's conduct. Furthermore, since public, private non-profit and private for-profit hospitals co-exist, their interests differ considerably, which has so far precluded the foundation of an effective organisation of hospitals. Smaller hospitals account for a rather large proportion of the market, so potential economies of scale are lost.

The Structural Health Reform Act of 1993 included a fundamental change in the system of hospital remuneration. In place of a system which covered costs incurred, from 1996, individual 'prices' were to be paid for specific services or diagnosis-related benefits (similar to DRGs). However, these 'prices' were to be negotiated between hospital associations and those of the health insurance funds at the federal and state levels. So no contracts were effected between individual funds and individual hospitals. Thus far, these 'prices' cover only about 30% of total hospital costs and the rest is still being financed by covering costs incurred. While increasing the incentives for hospitals to trade quality for possible profits, the introduction of pricing elements did not lead to significant cost reductions but rather to a significant decrease in the average length of stay.

Allowing hospitals to treat patients on an ambulatory basis before and after the actual period of stay, and opening hospitals for day case operations, increased competition between hospitals and ambulatory care physicians.

Pharmaceuticals

Every SHI patient is entitled to receive pharmaceuticals prescribed by an accredited physician or dentist, and these are dispensed in about 22 150 pharmacies in Germany. Physicians are not allowed to dispense pharmaceuticals in their private practices. Hospitals organise their own pharmaceutical supplies themselves without privately run pharmacies. According to the 'Red List' about 4000 substances are available on the market in more than 35 000 different pharmaceutical forms. The number of pharmaceuticals in Germany is one-tenth of the number of 40 000 that is often cited.

Appendix 2: Latest co-payment rules by types of benefit (Health System Modernisation Act – GMG – 2004)

Hospital and rehabilitation

The co-payment is €10 per day, for up to 28 days a year.

Ambulatory care

To consult a physician or a dentist a co-payment of €10 is required. It is to be paid directly to the provider, once in each quarter of the year when making a visit. No additional payment is required on referral by a family physician (who acts as gatekeeper) to a specialist.

Pharmaceuticals

Pharmaceuticals that are not prescribed by the physician in ambulatory care are excluded from reimbursement in SHI and must be paid for by the patient. For every other pharmaceutical, co-payment is 10% of the price, with an upper limit of €10.

Transportation

In future, transportation costs incurred for doctor's visits (ambulatory care) are no longer covered by SHI. Ten per cent of the costs incurred (minimum €5 and maximum €10) are to be paid for transportation to and from hospital when an ambulance car is being used.

Dentures

From 2005 on, SHI funds do not provide for dentures, crowns or bridges. Members of a SHI fund have to obtain obligatory insurance coverage by paying an extra premium either under SHI or PHI. For preventive dental visits and treatment (e.g. for fillings) no co-payment is required.

Sickness benefit

From 2006 on, the contribution for sickness cash benefits usually paid by SHI after six weeks of illness, has to be borne fully by the SHI-insured.

Appendix 3: Specific measures of various healthcare reform acts 1993–2003

1993: Health Care Structure Act ('Gesundheits-Strukturgesetz', GSG)

The trend towards ever-increasing health expenditure could not be reversed by repeated cost containment acts. This finally led to the enactment, in 1993, of the Health Care Structure Act, which tried to achieve two overall strategic policy aims:

1   To stabilise the precarious financial position of sickness funds and to prevent a major increase in contribution rates through increased efforts at cost containment (short-run measures). The latter had been the main policy focus since the mid-1970s.
2   To introduce structural reforms that would prove to be more effective in the long run than the short-term measures of cost containment of the earlier acts (long-run measures). Some of these measures were also designed to improve efficiency and equity, as well as control cost.

The short-run measures concentrated on budgeting overall expenditure, including incomes of ambulatory care physicians and dentists, hospital spending, and pharmaceuticals and medical and technical aids. While the self-administered organisations were to be involved in the budgetary process, these measures meant an increased government regulatory involvement in the healthcare sector. Originally, the process was limited to a three-year period (until 1995), after which time the structural reforms were expected to lead to increases in efficiency.

The long-run measures of the Health Care Structure Act concentrated on structural reforms as well as emphasis on the role of competition. If they had been successful, they would have obviated the necessity for a continuing sequence of short-term cost containment acts. But, in practice, they proved to be largely ineffective in curbing expenditure growth, as exemplified by the hospital and pharmaceutical sectors.

Additionally, the following measures were enacted:

• the introduction of a risk-adjustment system leading to large-scale transfers between SHI funds, together with an extension of the freedom to choose one's own health insurance fund
• the limitation of the number of doctors
• the introduction of a performance-related system of remunerating hospitals in lieu of comprehensive cover of costs
• first attempts toward greater integration of healthcare sectors, particularly of ambulatory care and stationary care (particularly in hospitals)
• a lowering of the remuneration of dentists
• a change in the form and the magnitude of co-payments for pharmaceuticals.

1997: The Reduction of Contribution Rates Act ('Beitragsentlastungsgesetz')

The aim was to lower contribution rates by 0.4%, increase co-payments for pharmaceuticals, lower sickness benefit ('Krankengeld'), reduce rehabilitation programmes in spas and cancel subsidies for spectacle frames.

For those born after 31 December 1978, dentures were almost completely eliminated from the benefit package.

1997: First and Second Health Insurance Restructuring Acts ('1. & 2. GKV-Neuordnungsgesetz')

These laws laid down the following measures:

- further increases in co-payments
- flat-amount subsidy for dentures
- introduction of elements of PHI
- (additional) special flat amount payment for hospitals ('Notopfer-Krankenhaus').

1999: Improvement of Solidarity Act ('GKV-Solidaritätsstärkungsgesetz')

The newly elected Red-Green Coalition passed several measures:

- budgets for the various sectors
- a reduction in co-payments for pharmaceuticals
- an extension of exemptions from co-payments (e.g. for the chronically ill)
- reintroduction of dentures in the catalogue of benefits for those born after 1978.

2000: Reform of the SHI 2000 Act ('Gesetz zur Reform der gesetzlichen Krankenversicherung ab dem Jahr 2000')

A series of measures was introduced with the aim of restrengthening structural reforms:

- greater weight to be accorded to stabilising contribution rates
- strengthening integrative measures aimed at close cooperation of sectors
- bolstering primary care
- reintroduction of measures aimed at primary prevention and health promotion
- promotion of self-help groups and counselling centres for patients through SHI funds
- augmenting benefits for rehabilitation
- introduction of a new (DRG-type) price system for hospitals (regulated further in the DRGs Financing Act 2000 ('DRG-Einführungsgesetz 2001')
- improved measures for quality assurance
- introduction of a 'positive list' of pharmaceuticals.

2001/2002: Laws for a New Order of Rights to Choose Among SHI funds and Risk Structure Compensation Amendment Act ('Gesetz zur Neuregelung der Krankenkassenwahlrechte und der Reform des Risikostrukturausgleichs (RSA)')

These Acts included:

- changes in the rules governing choice of SHI funds
- reform of the risk-adjustment process to include incentives for the introduction of disease-management programmes by SHI funds, the introduction of a system of pooling risks for especially expensive cases, and with effect from 2007, the reform of rules governing the transfers to be based on differential morbidity patterns of individual funds.

2003/2004: Health System Modernisation Act ('Gesundheits-Modernisierungs-Gesetz')

- improving the rights of patients and the insured
- improving quality of healthcare via an independent Institute for Quality and Economy in Healthcare, providing information and medical guidelines
- improved incentives for integrated systems of care
- reform of the remuneration system of ambulatory care doctors, replacing floating values by points (for services rendered) through fixed values, together with a degressive remuneration scheme for services provided over and beyond the ex-ante agreed-upon volume
- changes in the pricing system also for those patented pharmaceutical products which do not reflect noticeable therapeutic improvement, and exclusion of non-prescription drugs from the list of reimbursable benefits; mail-order delivery of pharmaceuticals becomes possible (under certain restrictions)
- reform of the organisational structure of SHI doctors' associations
- limits to administrative spending of SHI funds
- dentures shall be financed in future solely via income-related contributions of the employees (removing the employer's obligation to pay half of the contributions due); this measure is accompanied by an enhancement of the scope for choice between SHI and PHI funds
- a major restructuring of the financing process (including tax funding of maternity benefits); an additional 0.5 percentage point payable by employees (and no longer by the employers); elimination of cash benefits in case of death, delivery of a child, sterilisation (in future to be paid for privately); limitation of spectacles to children up to the end of their eighteenth year; exclusion of taxi and rental car charges for trips to the ambulatory care doctor; and major changes in co-payment rules (as described above).

This represents an extensive legislative process to steer the SHI system on a path of moderate expenditure growth (with, at best, moderate success) and to effect structural reforms to improve efficiency and equity (regarding which, there are still sizeable social class differences[6]).

References

1 Kupsch S, Kern AO, Klas C, Kressin BKW, Vienonen M, Beske F (2000) Health service provision on a microcosmic level – an international comparison – results of a WHO/ IGSF survey in 15 European countries. In: Institut für Gesundheits-System-Forschung (IGSF) (Hrsg) (eds) Schriftenreihe /Institut für Gesundheits-System-Forschung Kiel, Band 74, Kiel.

2 Breyer F, Haufler A (1999) Health care reform: separating insurance from income redistribution. Discussion Papers, University of Konstanz, No. 296.

3 Pfaff M (1997) Standortfaktor Gesundheit. In: Ministerium für Arbeit, Gesundheit und Soziales des Landes Nordrhein-Westfalen, Düsseldorf, pp. 81–126.

4 Kühn H (1995) Zwanzig Jahre 'Kostenexplosion' – Anmerkungen zur Makroökonomie einer Gesundheitsreform. *Jahrbuch für Kritische Medizin*. **24**: Argument.

5 Rosenbrock R (1998) *Gesundheitspolitik. Einführung und Überblick*. Publication series of the research unit Public Health Policy. Berlin: Wissenschaftszentrum Berlin, pp. 98– 203.

6 Pfaff M (1995) Funktionsfähiger Wettbewerb innerhalb und zwischen den gesetzlichen und privaten Krankenkassen. *Arbeit und Sozialpolitik*. **49**(9–10): 12–20.

7 OECD (2001) *OECD Health Data 2001*. Paris: OECD.

8 Association of Private Health Insurance Funds (2003) *Private Health Insurance – Facts and Figures 2002/2003*. Köln.

9 Schneider M (1994) Evaluation of cost-containment acts in Germany. In: OECD (eds) *Health: quality and choice*. Paris: OECD, pp. 63–81.

10 Busse R, Howorth C (1999) Cost containment in Germany. In: Mossialos EJ, Le Grand J (eds) *Health Care and Cost Containment in the European Union*. Aldershot: Ashgate, pp. 303–39.

11 OECD (1999) *OECD Health Data 1999: a comparative analysis of 29 countries*. Paris: OECD.

12 OECD (2003) *Health at a Glance – OECD Indicators 2003*. Paris: OECD, p. 128.

13 Pfaff M, Nagel F (1994) Gesundheitssysteme der Europäischen Gemeinschaft im Vergleich. *Das Gesundheitswesen*. **56**(2): 86–91.

14 Federal Bureau of Statistics (1997) Series **12**(2): p. 10.

15 Federal Bureau of Statistics (2002).

16 Pfaff AB, Langer BP, Mamberer FM, Freund F, Kern AO, Pfaff M (2003) Zuzahlungen nach dem GKV-Modernisierungsgesetz (GMG) unter Berücksichtigung von Härtefall- regelungen. Volkswirtschaftliche Diskussionsreihe der Universität Augsburg, Beitrag Nr. 253.

17 Federal Bureau of Statistics (2003).

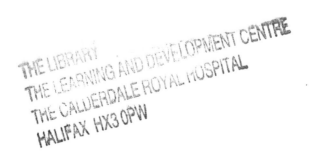

Chapter 11

The public–private mix in health services in New Zealand

Nicholas Mays and Nancy Devlin

Introduction

In the 1980s, when the first Nuffield *The Public–Private Mix* book was published, New Zealand's healthcare system was predominantly tax financed and administered mainly by elected area boards, funded via a weighted population formula. Public hospital services were free, but user charges applied to primary healthcare. A parallel privately financed sector provided supplementary access to health services, chiefly elective surgery, for those willing to pay for private health insurance or out-of-pocket.

Today, the healthcare system is predominantly tax financed and administered mainly by elected district boards, which receive funding according to a weighted population formula. Public hospital services are free, but user charges apply to primary healthcare (*see* Box 11.1). A parallel private sector provides supplementary access to services, chiefly elective surgery.

On the basis of this 'then and now' snapshot, one might conclude that New Zealand's healthcare system has remained remarkably free of dramatic (and analytically interesting) policy change. The opposite is true. Although the publicly financed health sector had escaped the widespread liberalisation of the New Zealand economy that occurred during the mid to late 1980s, in the early 1990s, a new government unleashed rapid, radical and (with the benefit of hindsight, perhaps ill-considered) restructuring of the publicly financed health system. The central element of this was an attempt to introduce competition between healthcare providers. Some of the more radical elements of the proposed reforms were never implemented; of those that were, most have subsequently been dismantled or attenuated.

This chapter describes the current complex mix of public and private finance and provision of healthcare in New Zealand. It then discusses the aims and consequences for the public–private mix of the short-lived experiment with supply-side competition within the public system and how, by the end of the 1990s, New Zealand had returned to a system remarkably similar to the 1980s. The chapter ends by exploring the parallels and differences between current healthcare issues and policies in New Zealand and the UK, and their likely effects on the future public–private mix of finance and provision.

Box 11.1 Key information on the New Zealand health system

- Total spending on health as a % GDP, 2000/01: 8.8% (9.2% including disability support/social care)
- Public spending on health as a % GDP, 2000/01: 6.8%
- Public spending as a proportion of total health spending, 2000/01: 76.7%
- Main source of public funds: general taxation (69% of total spending)
- Private spending as a proportion of total health spending, 2000/01: 23.3% (16.8% out of pocket; 6.2% private insurance)
- Publicly funded hospital services are largely 'free at the point of demand'; means-tested public subsidies plus user charges apply to primary health-care with the exception of GP visits for children under 6 years and maternity care
- Principal administrative units (2003): 21 district health boards (DHBs), comprising a majority of locally elected and the remainder government appointed members
- Provision of secondary healthcare services is dominated by publicly owned and managed hospitals with salaried staff; primary care is delivered by self-employed general practitioners and their support staff
- Comprehensive no-fault insurance is provided by the Accident Compensation Corporation (ACC), a social insurance scheme, for health, social care costs and loss of income arising from accident and injury (7.2% of total spending)
- Life expectancy at birth 76.9 years, close to OECD median (male 74.3; female 79.6; Mäori 69.4; Pacific 72.7; European/other 78.0)

Healthcare financing

The central principle underpinning New Zealand's health system, as in the UK, is universal access to services on the basis of need rather than ability to pay. Publicly financed healthcare and long-term care is mostly paid for out of general tax revenues which are allocated as a cash-limited budget by the Ministry of Health to subordinate territorial authorities, using a weighted capitation formula. The commitment to universal access is reflected in the absence of user charges for most publicly financed secondary care services (with rare exceptions – for example, assisted reproduction technologies), maternity care and, more recently, primary healthcare for children under 6 years.

Prices do, however, play a role in three important respects. First, general practitioner (GP) services and pharmaceuticals are only partially publicly subsidised, so user charges exert an important influence on demand.[1] GPs have maintained private for-profit status, with the vast majority receiving their income from fee-for-service. Second, where access to publicly financed services *is* denied (for example, by a patient failing to meet specified criteria of clinical need for elective surgery), patients have recourse to the private sector, where access is determined by their willingness and ability to pay for treatment by private insurance or out-of-pocket payments, as in the UK. Third, important categories

Table 11.1 Examples of how services are currently financed and provided in New Zealand

	Government provision	*Mixed provision*	*Non-government provision*
Public finance	Hospital inpatient and outpatient services; laboratory services for hospital inpatients and outpatients	Maternity services (often involves self-employed community midwives)	Community laboratory services GP services and pharmaceuticals for under-6s Rest home and long-term hospital care for older people with few resources
Mixed finance	Disability support services (DSS) – use of aids and equipment Hospital dental services for children and low income adults needing immediate treatment	Maternity services at Cornwall Suite, National Women's Hospital (free clinical services and extra amenities for a charge) – not permitted since 2000	GP services for adult Community Service Card (CSC) and High User Health Card (HUHC) holders Pharmaceuticals for over-6s DSS – Caregiver support
Private finance	Some elective surgery and diagnostic procedures – until 2000, but not permitted since		GP services for adults without CSC or HUHC Most dental services Significant amount of elective surgery Rest home and long-term hospital care for older people with sufficient resources

of services exist which are not financed publicly in any circumstances and for which consumers face the full costs. This includes, for example, most adult dental care and optometry. In these cases, demand is strongly influenced by price, as reflected in uneven distributions of spending across income groups.[2] The resulting complex relationship between public and private finance, and public and private provision that has arisen piecemeal over the past 60 years is summarised, using examples, in Table 11.1.

The role of user charges and subsidies for publicly financed services

Primary care

User charges in primary healthcare accompanied by partial public subsidies have long been a feature of the New Zealand system – in contrast to the NHS, where only pharmaceuticals attract a user charge. Anomalies arise from the co-existence of financial barriers to visiting GPs – the 'gatekeepers' to the rest of the system –

and 'free' secondary care. These include concerns about the inappropriate use of Accident and Emergency (A&E) services in hospitals and, more fundamentally, inequities in access to preventive and primary care (e.g. because GPs tend to practise in areas where they can make a living rather than where people most need their services).[3] Other anomalies include the fact that routine laboratory tests are free at the point of use in private ambulatory care settings, but adult dental and optometrical services attract no public funding. Ambulance services are publicly financed, but not in full, so patients are likely to be part-charged for emergency ambulance transport to hospital. Oddly, inter-hospital transfers of patients do not attract any part-charge.

In the 1990s, two initiatives attempted to address some of these issues. In 1992, there was an ill-fated effort to introduce user charges for hospital inpatients. These were abandoned just over a year later, following widespread public opposition and administrative problems.[4] Part-charges were also introduced for outpatients and day cases and set at a rate that reflected the likely charge patients would have faced had they visited their GP, in order to remove the incentive for people to use hospital A&E departments rather than their GP. These were removed in July 1997.

Second, universal primary care subsidies were replaced in 1991 by a system targeted according to patients' incomes and level of use of the service. With various adjustments to the eligibility criteria, these subsidies have persisted. The evidence on whether targeting subsidies to lower-income groups improved their access to services is inconclusive. Some studies show the expected result: that consultations increased for lower-income adults and decreased for higher-income adults. In contrast, other studies suggested that consultation rates fell both overall and for people on state benefits whose subsidy had risen.[4] An important problem was the low uptake of the Community Services Card (CSC) which entitles low-income holders to a GP visit subsidy. Reasons for this include: lack of knowledge about the eligibility criteria and benefits of having the card; the complexity of applying to obtain it; and problems assessing family income.[4] Around 40% of the population currently holds these cards; but an estimated one-quarter of the eligible population does not (and a further 5–10% have incomes just above the eligibility threshold).[5]

Problems with targeting subsidies effectively have led to a recent policy of giving subsidies to additional subgroups of the population and widening the scope of publicly financed services. New Zealand's first coalition government began this in 1997 by agreeing to pay GPs a subsidy sufficient at the time to enable them to make visits free for all children under 6. An evaluation of this scheme over the short term showed that, in terms of improved health outcomes and secondary costs averted, it was difficult to justify its $50 million per annum cost.[6] However, removing part-charges did have important effects on equity, improving access for those who did not qualify for the CSC and those whose incomes were just over the qualifying threshold.

The current Labour-led government is going still further towards a universal system of primary care,[3] with a plan to virtually eliminate user charges for primary healthcare over an 8–10 year period.[7] If this occurs, it will be the most significant change in the financing of the public system since its inception in the 1940s. The services provided by new primary health organisations (PHOs) (groups of self-employed primary care providers) will attract higher funding. To guard against the demand pressures which accompany the traditional fee-for-service mode of reimbursement, the increase in the proportion of public funding is being accompanied by an immediate shift to funding PHOs via capitation, using a risk-adjusted formula based on the characteristics of their enrollees. But during the lengthy transition between the former system of demand-led partial subsidies with co-payments and the new system of near-fully funded, capitated PHOs, GPs will continue to be able to levy user charges at a level to be negotiated between the local district purchaser (district health board, DHB) and the PHO with which the GP is affiliated. To avoid the financial incentive to under-serve the poor, the same level of co-payment will apply to all the patients enrolled with each PHO regardless of their income or other characteristics. Eventually, the subsidy for individuals on low incomes and high users can be removed.

If fully implemented, primary healthcare will shift from private provision with a minority share of public subsidy to private provision (PHOs are non-governmental organisations, NGOs) with a high proportion of costs met from public funding. The aim is an affordable service for all patients, though small user charges will probably remain. The plan to gradually reduce charges for services such as visits to the GP raises the question of whether and how co-payments for pharmaceuticals will be reduced. Currently, adults who are not on a high income, are not high users and who do not have a Prescription Subsidy Card, pay $15 per subsidised pharmaceutical, and more if the drug is not subsidised by the government's Pharmaceutical Management Agency (PHARMAC).

Disability support

Extensive user charges are also a feature of the disability support (social care) arm of the public health system since its origins lie in the 'social welfare' sector where user charges and demand-driven subsidies are commonplace, rather than in the health sector with its stronger tradition of universalism. In 1993, disability support services' funding was shifted into the health budget (Vote Health) and the budget capped.[8] It currently accounts for 25% of Vote Health. Long-stay care for disabled people under 65 years is effectively fully funded by government, since most recipients are on a state benefit, but long-term residential and hospital care of people over 65 years is income and asset-tested. People who are assessed as needing long-term care and whose assets are above the specified threshold (currently $15 000 for a single person) pay the full costs of their care up to a maximum of $636 per week, even if this is greater than their weekly income. In this situation, single people must either sell their assets to pay for care or get an interest-free loan from the government secured against their assets (usually their home). If a person's assets are within the threshold, they pay almost all their income towards their care up to the maximum of $636 per week. Their New Zealand Superannuation (state old age pension) is paid directly towards the cost of their care less a personal allowance. The current Labour-led coalition is committed to removing the asset test, but not the income test, from long-term residential care, but it has yet to decide how best to achieve this. Full removal of the asset test will require a considerable increase in the public share of the costs of long-term care.

The role of private health insurance and out-of-pocket payments for private services

Private insurance has a supplementary role in financing healthcare. Cover is largely purchased by individuals and there are no tax rebates for premiums. As in the UK, coverage is skewed towards middle- and upper-income groups, and private insurance is primarily used to access surgical and medical treatment in private hospitals (to avoid waiting for public treatment). Many policies also provide 'gap' cover for user charges in primary and other healthcare services, though this is becoming less common. Cover is available from 15 companies; one of these, Southern Cross, dominates with 75% of the market.[5] The private insurance industry is subject to few regulations (other than those that apply to insurance generally), reflecting its supplementary role.[9]

A curious feature of New Zealand's health spending trends is that in the 1980s when the public share of total health spending was at its highest, more New Zealanders (51%) held private insurance than at any point before or since.[i] During the past decade, two things are notable: the proportion of the population covered by private insurance has fallen considerably (it is currently about 35%); while the proportion of health spending financed by private insurance has more than doubled to about 6% (see Figures 11.1 and 11.2).[ii] Policies are increasingly held to cover major elective procedures rather than 'gap' cover in primary care. Out-of-pocket spending has also become more significant.

These trends are likely to be due, first, to 'adverse selection' in the private insurance market. During the 1980s many New Zealanders held private insurance (possibly reflecting low confidence in the public healthcare system), from which they presumably obtained some peace of mind, but claims were relatively low – and consequently premiums were also low. During the late 1980s and early 1990s, there was a substantial jump in claims, partly because of the ageing of the insured population. This was, in turn, accompanied by sharp increases in premiums, particularly for high-risk groups.[4] The outcome has been a reduction in the proportion of those aged under 60 years covered by insurance. By contrast, there has been relatively little reduction in the proportion of over-60s with insurance,[10] where claims for private elective surgery are likely to be highest (the average 65-year-old with insurance claims almost four times more per year than the average 30-year-old.[11]

In response to the rapidly worsening adverse selection problem (Southern Cross claims rose by an average of 7.6% in 2001 and in the four years up to 2002, the insurer paid out more in claims than it received in premiums), insurers have shifted from community rating to age-banding their premiums, substantially raising the price of insurance for older people and lowering the cross-subsidy from younger to older policy holders. It has also begun to negotiate inclusive, prospective prices with providers in an attempt to reduce the rate of increase of costs without having to control utilisation directly. Traditionally, private insurers have been relatively passive payers of bills presented by hospitals and specialists.

The second explanation for the smaller proportion of the population with private health insurance is simpler: the Fringe Benefit Tax, introduced in 1992, reduced the incentive for employers to offer insurance in lieu of wage increases. The Health Funds Association, representing the private medical insurance

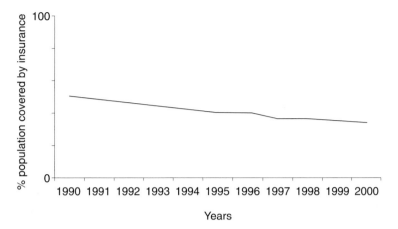

Figure 11.1 The proportion of the New Zealand population covered by private health insurance.

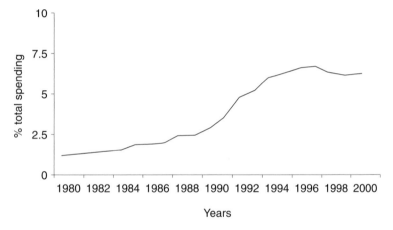

Figure 11.2 Proportion of total health spending in New Zealand accounted for by private insurance, 1980–2000.

industry, continues to press the government to introduce tax rebates to promote the uptake of health insurance, arguing that this will increase the resources available for healthcare, reduce pressure on the publicly financed system and reduce the amount of time people spend off work due to ill health. Since 1992, successive governments of both the Left and the Right have remained unmoved by these arguments. Tax concessions have opportunity costs the same as direct financing of healthcare, so it is unclear how they would necessarily 'lever' additional resources. Recent governments have preferred direct funding of health services that will be available to all, rather than subsidising access to services only available to people able to afford insurance. A major drawback of subsidising private medical insurance is that most of the extra spending will be devoted to people who already have insurance. It is also likely that an expansion of the private sector would simply divert staff from the public sector, particularly in the short term.

While private insurance accounts for a larger proportion of total spending in 2000 compared with 1980, the more important component of private spending continues to be out-of-pocket expenditure, which accounted for 16.8% of total spending in 2001 compared to 10.4% in 1980. More New Zealanders are opting out of private insurance because of adverse selection and the removal of tax incentives, and choosing to 'self-insure'. This makes sense, particularly for better-off people of working age.

The public–private mix of healthcare provision

Public hospitals account for just over half the total number of beds, including those in large tertiary hospitals. Between 1993 and 2001, the number of public hospital beds dropped by 22%, largely because of the closure of many small public hospitals. It was argued that it would be more efficient for the remaining large public hospitals to concentrate on their 'core business' of acute care. As a result, over the same period private hospital beds (many of which were for long-term care) increased by nearly 60% and now make up 48% of the bed stock.[5] In contrast to the NHS, there are no private beds in public hospitals, enabling a clear boundary to be drawn between the public and private sectors in hospital provision. The Labour-led government, in power since 1999, forbids public hospitals from engaging in any new private activity except where this leads to a *direct* benefit to public patients.[12] Income generation from private patients to be used subsequently for public patients, as in the UK NHS, is not sufficient justification, but a joint venture with a private provider (e.g. installation of a privately owned CT scanner in a public hospital) would be permitted if it led to a clear improvement for public patients in the quality or accessibility of a necessary service. Public providers are not permitted to offer non-clinical 'extras' to their patients for a charge (i.e. services that are not part of the range and standard of services generally available from public funds) (*see* Table 11.1).

There is no clear distinction in New Zealand between acute and long-term care beds, so OECD time series statistics are not available.[5] Consequently, the public–private mix of total beds disguises the dominant role that public providers have in the delivery of medical and surgical services. The vast majority of secondary care is still provided by public hospitals, although DHBs, in their role as local purchasers, are now required to choose the most effective provider irrespective of whether this is publicly or privately owned. Since they own and run the public hospitals, some non-government providers are critical of their unbiased ability to do this consistently, particularly in relation to hospital services. For many non-hospital services, contracts with private for-profit and non-profit organisations are the norm (e.g. primary healthcare). As in the UK, published information on the relative prices of public and private provision of comparable services is scarce.

Most specialists split their time between salaried positions in the public sector and fee-for-service work in the private sector.[13] The perverse incentives arising from this practice have long been noted in New Zealand,[14] as they have in the UK, without being addressed. On the other hand, this arrangement may make it easier for employers to contain wage costs in the public sector.

As in the UK, private hospitals fall into two main categories: those providing elective surgery; and those providing long-stay geriatric care.[15] There is limited private sector involvement in other types of services, such as mental health and maternity services. Since public hospitals do not accept private patients, the surgical services funded by out-of-pocket payments and private insurance are provided exclusively by the private sector. The latest available data on the split of elective surgery between public and private providers is for 1994 and 1995, and shows that private hospitals were performing 46% of total elective surgery in those years.[16] This share may have declined subsequently, since there was a significant increase in public funding earmarked for electives in the second half of the 1990s. In general, private surgery tended to be concentrated in the less complex procedures and in specialties such as orthopaedics and plastic/cosmetic surgery. Private surgical patients are more likely to be of working age and less likely to live in deprived areas, suggesting that a combination of insurance coverage and income influences people's ability to use the private surgical sector. This is similar to the public–private pattern in Britain.[17]

Scott[9] estimated that 38% of government spending for age-related disability support services went to public and 62% to private providers; other (non-age related) health and disability support services were 46% public and 54% private.

Provision of primary care is predominantly from private sector GPs, tradition-ally paid on a fee-for-service basis (until recently, a typical GP would receive 60% of their income from private payments, but now, as described above, they are increasingly grouped in capitated PHOs with increasing public finance). Dental care is paid for in a number of different ways: children's dental services are provided free of charge by salaried dental nurses working in the School Dental Service (a public provider); dental care for adolescents up to 18 years is fully subsidised and provided by private, self-employed dentists contracted to the state (paid using a mixture of capitation and subsidies per service); while most adult dental care is both provided and paid for privately. Optometrical services are provided by self-employed optometrists and paid for privately.

The quasi-market and the public–private mix, 1993–99

Nature of the quasi-market reforms

Throughout the 1980s and early 1990s, dissatisfaction with New Zealand's healthcare system – which at that stage comprised 14 area health boards (AHBs), both funding and providing hospital and some other services in their regions – was rife.[18] A succession of reports pointed to inefficiencies, poor management, budget overruns and badly eroded assets in public hospitals.[19] Waiting lists were increasing and a decline in public confidence in the system was associated with a growth in private insurance (*see* Figure 11.2). AHBs were criticised for facing no clear incentives to be efficient or responsive to patients and for weak accountability for their use of public resources.[4]

In 1993, the pro-market philosophy of the prevailing government led to an attempt to introduce the perceived advantages of a competitive market into the publicly financed healthcare sector. Central to this model was the full separation of purchasing from provision, aiming to increase efficiency, contain expenditure and reduce waiting lists.[20] Purchasing was undertaken by four ministerially appointed regional health authorities (RHAs). Hospitals became state-owned companies called Crown Health Enterprises (CHEs), subject to normal company law and required to be as successful and efficient as comparable private businesses while still operating in a socially responsible way. They were allowed to borrow privately for capital investment as long as they had income to cover repayments and interest. Any profits were to be returned to the two 'shareholding' Ministries of Health and Finance for reinvestment in the public health system, including in the CHEs themselves. The CHEs employed all the existing hospital staff, but on local pay and conditions. Contracts between purchasers and public hospitals were legally binding and most were diagnosis-related group (DRG)-based cost-and-volume contracts.

The impact of the quasi-market

According to most commentators, the impact of the experiment with competition between providers was in stark contrast with the expectations of its proponents,[21] though there was little explicit evaluation of the reforms and so limited evidence on which to base conclusions about their effects. Table 11.2 summarises the performance of the changes against key government goals, insofar as these can be discerned. Evaluation is further complicated by changes in the overall funding available and by secular trends such as increases in the levels of outputs and increased productivity, which pre-dated the quasi-market and continued during the period.[4] Similarly, longstanding improvements in population health, such as longer life expectancy at birth, which had been increasing steadily since the early 1960s, continued, but it is problematic to attribute these to the performance of the health system before or after 1993. On the other hand, Ministry of Health analysis of trends in mortality rates for 'avoidable' and 'unavoidable' causes of death shows a steady decline in the former since 1980, and particularly since 1986, and little or no change in the latter,[22] suggesting that healthcare has made a positive difference to health in the past 20 years, but even this is hard to relate to the changes made to the healthcare system.

Notwithstanding difficulties in measurement and lags between cause and effect, it is clear that some consequences can be plausibly related to the quasi-market. Little competition occurred between providers, especially hospitals. Many CHEs inherited and continued to post deficits and none returned any profits to the Crown. Barriers to entry limited contestability. Purchasers were conservative and dominated by providers, and barriers to exit (the government propped up deficit-ridden CHEs) arguably weakened economic incentives. Purchasers and providers struggled to establish contractual relations, transition and transactions costs were high, and the expected savings did not occur.

While there are no comprehensive figures on the transactions costs of the purchaser–provider split, these are believed to have been 'higher than expected'.[4] Contracting would have been *expected* to incur higher costs because transactions that were previously internal within a largely integrated system were now dealt with by negotiating, writing, monitoring and enforcing contracts between legally separate entities. However, it appears that these costs were particularly high in New Zealand due to the poor information systems that existed before the reforms; the tendency to take a legalistic 'completely specified' approach to contracting; and the adversarial relationships between purchasers and providers.[4] The higher

Table 11.2 Assessment of quasi-market reforms, 1993–9, against objectives

Criteria for evaluation	Effects predicted/ objectives	Positive effects (benefits)	Negative effects (costs)
Efficiency, responsiveness, quality	Supply-side competition leading to greater overall efficiency	Better information on services provided and resources used to provide them, allowing better informed purchasing decisions[44]	Little competition between hospitals due to local monopoly position and political concerns about hospitals going out of business – purchasers relatively weak[50,51]
		Long-term trends of increased level of outputs and increased productivity continued, but probably did not accelerate and may have decelerated early in the reform period;[45–47] with likely slower rates of improvement in productivity during the 1990s compared to the AHB period	
		Some competitive tendering led to savings in hospital services,[48] while benchmark price competition between non-hospital providers for service contracts is held to have improved efficiency[49]	
		Improved efficiency in use of pharmaceutical budgets[33]	
		Difficulties in rewarding efficient providers with additional work because of equity concerns	
	Less variation between providers in efficiency (e.g. unit costs)		Still substantial variation between providers in resource use, treatment patterns[25]
	Greater responsiveness to needs of particular patient subgroups	Wider range of non-hospital providers entered system (e.g. PHOs, Māori providers) which may offer more responsive service to particular communities[25,52]	Cases of major failure in service quality at specific providers attributed to reforms[53]

Table 11.2 (*cont.*)

Criteria for evaluation	Effects predicted/ objectives	Positive effects (benefits)	Negative effects (costs)
	Improved integration of budgets and services leading to better value for money	Some limited experiments and pilots showed some potential[54]	
Choice	Improved choice for service users in both primary and secondary care	See above under responsiveness; some limited choice of additional private providers as a result of tendering[48]	
Equity of access	More consistent levels of access to particular services	Elective surgical booking system may have increased consistency of access criteria, though not specifically a product of quasi-market	
	Reduced waiting times	Numbers on waiting lists increased between 1993–6; changes in recording and targeted expenditure make further comparisons difficult	
	Better access for Mäori and other minority groups	Increase in range of NGO providers, particularly 'by Mäori, for Mäori'[45]	Continued problems in access to healthcare for rural populations
Accountability	Clearer accountability as purchase, provision and regulatory roles separated	Lines of accountability and delineation of functions between agencies improved[4]	Difficulty in reconciling purchasers' and providers' interests
			Increased conflict between managers and staff and between providers
			Public anxiety about system remained high
	Providers more strongly accountable through performance to agreed contracts	Contracts allowed clearer specification of what was to be provided	Contracts criticised for not giving enough attention to quality
Financial management/ cost containment	Lower rate of increase of overall health spending	Increased use of capitation and budget holding by PHOs (e.g. IPAs) led to savings (e.g. in laboratory spending)[25]	

Table 11.2 (*cont.*)

Criteria for evaluation	Effects predicted/ objectives	Positive effects (benefits)	Negative effects (costs)
	Ability to deliver more services with same budget or same services with less funding ('savings') and make a surplus to be used either to provide more services or to be returned to government		Hospitals in deficit before and after reforms – access to equity support from government weakened incentives to contain costs
			No sign of 'savings' since any spare capacity immediately used
	Higher management costs but expected offset by efficiency gains		Increase in transaction costs due to lengthy contract negotiations[55] and large number of contracts – by 1997/8, 4580 contracts in the sector
			Likely higher management costs though little data

AHB: Area Health Board; NGO: non-governmental organisations

Source: Cummings and Mays, 2002.[56]

costs did not appear to generate corresponding benefits (though evaluation was scant).

The evidence suggests that the quasi-market model did not obviously achieve greater efficiency largely because it was so highly regulated. In 1996, a Treasury briefing to the incoming minister of CHEs stated:

> *The reforms have yet to yield the original expectations. By a range of measures . . . the pace of performance seems, if anything, to have weakened since the advent of the reforms* (quoted in Ashton, 1999).[4]

There were further concerns. The model emphasised the increased production of health service *outputs* in the public sector reform jargon of the day (i.e. more activity), which, it is argued, led to insufficient attention being paid to the quality of services and their effects on health *outcomes* (though purchasing for outcomes has eluded most health systems and broad measures of population health such as life expectancy at birth continued to improve). A major inquiry into quality of care and patient safety at one public hospital went as far as to argue that the quasi-market had contributed directly to specific instances of poor care,[23] although since the quasi-market also overlapped with the introduction of general management in the hospitals, this may have been the more fundamental cause of difficulties. Further, there was a crucial lack of 'buy-in' among health professionals and the general public, particularly to the idea that supply-side competition within a public service could improve quality and efficiency. The health workforce felt demoralised and disempowered as a result of tensions arising from the clash of managerial and clinical cultures.[13,24]

There were some positive trends, though in each case whether they were because of, despite, or unrelated to, the quasi-market is a moot point. Activity rates continued to increase and unit costs to fall.[22] But the discharge rate for conditions that could be treated by primary care continued to rise throughout the 1990s from 2000 per 100 000 in 1988/9 to 3000 per 100 000 in 2000/1, suggesting an increase in rates of chronic illness and/or a failure of primary care to reach certain sections of the population (e.g. low-income and Māori/Pacific Island peoples). Initiatives to reduce waiting times for elective surgery increased levels of non-urgent surgery from the mid-1990s. Lengths of stay had been falling during the 1980s and continued to fall in the 1990s, albeit at a slower rate. For example, average length of stay for general medicine was 10 days in 1988/9, 6 days by 1993/4 and had reached an apparent plateau of 4 days by 1998/9. Day case rates, which had been rising rapidly in the late 1980s, continued to rise, but much more slowly.

Better information systems facilitated greater accountability and better management of capital. Māori co-purchasers and providers were better able to attract funding to provide culturally appropriate services. GPs organised into groups – Independent Practitioner Associations (IPAs) – to contract with purchasers, many opting to become 'budget holders' with responsibilities for pharmaceutical and laboratory services. Some savings resulted from changes in prescribing behaviour and particularly in laboratory referrals.[25]

Nonetheless, these gains were overshadowed by the perceived failure of the quasi-market, particularly in relation to its ambitious efficiency goals. New Zealand's first proportionally elected, right-of-centre, coalition government responded in 1996 by symbolically renaming CHEs as more neutral 'Hospital and Health Services (HHSs)' and removed their for-profit status. 'Cooperation' replaced 'competition' as the new political watch-cry and the RHAs were replaced by a single, national purchaser, the Health Funding Authority (HFA). Thus, by 1996, key parts of the 1993 market model had already been discarded by the party which had introduced it.[18]

Dismantling the quasi-market?

A new, left-of-centre, coalition government was elected in late 1999. It moved quickly to honour its pre-election pledge to dismantle the remaining elements of the quasi-market model and to 'put the public back into the public health system'. The system was shifted towards its earlier, pre-1993, local, political origins and away from a 'corporate rationalist model',[26] although some features of the quasi-market period remain (e.g. the emphasis on upward accountability of health sector agencies to the Minister of Health and the contracts between public purchasers and non-governmental providers).

HFAs were abolished and most of their functions were transferred to 21 district health boards (DHBs), comprising a majority of locally elected and a minority of ministerially appointed members. DHBs plan most health and disability support (social care) services and are responsible for the level, mix and quality of services, including meeting the health goals, targets and standards set by the Minister of Health. Public hospitals are owned and managed by the DHBs, so that the local purchase function and public hospital provision are once again integrated vertically within a single organisation. Funding for the DHBs is determined by a weighted capitation formula, as was also the case for the AHBs of the 1980s and the RHAs. The formula is designed to effect a fair distribution of the available resources between DHBs according to their relative needs, measured by their share of the projected population and adjusted according to the national average cost of health and disability support services used by different demographic groups (by gender, age, ethnicity and deprivation status).

The effect of the quasi-market on the public–private mix of finance

Despite the tremendous structural and organisational upheaval they generated, the effects of the above twists in policy are not easily detected from trends in real expenditure per person, nor in the mix of public and private finance (*see* Table 11.3 and Figure 11.3). In part, this is because the changes of the 1990s were not primarily directed at changing the sources of finance for healthcare. Public and private spending have risen in real terms in most of the past 20 years. When it has not, this has generally been in periods of economic recession affecting both public and private financing (*see* Figure 11.4). The proportion of total spending accounted for by public sources fell between 1990 and 1998; however, it had been falling gradually since 1980 when it stood at 88%. It is currently around 78%.

The quasi-market reforms do not appear to have disturbed the public–private mix in finance directly – perhaps because competition was restricted to the *provision* of publicly financed services. The principal means by which finance was raised for the health system – general taxation – remained unchanged (*see* Table 11.4). The reduction in the public share of overall health spending was more obviously a product of the government's desire to contain public spending as a whole, particularly in the mid- to late 1980s before the quasi-market when private health costs were rising (*see* Figure 11.3).

In real per capita terms, public spending increased over the period of the quasi-market experiment in the 1990s (Table 11.3 and Figure 11.3), although the genuine increases in public expenditure were not always consistent, particularly not as a share of GDP, though they did not fall as a percentage of GDP (Figure 11.5). By 2000/1, public health spending accounted for 6.8% of GDP (up from about 5.5% in 1993/4) together with a rising share of public spending.

In other words, contrary to expectations, the quasi-market did not obviously contain spending. For example, funding the deficits incurred by CHEs accounted for over $200 million per annum of public spending over the period 1993/4 to 1997/8.[10] The CHEs found it relatively easy to borrow privately, but did not always have sufficient income to support their investments. In theory, private lenders should have exerted considerable commercial discipline on public hospitals operating as ordinary companies, but it became apparent that the Crown would not allow CHEs to go bankrupt, thereby allowing lenders to charge a risk premium without necessarily having to bear the risk.

Table 11.3 Expenditure trends in New Zealand, 1980–2000

| | Total expenditure ($ million 1999/2000) | | | Expenditure per capita ($ million 1999/2000) | | | | | | | | |
| | | | | 'Usually resident' population | | | 'Resident' population | | |
	Public	Private	Total*	Public	Private	Total*	Public	Private	Total*
1979/80	4028	549	4577	1306	178	1484	n/a	n/a	n/a
1980/81**	4189	570	4759	1320	179	1500	n/a	n/a	n/a
1981/82	4170	565	4735	1316	178	1495	n/a	n/a	n/a
1982/83**	4143	593	4736	1356	193	1549	n/a	n/a	n/a
1983/84	4236	633	4869	1317	197	1514	n/a	n/a	n/a
1984/85	3854	626	4480	1190	193	1383	n/a	n/a	n/a
1985/86	4244	674	4918	1301	207	1507	n/a	n/a	n/a
1986/87	4489	657	5146	1366	200	1566	n/a	n/a	n/a
1987/88	4902	824	5726	1482	249	1731	n/a	n/a	n/a
1988/89	5097	842	5939	1531	253	1784	n/a	n/a	n/a
1989/90	4957	1057	6014	1479	315	1794	n/a	n/a	n/a
1990/91	5113	1104	6217	1516	327	1843	n/a	n/a	n/a
1991/92	5108	1355	6463	1501	398	1899	1461	388	1848
1992/93	5057	1542	6599	1468	447	1915	1431	436	1867
1993/94	5427	1574	7001	1554	451	2005	1516	440	1956
1994/95	5499	1627	7126	1551	459	2010	1515	448	1963
1995/96	5581	1697	7278	1550	471	2021	1514	460	1974
1996/97	5941	1745	7687	1627	478	2105	1588	467	2055
1997/98†	6279	1873	8153	n/a	n/a	n/a	1661	496	2157
1998/99†	6733	1911	8643	n/a	n/a	n/a	1770	502	2272
1999/2000	6984	1968	8952	n/a	n/a	n/a	1827	515	2342
RAAGR††	2.8%	6.5%	3.4%				2.8%	3.6%	3.0%

* Totals may not always add up due to rounding.
** Estimated.
† 1997/8 and 1998/9 expenditure has been revised.
†† Real annual average growth rate (RAAGR) between 1979/80 and 1999/2000 for total funding, and between 1991/2 and 1999/2000 for per capita funding.

Source: Ministry of Health (2001).[57]

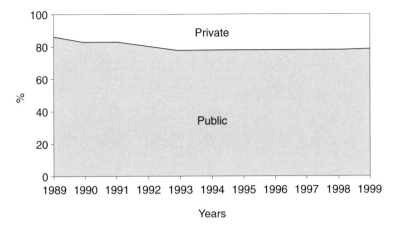

Figure 11.3 The public–private mix in New Zealand healthcare expenditure, 1989–99.

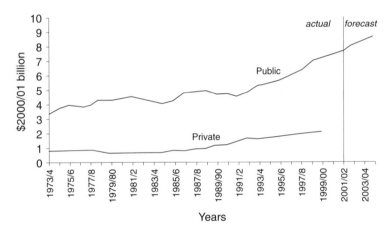

Figure 11.4 Real health expenditure in New Zealand, 1973/4 to 2004/5 ($2000/01 billion). *Source*: The Treasury, Health Expenditure Trends.[57]

The effect of the quasi-market on the public–private mix in provision

As with finance, the quasi-market appears to have had surprisingly little direct impact on the mix of provision, even though provider competition had the potential dramatically to alter the mix of provision. Reports commissioned by the government indicated substantial amounts of inefficiency in some public hospitals, such that overall costs could be lowered by 24–32%, were performance lifted to that of the best.[19] A further report (commissioned by the private insurer, Southern Cross) concluded that 'private hospitals perform selected specialties for approximately two-thirds of the cost of similar operations performed in public hospitals'.[27] This suggested that competition between public hospitals, and between public and private hospitals (with contracts being awarded to the most technically efficient bidder) would substantially change the mix of providers.

In practice, although the RHAs were required to encourage competition between providers, the barriers to entry and exit described earlier meant

Table 11.4 Health spending in New Zealand by source of funds (%) 1980–2001

	Vote Health	CHE/HSP deficit financing	ACC	Other government agencies	Local authority	Total public funding*	Private household	Health insurance	Not-for-profit organisations	Total private funding*
1979/80	80.5	n/a	0.7	6.6	0.3	88.1	10.4	1.1	0.4	11.9
1980/81	n/a	n/a	n/a	n/a	n/a	n/a	n/a	n/a	n/a	n/a
1981/82	81.7	n/a	0.9	5.1	0.4	88.1	10.2	1.3	0.4	11.9
1982/83	n/a	n/a	n/a	n/a	n/a	n/a	n/a	n/a	n/a	n/a
1983/84	79.0	n/a	2.5	5.2	0.3	87.0	11.0	1.5	0.5	13.0
1984/85	78.9	n/a	2.8	4.9	0.3	86.0	10.8	1.8	0.4	13.0
1985/86	78.2	n/a	3.1	4.7	0.3	86.3	11.4	1.9	0.5	13.7
1986/87	80.4	n/a	2.9	3.7	0.3	87.3	10.4	2.0	0.4	12.8
1987/88	78.4	n/a	3.0	3.9	0.3	85.6	11.6	2.4	0.4	14.4
1988/89	77.8	n/a	3.8	3.9	0.3	85.8	11.4	2.4	0.4	14.2
1989/90	72.7	n/a	4.4	4.8	0.5	82.4	14.5	2.8	0.3	17.6
1990/91	73.9	n/a	3.5	4.3	0.5	82.2	13.9	3.5	0.3	17.7
1991/92	67.9	n/a	6.6	4.0	0.5	79.0	15.9	4.8	0.3	21.0
1992/93	66.3	n/a	6.0	3.9	0.5	76.6	17.9	5.2	0.3	23.4
1993/94	64.9	3.1	6.0	3.0	0.5	77.5	16.1	6.1	0.3	22.5
1994/95	65.0	3.2	5.4	2.9	0.6	77.2	16.2	6.4	0.3	22.8
1995/96	65.2	2.6	5.4	2.9	0.7	76.7	16.3	6.7	0.3	23.3
1996/97	66.1	3.0	4.9	2.7	0.6	77.3	15.6	6.8	0.3	22.7
1997/98**	65.8	2.4	5.2	3.0	0.6	77.0	16.3	6.4	0.3	23.0
1998/99**	68.1	0.5	5.7	2.9	0.7	77.9	15.5	6.2	0.4	22.1
1999/2000	68.0	0.1	6.5	2.8	0.7	78.0	15.4	6.3	0.4	22.0
2000/01	65.5	0.6	7.2	2.9	0.6	76.7	16.8	6.2	0.3	22.0

* Totals may not always add up due to rounding.
** 1997/8 and 1998/9 figures have been revised.

Source: Ministry of Health (2001);[57] Ministry of Health (2002).[10]

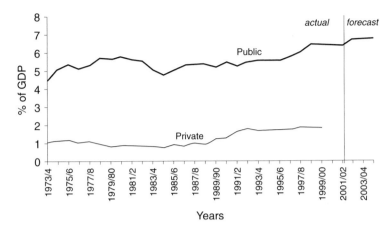

Figure 11.5 Health expenditure in New Zealand as a proportion of GDP, 1973/4 to 2004/5. *Source*: The Treasury, Health Expenditure Trends.[57]

historical spending patterns were resistant to change.[9] Most contracts were with the local CHEs, which effectively had local monopolies in the provision of most services.[15] Two years after the purchaser–provider split was introduced, the Ministry of Health (1996) commented that:

> *Competition for the provision of publicly funded healthcare appears to be increasing, but to a limited extent so far.*[28]

In 1997, 5865 publicly funded procedures were purchased from the private sector – just 1% of total discharges – although this represented more than double the number of discharges in 1993/4.[29] [iii] By 2000/1, the proportion of publicly funded medical and surgical discharges had shown a steady increase, but had still only reached 2.8% of the total.[22]

There are two explanations for the lack of major change in the mix of hospital provision. First, the original evidence on the relative inefficiency of public hospitals was questionable, so the scope for poor performers to improve efficiency in response to competitive pressure may have been overstated.[30] Second, barriers to entry and risk-averse purchasers severely limited contestability. In practice, patients generally received care from the same local hospital that they always had.

On the other hand, the separation of purchase from provision had clarified the responsibilities of different agencies and improved governance arrangements, enabling more explicit public accountability. The establishment of CHEs and HHSs as Crown-owned companies also facilitated the introduction of commercial practices, such as a regime of capital charges and accrual accounting, which are generally associated with more efficient use of income and assets by public bodies.

While the quasi-market period was not associated with any significant changes to the public–private mix of hospital services, it was marked by a large increase in the number of 'bulk-funded', non-governmental providers of primary and related ambulatory care, serving predominantly low-income, Māori and Pacific Island populations. The period was also marked by the spontaneous emergence of IPAs, as groups of GPs organised themselves in anticipation of negotiating contracts with RHAs and the HFA (e.g. in order to manage pharmaceutical spending for their patients).[25] It seems unlikely that this growth of non-government providers would have occurred without the separation of purchase from provision. Some of these organisations have formed the basis for the recently established PHOs through which the move towards a near-universal primary healthcare system will be implemented (see above).

Rationing publicly financed services

Traditionally, the rationing of publicly financed healthcare in New Zealand, as in the UK, has been largely implicit, often through the actions of individual clinicians faced with resource constraints. The alternative is the development of priority-setting rules and decision-making processes to produce explicit decisions about 'who gets what'. In principle, the advantages of explicit rationing are that decisions are more likely to be consistent and transparent, and decision makers can be held accountable for them. Private insurers and private providers have tended to advocate explicit rationing in the form of a clear definition of which services are inside and outside the public 'package' of entitlements, so that they can market their services as meeting the gap between individuals' demands and what society is prepared to pay for, collectively. There have been two notable initiatives in explicit priority setting in New Zealand in the recent past.

Prioritisation between services

First, there have been attempts to make explicit decisions about what services are (and are not) to be publicly funded. Under the quasi-market, this took the form of a failed attempt to define a simple list of 'core health services' which the RHAs were to purchase (to enable them, eventually, to behave like 'health plans' and compete on level terms for enrollees). A National Committee on Core Services considered, and then rejected, a number of possible approaches to defining the core: a positive list of services *in* the core; a negative list of services *not* in the core; and a priority-ranked list (like Oregon's). In 1998 the HFA built on these efforts by developing a prioritisation framework, which incorporated Programme Budgeting Marginal Analysis (PBMA) to determine those services 'at the margin'. These were then to be appraised against each of five principles: effectiveness; cost; equity; acceptability; and consistency with honouring the Treaty of Waitangi.[31 iv] Costs and effectiveness were, where possible, to be evaluated using cost-utility analysis.[32] Although the HFA was disbanded when a left-of-centre coalition replaced a right-of-centre government, and before its proposed process had become standard practice, its approach marked an important step forward in allocating resources, since cost-utility analysis continues to be used routinely by PHARMAC, a statutory corporation which manages the purchase of GP pharmaceuticals on behalf of the DHBs.

PHARMAC was set up in 1993 in response to government concern at the growth of public spending on pharmaceuticals and with the principal objective of securing the best health outcomes for people in need of GP-prescribed pharmaceuticals from the budget available. It does this, first, through managing access to a schedule of subsidised pharmaceuticals using evidence on the effectiveness and cost of each product (based on its projected cost per quality-adjusted life-year gained), in conjunction with other criteria, such as whether the product is likely to be of particular benefit to the health of Māori people or corresponds to a government health priority. Second, it uses reference pricing to decide the level of subsidy which products on the schedule will attract. All drugs within a given therapeutic subgroup are subsidised at the level of the lowest-priced pharmaceutical in that subgroup. From the patient's point of view, this generally means that GP prescription charges are $15 for a 'fully subsidised' pharmaceutical. PHARMAC also negotiates package deals and tenders sole or preferred supply arrangements with individual companies in order to obtain the best possible price for the tax payer and promotes best practice in prescribing to doctors. In September 2001, PHARMAC was given the further responsibility of managing the purchasing of hospital pharmaceuticals on behalf of the DHBs.

PHARMAC has been extremely successful in slowing the rate of growth of GP pharmaceutical expenditure while extending the scope of the schedule. Between 1979/80 and 1997/8, expenditure grew at an average of 10.1% per year. Between 1997/8 and 2001/2, it declined by 0.5% per year while the volume of drugs prescribed rose by 4.5% per year between 1993 and 2002. PHARMAC argues that without its intervention, growth in spending would have averaged about 9% since 1993 and without any better access to subsidised pharmaceuticals.[33] In the same period, Australian spending, for example, has generally risen by at least 10% per annum.[34]

Prioritising patients for surgery

The second initiative related to explicit priority setting was introduced to decide which patients should be given priority among those waiting for the commonest elective procedures. For the most part, patients are assessed on clinical criteria, scored between 0 and 100 and ranked in terms of their 'need' and ability to benefit. A 'clinical threshold' score determines which patients *can* benefit clinically from surgery; a 'financial threshold' score determines which patients in practice *will* be offered surgery from available resources.[35] Those whose scores are above the financial threshold are given certainty of treatment, and a guaranteed maximum wait for surgery (the current goal is no more than six months). Those whose scores fall below the threshold are told that they will not receive publicly funded treatment, but will be reassessed at a later date. This system provides a relatively sophisticated way of managing waiting lists compared with 'first-come-first-served', though it took time to achieve tolerable levels of consistency between clinicians in their scoring.

On its introduction in 1997, the system immediately revealed important disparities between regions in patients' access to services for a given level of clinical 'need' (something which otherwise would have gone unmeasured and unnoticed). The gap between the clinical and financial threshold regionally, and between surgical procedures, promoted public debate over the adequacy of funding which led to an increase in the proportion of public funds devoted to elective surgery. This 'booking system', plus the extra resources, increased the number of operations and reduced the numbers waiting more than six months (one of the government's targets) from 35 000 to 6000 between 1998/9 and 2001/2.[22]

Prioritisation in the future

The devolution of the planning/purchasing function since 2000 means that resource allocation is now in the hands of 21 DHBs. It is unclear whether they will have the capacity to build on the HFA's prioritisation methods – although at least one has started to develop a similar, principles-based prioritisation process,[36] while others have adopted different approaches. Devolution may be seen as incompatible with a national surgical booking system based on a single set of clinical criteria and has coincided with a major change in the electives points scheme. It has recently evolved into a simple 'integrated scoring system' based on a 1–5 point scale used across all surgical areas to determine patient priorities. This is no longer an explicit system, but merely an extension of the usual implicit clinical judgements. Clinicians' judgements of clinical need will be made relative to other patients they typically see – not measured in a manner that enables comparisons with patients elsewhere, which could perpetuate rather than reduce inter-regional inequities in access.[37]

The overall picture suggests a retreat from previous bold and widely heralded initiatives to prioritise explicitly, both in terms of resource allocation between services (HFA) and between patients (electives), in face of the difficulty of reconciling objectivity with the flexibility required to deal with complex aggregate and individual rationing decisions.

The public–private mix in NZ and the UK: parallels, differences and future prospects

While New Zealand is a much smaller (and somewhat poorer) economy than the UK, the two health systems share common objectives and both still use general taxation as the principal means of finance, presenting opportunity for comparison. Both countries have recently attempted to project the effects of changes in demography, medical technology and public expectations on future spending[38,39] and concluded that these pressures can be accommodated within a publicly-financed system (albeit at higher levels of public spending). Greater certainty over future spending paths has been provided in both countries – in the UK, by unprecedented planned growth in NHS spending, financed by an increase in National Insurance contributions (a form of proportional income tax in all but name); in New Zealand, more modestly, by the Government committing to a three-year funding package (2002/3–2004/5) for Vote Health (the non-injury-related public health system), which will amount to a 15% real-terms increase over three years. Both countries are planning for public health service spending to take an increasing share of public spending and of GDP, at least for the next few years. In New Zealand, it is hoped that this will enable a widening of the scope of the public system to include far more of primary care; in the UK, it is planned to use the additional resources to improve the accessibility and timeliness of treatment.

The UK has recently considered, and rejected, the possibility of shifting to an alternative means of generating funds for its public health system, such as social insurance. The Wanless report reiterated that general taxation remained the most efficient and fair means of generating revenue.[39] Similarly, there seems little enthusiasm in New Zealand for moving away from taxation, although the Labour-led government has stated its intention to explore the feasibility of an earmarked 'health tax' to pay for Vote Health rather than relying on general taxes. Unlike the UK, there are no plans to link this to an increase in overall taxation. One possible approach would be simply to ring-fence a proportion of current income tax to pay for Vote Health. By contrast, a recent international review concluded that general taxation remains the most efficient and fair means of raising finance for a public system.[40]

A key difference between New Zealand and the UK has been the presence of user charges for primary healthcare, although New Zealand has begun a long-term process of increasing the public share of primary healthcare finance. Likewise, the intention to remove the asset test from long-term care of older people will increase the public share of disability support funding. The renewed commitment to the publicly financed health system generally in both countries suggests that the share of healthcare accounted for by public sources will be maintained, at least – and possibly increased – in the future.

Ostensibly, both countries have devolved responsibility for budgets and planning from more centralised systems to local levels, while attempting to maintain or even improve equity of access. In New Zealand, the principal administrative unit is the DHB, with boundaries defined by the catchments of *hospitals*. It funds both the hospitals it runs and the primary healthcare services provided by new PHOs. In contrast, the NHS in England and Wales[iv] is now organised around primary care trusts (PCTs), which commission most of the secondary care and other services for their populations.

Both countries embarked on market-inspired reforms in the 1990s. In the UK, the purchaser–provider split took the form of an 'internal market', mostly within the public sector, whereas in New Zealand the split was potentially more ambitious.[9] In both cases, the use of price competition has been rejected – although the use of non-price competition continues to hold appeal for English policy makers. England is set to encourage competition between NHS and private providers – using Health Resource Groups (a DRG-like system) to set national prices that PCTs will use to commission services. In New Zealand, publicly financed hospital services will remain largely within the DHBs' own hospitals. Given the New Zealand government's renewed commitment (since 1999) to a truly 'public' health system and New Zealanders' weariness (and wariness) of reform, it seems likely that the current approach to provision will remain unchanged, with no explicit market incentives to efficiency. Instead, the Minister of Health negotiates a funding agreement with each DHB, through which it receives its weighted capitation budget in return for delivering an agreed range of services to national standards and pursuing the government's performance expectations.[41] DHBs are required to report regularly against each of the performance indicators, though their funding is not performance-related. Though most of the indicators are input-, process- or activity-related (e.g. ensuring the delivery of agreed volumes of elective surgery), some are more outcome- or quality-focused (e.g. low birth weight rate, repeat admissions among children with asthma, number of people waiting more than six months for coronary by-pass grafting). Currently, there are few quantitative targets with timelines attached, unlike in the UK NHS. Elective surgery is a partial exception, with clear waiting time targets, if not specific delivery dates. DHBs are also required to demonstrate that they are encouraging a comprehensive approach to quality improvement.

The prospects for the future public–private mix in *provision* are thus different between the two countries. The provision of NHS-funded healthcare, at least in England, seems likely to tip towards more use of the private sector for at least three reasons. First, the increases in public funding for healthcare[42] and likely bottlenecks in supply mean more use of the private sector both as a stop-gap and a planned supplier. Second, the private sector is increasingly being used to improve service quality – in particular, to meet increasingly ambitious waiting times targets. Related to this are NHS initiatives to improve patient choice: patients who have waited for six months for elective surgery will be offered a choice of treatment in an alternative NHS hospital, a UK private hospital or a hospital elsewhere in Europe. Third, the proposal to permit high-performing NHS hospitals to become 'Foundation Trusts' in the form of public interest, not-for-profit entities at arm's length from the NHS represents another partial shift away from state-owned provision.[v]

In contrast, lower planned spending increases in New Zealand have not created the same supply pressures to use private providers; nor, arguably, do the same opportunities (or pressures) exist from the availability of easily accessible services overseas. There is likely to be an increase in publicly financed care delivered in the private sector in New Zealand, for other reasons, since the new PHOs are non-governmental organisations, albeit not-for-profit and with significant community governance.

Finally, a fundamental question in any cash-limited, tax-financed system that aims to deliver services on the basis of need (rather than ability to pay) – and a question that persists regardless of the amount of vigorous structural change that takes place – is how to ration scarce resources. With refinement, New Zealand's economics-based approach to prioritising services, combined with its 'points system' to determine access to surgery at the patient level, had the potential to provide the most comprehensive, explicit rationing strategy of any country. The 'points system' was a quantum improvement over crude methods of managing waiting lists, such as waiting list and waiting times targets, which continue to be popular in the UK despite their known problems.[35] Similarly, although the inter-service prioritisation process was barely up and running before the HFA was dismantled, its foundation in PBMA offers great potential for other countries to build on. It avoids, for example, the weakness of England's National Institute for Clinical Excellence, which focuses principally on new technologies, leaving the cost-effectiveness of existing practices largely unexamined. Addressing 'who gets what' remains a central challenge for both countries.

Conclusions

New Zealand's attempt to use market forces in publicly financed healthcare had little direct effect on the public–private mix of finance or provision. It also failed to achieve its stated aims. Arguably, this was because it is impossible to mimic the dynamism of a private market when public ownership of providers and political accountability for public funds prevents governments from allowing poor performers either to be taken over by competitors or to go out of business. One plausible verdict is that the quasi-market 'failed' because it was never really implemented, in the same way as its UK counterpart.[43]

The main modest public–private change since 1993 has been in provision – not financing – with the emergence of IPAs and large numbers of Māori and Pacific Island-owned providers of primary care during the quasi-market period in the 1990s. This trend seems likely to continue, as the government's primary care strategy is implemented. It is likely to produce an increasing public share of primary care funding which should, in turn, raise the proportion of public health spending devoted to primary care as well as increasing the public share of total health spending. It remains to be seen whether reduced user charges for primary healthcare, delivered through capitated organisations, will improve equity of access, reduce avoidable admissions and improve management of chronic disease, thereby improving health and reducing health inequalities, as hoped. However, it will bring the contours of New Zealand's public–private mix much closer to those of other countries with similar systems.

The overall performance of New Zealand's publicly financed system probably continued to improve in the 1990s despite the furore over the quasi-market and the disappointing lack of transformative enhancement in efficiency. Although there are still problems of overspending, variations in quality, efficiency and equity of access, there have been improvements on important dimensions such as waiting times for electives, access to pharmaceuticals, infant mortality and life expectancy. Perhaps the most challenging issue for the future relates to the outstanding health differences between socioeconomic and ethnic groups, driven by wider societal influences. Better and more accessible primary care may reduce – but is unlikely to remove – these disparities, which exist in many advanced countries, including those with universal primary healthcare.

Thanks to Grant Johnston, New Zealand Treasury, for helpful comments on an earlier draft of this chapter.

References

1 O'Dea D, Szeto K, Dove S, Tilyard M (1993) *The effect of changes in user charges on visits to New Zealand GPs*. Paper delivered to the New Zealand Association of Economists Conference, Lincoln, Christchurch.

2 Devlin N, Richardson A (1993) The distribution of household expenditure on healthcare. *New Zealand Medical Journal.* 106(953): 126–9.

3 Minister of Health (2001) Primary Health Care Strategy. Wellington: Ministry of Health. Available from URL www.newhealth.govt.nz/primaryhealthcare.htm

4 Ashton T (1999) The health reforms: to market and back? In: Boston K, Dalziel P, St John S (eds) *Redesigning the Welfare State in New Zealand: problems, policies, prospects.* Auckland: Oxford University Press, pp. 134–53.

5 French S, Old A, Healy J (2001) *Health Care Systems in Transition: New Zealand.* Copenhagen: World Health Organization Regional Office for Europe.

6 O'Dea D, Penrose A (1999) *Free child healthcare: economic evaluation of a New Zealand*

experiment. Paper to Inaugural Australia-New Zealand Health Services Research and Policy Conference, Sydney.

7 Minister of Health (2002) Implementing the primary care strategy and improving access to primary care services. Memorandum to Cabinet Social Policy and Health Committee. Available from URL www.executive.govt.nz/minister/king/cabinet02–03/index.html

8 Ashton T (2000) New Zealand long-term care in a decade of change. *Health Affairs.* 19(3): 72–85.

9 Scott C (2001) *Public and Private Roles in Healthcare Systems.* Buckingham: Open University Press.

10 Ministry of Health (2002) *Health Expenditure Trends in New Zealand, 1980–2000.* Wellington: Ministry of Health. Available from URL www.moh.govt.nz

11 Health Funds Association of New Zealand Inc. (2001) *An Insight into the New Zealand Health Insurance Industry.* Wellington: Health Funds Association.

12 Minister of Health (2000) District Health Boards and the non-government health sector. Memorandum to Cabinet Social Policy and Health Committee. Available from URL www.executive.govt.nz/minister/king/cabinet11–00/index.html

13 Vaithianathan R (1999) The failure of corporatisation: public hospitals in New Zealand. *Agenda.* 6(4): 325–38.

14 Health Boards New Zealand Inc. (1991) *Study Tour.* Wellington: Health Boards New Zealand.

15 Devlin N, O'Dea D (1998) Hospitals. In: Pickford M, Bollard A (eds) *The Structure and Dynamics of New Zealand Industries.* Palmerston North: The Dunmore Press, pp. 287–322.

16 Johnston G, Lynn R (2001) Cuts both ways: elective surgery in private and public hospitals. Wellington: The Treasury and Ministry of Health, unpublished draft.

17 Keen J, Light D, Mays N (2001) *Public–Private Relations in Health Care.* London: King's Fund Publishing.

18 Devlin N, Maynard A, Mays N (2001) New Zealand's health sector reforms: back to the future? *British Medical Journal.* 322(7295): 1171–4.

19 Hospital and Related Services Taskforce (1988) *Unshackling the Hospitals.* Wellington: Hospital and Related Services Taskforce.

20 Upton S (1991) *Your Health and the Public Health: a statement of Government policy.* Wellington: Minister of Health.

21 Hornblow A, Barnett P (2000) A turbulent decade: lessons from the 'health reforms'. *New Zealand Medical Journal.* 113(1108): 133–4.

22 Ministry of Health (2002) Health and independence report, 2002. Wellington: Ministry of Health. Available from URL www.moh.govt.nz

23 Stent R (1998) *Canterbury Health Limited: report by the Health and Disability Commissioner.* Auckland: Health and Disability Commissioner.

24 Hornblow A (1997) New Zealand's health reforms: a clash of cultures. *British Medical Journal.* 314(7098): 1892–4.

25 Malcolm L, Wright L, Barnett P (1999) *The Development of Primary Care Organisations in New Zealand.* Wellington: Ministry of Health. Available from URL www.moh.govt.nz

26 Alford R (1975) *Health Care Politics.* Chicago: Chicago University Press.

27 Moore C, Frater P (1986) *Report on a Study of Private and Public Hospital Surgical Care and Private Medical Insurance.* Wellington: Business and Economic Research Limited.

28 Ministry of Health (1996) *Purchasing For Your Health, 1994/95: a performance report on the second year of the Regional Health Authorities and the Public Health Commission.* Wellington: Contract Monitoring Unit, Ministry of Health.

29 Ministry of Health (1998) *Purchasing For Your Health, 1996/97.* Wellington: Performance Management Unit, Ministry of Health.

30 Easton B (1997) *The Commercialisation of New Zealand.* Auckland: Auckland University Press.

31 Health Funding Authority (1998) *How shall we prioritise our health and disability support services?* A Discussion Paper. Wellington: Health Funding Authority.

32 Ashton T, Devlin N, Cumming J (2000) Priority setting in New Zealand – translating principles into practice. *Journal of Health Services Research and Policy.* **5**(3): 170–5.

33 Pharmaceutical Management Agency (PHARMAC) (2002) Statement of intent, 1 July 2002 to 30 June 2003. Wellington: Pharmaceutical Management Agency. Available from URL www.pharmac.govt.nz/pdf/SOI2003.pdf

34 Pharmaceutical Benefits Scheme (2002) Cost to Government of Pharmaceutical Benefits. Canberra: Department of Health and Ageing. Available from URL www.health.gov.au/pbs/pbs/phbeninf.htm

35 Derrett S, Devlin N, Harrison A (2002) Waiting in the NHS: Part 2 – a change of prescription. *Journal of the Royal Society of Medicine.* **95**(6): 280–3.

36 Adam B, Devlin N, Buckingham K (2002) Developing an integrated approach to priority setting and planning in the new health system. *Health Manager.* **8**(4): 4–6.

37 Derrett S (2002) Surgical prioritisation and rationing: some recent developments. *New Zealand Bioethics Journal.* **2**(3): 3–6.

38 Johnston G, Teasdale A (1999) *Population ageing and health spending: 50-year projections.* Occasional Paper No. 2. Wellington: Ministry of Health.

39 HM Treasury (2002) *Securing our Future Health: taking a long-term view – final report.* Chair: Sir Derek Wanless. London: HM Treasury.

40 Mossialos E, Dixon A, Figueras J, Kutzin J (eds) *Funding Health Care: options for Europe.* Buckingham: Open University Press.

41 Ministry of Health (2003) Operational policy framework, effective 1 July 2003. Wellington: Ministry of Health. Available from URL www.moh.govt.nz

42 Chancellor of the Exchequer (2002) The Budget. London: HM Treasury.

43 Le Grand J, Mays N, Dixon J (1998) The reforms: success or failure or neither? In: Le Grand J, Mays N, Mulligan J-A (eds) *Learning from the NHS Internal Market: a review of the evidence.* London: King's Fund Publishing, pp. 117–43.

44 Ashton T (1996) *Contracting for health services in New Zealand: early experiences.* Paper to International Health Economics Association Inaugural Conference, Vancouver.

45 Mays N, Hand K (2002) A review of options for health and disability support purchasing in New Zealand. Treasury Working Paper 00/20. Wellington: The Treasury. Available from URL www.treasury.govt.nz/workingpapers/2000/00–20.pdf

46 Organisation for Economic Cooperation and Development (1996) *New Zealand.* Paris: OECD.

47 Ministry of Health (2001) *Health and Independence Report, 2001.* Wellington: Ministry of Health. Available from URL www.moh.govt.nz

48 Ashby M (1996) *Performance improvement in the health sector.* Paper to New Zealand Institute of Management Conference.

49 Organisation for Economic Cooperation and Development (2001) *OECD Health Data 2001: a comparative analysis of 30 countries.* Paris: OECD.

50 Ashton T, Press D (1997) Market concentration in secondary health services under a purchaser-provider split: the New Zealand experience. *Health Economics.* **6**(1): 43–56.

51 Ministry of Health (1997) *Purchasing For Your Health, 1995/96.* Wellington: Ministry of Health.

52 Ministerial Inquiry into the Under-Reporting of Cervical Smear Abnormalities in the Gisbourne Region (2001) *Report.* Wellington: Ministerial Inquiry into the Under-Reporting of Cervical Smear Abnormalities in the Gisbourne Region.

53 Russell M, Burns P, Gilbert A, Slack A, Gendall K, Cangialose C *et al.* (2001) *Evaluation of Ten National Demonstration Integrated Care Pilot Projects. Ten reports to the Ministry of Health.* Wellington: Health Services Research Centre, Victoria University of Wellington.

54 Lovatt D (1996) Lessons from contestability. *Health Manager.* **3**: 12–15.

55 Ashton T (1998) Contracting for health services in New Zealand: a transaction cost analysis. *Social Science and Medicine.* **46**(3): 357–67.

56 Cumming J, Mays N (2002) Reform and counter-reform: how sustainable is New Zealand's latest health system restructuring? *Journal of Health Services Research and Policy.* **7**(Suppl): 46–55.

57 Ministry of Health (2001) *Health Expenditure Trends in New Zealand 1980–2000.* Wellington: Ministry of Health. Available from URL www.moh.govt.nz

Endnotes

i This can be explained principally by people buying 'gap' insurance to meet their out-of-pocket GP visit and prescription expenses.

ii In 1999/2000 dollars, spending on healthcare funded by private insurance *per person covered* was $98 in 1989/90 compared with $432 in 1999/2000 (derived from MoH 2002, Table 4B; coverage assumed to be 51% and 34% respectively).

iii The NHS in Scotland and Northern Ireland is organised differently at local level without primary care-led purchasing.

iv The Treaty of Waitangi is an agreement between Māori (the indigenous people of New Zealand) and the Crown. Honouring the Treaty is an important goal of economic and social policy. It is particularly important in health policy because the health of Māori is poor relative to that of non-Māori New Zealanders.

v If anything, the trend in relation to NZ's public hospitals is in the opposite direction after a period in the 1990s when public hospitals were set up and treated as autonomous publicly owned companies. For example, the extent of their freedom to raise private debt has been progressively reduced in the past few years just as the NHS is experimenting with giving some of its hospitals greater financial freedoms. The NZ rationale for this appears to have had little influence on the debate in the UK.

Chapter 12

The role of the private sector in the Australian healthcare system

Jane Hall and Elizabeth Savage

Introduction

The Australian healthcare system presents a complex set of arrangements and interactions between the public and private sectors. Government health policy objectives include the provision of tax-financed medical services, medicines and acute healthcare for all Australians under Medicare. Most Australians interpret this as meaning no substantial barriers to the use of health services. Alongside this sits another government goal that explicitly supports the private sector, 'Choice through private health: a viable private health industry to improve the choice of health services for Australians'.[1] Perhaps it is not surprising that the relationship between the two sectors is complex and at times uneasy.

Since 1996, the Australian government has designed and implemented a strategy to support and expand the role of private health insurance. The result has been that that the proportion of the population covered by private health insurance has grown from just over 30% to 45% of the population in a surprisingly short time. This is remarkable, taken in the context of a very limited role for private health insurance (it covers only private in-hospital treatment and some ancillary services) and universal access without user fees to public hospitals. Yet the history of the Australian health system demonstrates a private sector developing from within, and often protected by, government; private practice publicly supported, as one commentator has described it.[2] At the beginning of European settlement in Australia, there was no private sector; salaried medical practitioners were employed to provide for convicts and the military, within government-owned and operated hospitals. Since then, healthcare providers have sought to influence public policy and to encourage the growth of the private sector in healthcare.[3]

Here we consider the interplay of the public and private sectors in the Australian healthcare system. First we describe the overall structure and funding flows, focusing on hospitals, private insurance, pharmaceuticals and general practice. Developments in private health insurance cannot be understood without some sense of the role and funding of hospitals. We then explain the development, implementation and impact of health insurance policy in the past seven years. The Pharmaceutical Benefits Scheme (PBS) has captured worldwide attention, since the introduction of the requirement that new products are demonstrated to be cost-effective before being accepted into the scheme. There have been several strategies employed to restrict the growth in pharmaceutical expenditure, but nonetheless, this remains the fastest-growing area of the health budget. Finally, the supply of medical services, particularly general practitioners (GPs), has become a major policy issue during 2003. Whereas only two years ago, the number of GPs was considered in excess of requirements, there is now widespread acceptance that there is an absolute shortage, and that remuneration for non-specialist medical services has fallen in real terms and is inadequate. The Government response addresses not only fee levels but also measures that would change the structure and funding of medical care, by allowing for private insurance coverage of some part of medical costs.

Background: structure and funding

In 2001–2, total Australian health expenditure was estimated at $66.6 billion, or 9.3% of GDP.[4] Australia is a federation of states and territories, in which the Commonwealth Government funds 46% of total (recurrent and capital) health spending, the six state and two territory governments 22.3%, bringing the government total share close to 70%. Figure 12.1 summarises the structure and major flow of funds in the Australian system.

The Australian Government has responsibility for medical services and pharmaceutical benefits. The six State and two Territory governments own and operate public hospitals, but there is a significant Commonwealth contribution to public hospital operating costs, negotiated through five-yearly agreements (previously the Medicare Agreements and now known as the Australian Health Care Agreements). The overall financial implications of the complex interactions between public and private sectors and different levels of government are shown in Table 12.1 for the year 2001/2. The net private health insurance contribution to total recurrent expenditure, at 8.1% of total recurrent spending, was about one-quarter of the private finance component, the remainder being primarily individual out-of-pocket expenses.[4]

Most medical services are provided by private practitioners, paid by fee-for-service with a fixed rate of reimbursement from the Commonwealth government through Medicare. There is no control of fee levels, but in fixing the Medical Benefits Schedule (MBS), the Australian government effectively determines a floor price for medical services. Practitioners may direct-bill Medicare (known as bulk-billing in Australia) for out-of-hospital services. In this case they receive 85% of the MBS fee, and the patient incurs no out-of-pocket charge. If the practitioner does not bulk-bill, the patient must pay the total fee upfront and claim the Medicare rebate from the government. Any charge above 85% of the MBS fee is met by the patient as a co-payment and, for out-of-hospital services, this cannot be covered by insurance. The levels of co-payment vary by area of residence and specialty (rural and remote area residents and patients requiring specialist surgical, medical, obstetrics and anaesthetics tend to face higher co-payments). GPs play an important gatekeeping role in the system, as referral is essential for any reimbursement of specialist services, including diagnostic tests, and therefore most hospital admissions. Consumers are able to choose their own medical provider. GPs comprise 40% of active medical practitioners. In 1998, 14.5% of GPs worked in solo practices, and of practices, 40.5% had one and

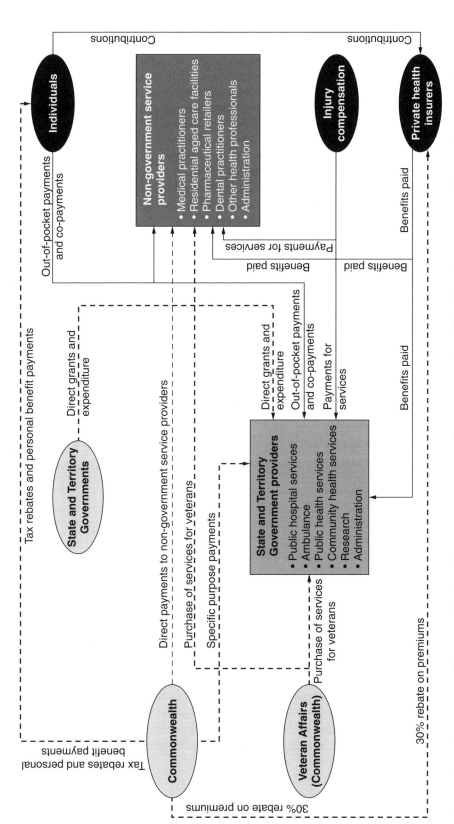

Figure 12.1 The structure of the Australian health system. *Source:* Australian Institute of Health and Welfare (2002) *Health Expenditure Australia 2000–2001*, Figure 1, p. 4.

Table 12.1 Percentage distribution of recurrent expenditure by funding source: 2001/2

Area of expenditure	Commonwealth	Other Government	Private insurance	Individual out-of-pocket	Other	Total
Public hospitals	12.7	12.3	0.4	0.4	0.8	26.6
Private hospitals	2.7	0.0	3.9	0.5	1.1	8.2
Public psychiatric hospitals	0.0	0.6	0.0	0.0	0.0	0.7
Residential aged care	4.9	0.3	0.0	1.3	0.0	6.6
Ambulance	0.2	0.8	0.2	0.4	0.1	1.7
Medical services	14.4	0.0	0.7	1.9	0.8	17.8
Other professional services	0.9	0.0	0.5	2.3	0.4	4.0
Benefit-paid pharmaceutical	7.6	0.0	0.0	1.3	0.0	8.9
All other pharmaceuticals	0.1	0.0	0.1	5.1	0.1	5.4
Aids and appliances	0.3	0.0	0.4	3.1	0.1	3.8
Community and public health	1.0	4.3	0.0	0.0	0.0	5.3
Dental services	0.5	0.6	1.1	3.7	0.0	5.9
Administration	1.6	0.6	0.8	0.0	0.0	3.0
Other (nec)	0.0	0.0	0.0	0.0	0.0	0.0
Research	1.3	0.3	0.0	0.0	0.4	2.0
Total recurrent expenditure	48.5	19.7	8.1	20.0	3.7	100.0

Source: Australian Institute of Health and Welfare, Health Expenditure Australia 2001–2002, Table M, p. 76.

41.3% had two to four practitioners. In the same year there was an average of 6.4 GP consultations per person.[1]

Medical services provided to private hospital inpatients are also billed on a fee-for-service basis, by the medical practitioner, with Medicare benefits covering 75% of the MBS fee set by the government. The gap between 75% of the MBS fee and the amount charged by the doctor is either funded by private insurance or paid by the patient as an out-of-pocket expense. Prior to 2000, regulations prevented private health insurance from insuring the gap between the doctor's charge and MBS fee. Public hospitals treat private as well as public patients, with medical services funded in the same way as private hospital patients.

All Australian residents are entitled to free public hospital treatment anywhere in Australia. Public patients treated in public hospitals forego choice of medical provider (in theory) and are treated by specialists paid by the hospital. These specialists may be private practitioners, in which case they are paid on a sessional (or hourly) basis for treatment of public patients, or salaried staff specialists who also have rights to private practice and to access the MBS income derived from it.

Dental services are almost entirely privately provided, under fee-for-service private practice arrangements. State and territory governments operate some public dental services with an emphasis on emergency care for low-income groups. The Commonwealth initiated a public dental health programme for prevention and treatment for the same target group in 1994 but it was discontinued in 1996.[5]

Private insurance was established first by the hospitals, in 1932, and then by doctors, in 1946, as a means of reducing the problem of bad debts. Insurance is now highly regulated. Community rating, namely that premiums are not related to age or experience, has been a feature of Australian health insurance since the 1950s, though recent developments have weakened this provision, as described further below. Insurance funds (with a few special funds excluded) must accept all purchasers for each policy type offered. In addition, all increases in premiums must have government approval and applications for increases are considered once each year.

Private health insurance is limited to covering private treatment in either a public or private hospital, to a portion of the medical fees charged for private in-hospital treatment, prostheses and devices provided to private inpatients, and to ancillary services, which include dental care, allied health services such as physiotherapy, complementary care such as chiropractic and acupuncture, and some associated preventive activities such as gym membership and sports equipment. Annual premiums vary depending on the extent of cover, the front-end deductible and the state of residence. Private health insurance coverage of the population is currently 43.4% (June 2003); it reached its highest rate of 68% in 1981 but it has not fallen below 30% since 1984 and the introduction of universal free public hospital treatment.

Hospitals – the interplay of public and private interests

Hospitals developed from charitable institutions, which operated nursing facilities for the care of the poor and in which medical practitioners provided their services for free. Honorary medical officers were specialists otherwise in private, fee-for-service practice and had the highest standing in the medical profession. Developments in the effectiveness of medical and nursing care had two effects: a growth in costs, for which the charities turned to state governments for assistance; and a growth in clientele for whom charges were introduced: an intermediate level of care for the respectable working class, and private care for those who could afford (relative) luxury.

Once the Commonwealth government gained the power to raise income taxes (1942), it had greater revenue-raising capacity than the states. What followed (in 1945) was the provision of Commonwealth funds to the states to support their public hospitals, and the five-yearly agreements on hospital funding between the Commonwealth and the states and territories continue as the basis for the Commonwealth contribution to the public hospital component of Medicare.

Complex incentives can arise from the payment contracts for medical practitioners in hospitals. For example, staff specialists in New South Wales (NSW) public hospitals, although paid a salary by the public hospital, have the right of private practice. The hospital bills the Commonwealth government for the MBS fee in the name of the staff specialist. MBS fees are paid into a trust fund nominated by the specialist. The hospital charges a management and facility fee and the remaining funds can be spent by member specialists of the trust fund either on service-related items, such as specialised equipment, conference expenses and the employment of research staff, or drawn as additional salary. Arrangements vary from state to state, but in NSW the government offers five different schemes allowing specialists to forego varying amounts of salary in return for access to a specified maximum amount of income from the trust fund. For example, a staff specialist may elect to forego 14% of salary in return for a maximum draw of 24% of salary from the trust fund. If there are insufficient funds in the trust to pay the contracted amount, within certain bounds the hospital will top up the payment by reducing the facility fee drawn from the trust fund.

While state and territory governments determine, and can cap, public hospital operating budgets, private patients generate additional revenue for public hospitals from private insurance funds and out-of-pocket charges. As this revenue is treated more flexibly than state-provided budgetary funds, the state and territory governments, the public hospitals and the medical practitioners have an incentive to treat private patients at the margin.

Developments in the hospital sector

In 2001–2, the private hospital sector was responsible for 28% of all hospital bed-days and 36% of separations, up from 32% in 1996–7. Since 1996–7, total hospital separations have increased by 20%, with a 4% increase in bed-days. The use of private hospitals has increased since the implementation of the insurance incentives, though the extent to which increased usage of private hospitals has displaced public hospital activity is not clear. In the four years from 1996–7 to 2001–2, public-patient separations in public hospitals grew by 12%; the corresponding growth rate for private separations in private hospitals was 39%. Figure 12.2 shows trends in patient numbers over a longer period. It shows small annual increases in the total number of patients treated in public hospitals in recent years, with private patient numbers falling.

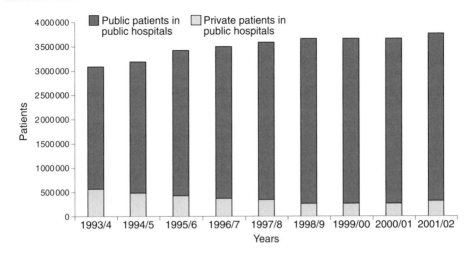

Figure 12.2 Public hospital separations by patient type, 1993–2002. *Source*: Australian Institute of Health and Welfare (2003) *Australian Hospital Statistics 2001–02*, Table 6.5 and earlier issues. *Note*: Excludes separations for status not reported, those ineligible for Medicare, and compensable and Department of Veterans Affairs separations.

Figure 12.3 shows private-patient separations over the same period. There has been a fall in the number of private patients treated in public hospitals over time but this has been outweighed by the increase in those treated in private hospitals. Further, the share of acute hospital activity contributed by private hospitals had been increasing steadily prior to the private health insurance incentives; for the ten years prior to 1995–6 separations had increased by 80% (compared to 46% in the public sector), and bed-days by 24% (compared to 3% in the public sector).

The ownership of private hospitals is for-profit, publicly listed corporate groups (41% of beds); not-for-profit, religious or charitable bodies (37% of beds);

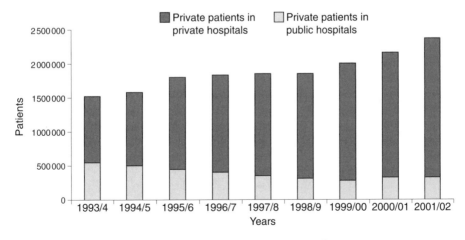

Figure 12.3 Private patient hospital separations by hospital type, 1993–2002. *Source*: Australian Institute of Health and Welfare (2003) *Australian Hospital Statistics 2001–02*, Table 6.5 and earlier issues. *Note*: Excludes separations for status not reported, those ineligible for Medicare, and compensable and Department of Veterans Affairs separations.

independent for-profit (8%); for-profit groups but not publicly listed (7%); and other not-for-profit (7%). The size and nature of the private hospital sector has changed quite significantly over the past 15 years. For-profit corporate ownership has expanded (from 5% of beds) and become the major form of private hospital ownership, overtaking the religious hospitals. These corporations are large national and international private healthcare interests; Mayne has 50 private hospitals and there are four other groups with between 12 and 17 hospitals each.[6] They are also expanding through vertical integration. For example, Mayne's pathology and radiology interests generate turnover from diagnostic services of $300 million annually, and they have also been buying private general practices. Some private hospitals have developed the capacity to treat complex cases with sophisticated diagnostic and therapeutic technology, and some now operate emergency departments.

There have been a number of new private hospitals located in the grounds of major public hospitals, although the pace of development seems to have slowed. These facilities, with hotel-style amenities, provide a marked contrast to the often run-down state of the public hospital. The private hospitals concentrate on profitable elective surgical care; day surgery comprises 50% of their workload. What evidence there is does not suggest that the private hospitals are more efficient than public hospitals; costs per case, lengths of stay and procedure rates are higher in the private compared to the public sector. The co-location of public and private hospitals seems of most benefit to the doctors, enabling them to combine private and public practice more easily.

There have also been attempts to use private-sector finance and expertise in the building and operating of public hospitals. The first development was in NSW at Port Macquarie in 1994, when the Hospital Corporation of Australia (later Mayne) was contracted to build and operate a new public hospital. The NSW government predicted cost savings in both building and running the hospital and that the use of private finance would enable an earlier start to the building. However, an independent report by the Auditor-General in 1996 concluded that the arrangement would cost an additional $143 million over 20 years, by which time the ownership of the buildings and the land would have been lost. Not only were the arrangements more expensive from the state government perspective, costs were also transferred to the Commonwealth government through shifting to fee-for-service private practice. Similar findings have been reported from Victoria, South Australia and Western Australia experiments.[6]

Commonwealth funding to private hospitals now represents 2.7% of total recurrent healthcare expenditure, principally through insurance subsidies. Direct private health insurance payments still represent private hospitals' major revenue source, although their share has fallen markedly. In 1994–5, the private insurance share of private hospital recurrent funding was over eight times the Commonwealth's contribution; by 2001–2 it had dropped to only 1.5 times this figure.

The relationship between private and public specialist medical practice has been further complicated by recent developments in medical indemnity insurance. Most specialist practice combines both public treatment (through public hospitals) and private practice, which may occur in consulting rooms, private hospitals or day surgery facilities, or public hospitals or any combination. During 2002, the largest insurer for medical practice went into liquidation, primarily because premiums charged did not fund exposure to claims, leaving many practitioners without insurance not only for their current practice but also for any previous claims. This was not the only insurance fund failure in the poorly regulated Australian market at the time – the building industry was similarly hardly hit – and it offers an interesting case study of how different healthcare is considered to be. State and territory governments moved quickly to accept liability for all public hospital work, and the Commonwealth government provided guarantees for the continuation of current malpractice cover. What has remained at issue is the liability 'tail', for claims not yet registered for which the amount is unknown and unfunded. The government response that doctors be levied to meet the shortfall has received a hostile reaction from the profession. At the time of writing, non-salaried specialists were refusing to renew their contracts with public hospitals, precipitating a medical staffing crisis and the image of hospitals cancelling urgent surgery and turning away patients. The Commonwealth government is taking responsibility for resolving the problem, and has promised interim funding arrangements and further negotiations to get the doctors back to work.

Private health insurance

About 43% of the Australian population was covered by private health insurance at the end of June 2003.[7] Sixty per cent of those are covered by insurance policies with front-end deductibles (FED). There are currently 44 registered health insurance funds, 38 of which are not-for-profit. Community rating has been a feature of Australian private health insurance since the post-World War II period; this requires that individuals pay the same premium for the same level of cover, irrespective of risk class, and that families pay double the corresponding single premium. Recent changes under the private health insurance incentives have weakened this provision (as explained further below), but the principle that individuals should pay the same over the life cycle, irrespective of risk factors, remains.

The current impact of insurance premiums across families is illustrated in Table 12.2. In general, the premiums comprise small shares of income except for the median-income single person aged over 65. However, out-of-pocket expenditure as a proportion of income is considerably higher for 1998–9, the year of the most recently available Household Expenditure Survey (Figure 12.4). Out-of-pocket expenditure was over 10.5% of income in the lowest quintile, falling to 2.5 for the top 20% of households. Figure 12.4 also shows the value of publicly provided health services as a percentage of income for each income quintile, estimated by the Australian Bureau of Statistics according to average utilisation rates for location and the age and sex of household members. The regressive nature of out-of-pocket expenditure contrasts with the progressive nature of public health benefits. For the lowest income quintile, the average value of imputed indirect health benefits arising from public sector expenditure is approximately 50% of income, while for the top quintile it is 4% of income, reflecting the concentration of those aged above 65 at lower income levels. Figure 12.5 shows how total health benefits for each quintile are broken down between those privately and publicly provided.

Table 12.2 Health insurance premiums as a percentage of income for selected households, 2002

| Family type | Median income $A/year | Hospital cover | | | Ancillary cover | |
		Basic no FED (% income)	Top no FED (% income)		Narrow (% income)	Broad (% income)
Single person, aged <35	26 783	2.4	2.9		1.0	1.5
Single person, aged >65	11 910	5.4	6.6		2.3	3.3
Couple with dependants, youngest <5	54 612	2.4	2.9		1.0	1.4
Couple with dependants, youngest 15–24	73 712	1.7	2.1		0.7	1.1

Source: Australian Bureau of Statistics website (www.abs.gov.au) AusStats: Income and Welfare – Household Income from 1999–2000 Survey of Income and Housing Costs, indexed to 2003 using Average Weekly Earnings series of All Employees Total Earnings.

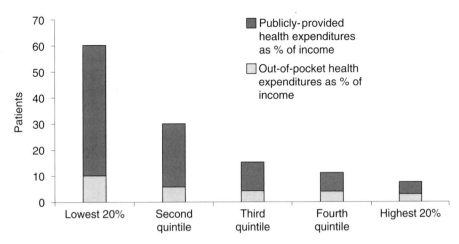

Figure 12.4 Out-of-pocket health expenditures and publicly provided health benefits as a percentage of income by income quintile, 1998–9. *Source*: *ABS Household Expenditure Survey 1998–9.*

The purchase of private insurance coverage is strongly related to income. Table 12.3 presents insurance coverage by income quintile of the population for 1998–9 and also shows the coverage in 2001 for the lowest and highest quintiles. The coverage rate in the top quintile of the distribution was 76% in 1998 and 80% in 2001, while that in the lowest quintile was 20% in 1998 and 26% in 2001. Major growth has been in the middle quintiles. The insurance coverage of households in the top quintile was very high before the incentives, reflecting much higher levels of income. The average income of the top quintile is almost double that of the next highest quintile and approximately 12 times that of the lowest 20%.

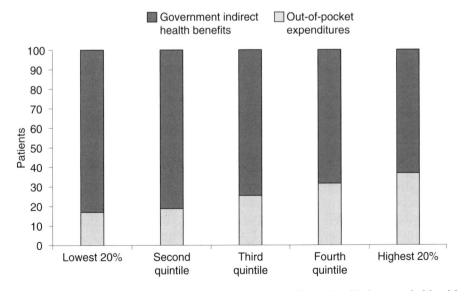

Figure 12.5 Percentage breakdown of out-of-pocket health and publicly provided health benefits by income quintile, 1998–9. *Source*: *ABS Household Expenditure Survey 1998–9.*

Table 12.3 Insurance coverage of the population by income quintile

	Quintile				
Year	1	2	3	4	5
1998*	20%	27%	40%	50%	76%
2001†	26%	–	–	–	80%

* 1998 data from *ABS Household Expenditure Survey 1998–9.*
† 2001 data for quintiles 1 and 5 from *National Health Survey Summary of Results 2001*, Table 24, p. 61.

Prior to 1975, government-subsidised voluntary private health insurance for both hospital and medical benefits covered most of the population. Free treatment at public hospitals and by primary care medical practitioners was means tested. Publicly funded insurance was introduced in 1975 (Medibank), then successively dismantled until most people were again covered by tax-subsidised private insurance and free public services were means tested. In 1984, universal public insurance was re-established. Prior to Medibank and between Medibank and Medicare, around 70% of the population held private health insurance, with 15% eligible for public treatment, and the remainder with no insurance against healthcare costs. The proportion of the population with insurance for private hospital treatment had been dropping steadily since the beginning of the 1980s, i.e. even prior to Medicare, and by the mid-1990s it had fallen below 40%. Between 1989–90 and 1995–6, premium costs had risen by 9.8% per annum, while the corresponding CPI increase was 2.8%.[8] Not only were costs rising rapidly but also those people who actually used it found themselves facing unpredictable and sometimes large out-of-pocket expenses from practitioners who charged above the MBS fee.

At the same time, public hospitals were under increasing pressure. Two of the three major components of the Australian healthcare system, medical care and pharmaceuticals, are open-ended in terms of expenditure. Public hospital expenditure, under the budgetary control of the state/territory governments, could be capped, and this is what governments did during the 1980s and 1990s.

Developments in private health insurance

The Australian government acted to stem falling insurance coverage by introducing incentives for low-income individuals/families to take out private cover and a tax surcharge for high-income earners without it. At the same time, the state of the private health insurance industry was referred to the Industry Commission.[8] Their analysis of the industry indicated that the largest component of the increase in premiums (40%) was contributed by increases in private hospital benefits per bed day, followed by a shift by the insured to obtaining treatment in private, rather than public, hospitals (27%) As the coverage rate declined, the average age of the insured population was increasing. It would seem that private health insurance was faced with a classic adverse selection problem, and that was certainly the diagnosis accepted by the Commission in its review. Its findings established the context for a further two stages of incentives to support private insurance.

The current strategy has been refined through three major stages. The first step, introduced in July 1997, was labelled the carrot-and-stick policy, as it used incentives and penalties. The carrot involved an income-tested rebate, which made private health insurance more affordable for those with low income. The maximum rebate ranged from $100 for a single person with hospital-only cover to $450 for a family with both hospital and ancillary cover. The taxable income thresholds were $35 000 for a single person and $70 000 for a couple. The threshold increased by $3000 for each dependent child after the first. The stick focused on high-income groups who were penalised though a Medicare levy surcharge for not having private insurance. Those without hospital insurance had their tax increased by an additional 1% of taxable income, a levy imposed on single taxpayers with annual taxable incomes greater than $50 000 and families with combined taxable income greater than $100 000. The threshold increased by $1500 for each dependent child after the first. High-income individuals face a negative effective premium if their tax surcharge exceeds the insurance premium.

In January 1999 the means test was removed and anyone purchasing private insurance received a 30% subsidy, paid either as a tax rebate or as a reduced purchase price of insurance. The rebate applied to expenses for ancillary services (dental, optical, chiropractic, etc.) as well as to hospital care. The final step was the introduction, in July 2000, of what is known as Lifetime Health Cover. Until then, all private health insurance had been community rated, i.e. anyone could purchase the same cover at an identical price irrespective of age, gender or other risk factors. Under Lifetime Health Cover, the base premium is applied to those purchasing insurance up until the age of 30. Those who have continuous private health insurance cover from 30 on continue to pay the base rate, but individuals joining beyond 30 pay an age-related premium calculated at 2% on top of the base premium for every year of age, up to the age of 65.

The government's solution to the private health insurance problem was to secure a reduction in the costs of premiums (the 30% rebate), limit the out-of-pocket costs faced by the insured patient (the introduction of no gap policies), and encourage younger people to join and maintain their fund membership (Lifetime Health Cover).

Voluntary health insurance can be regarded as supplementary where it provides higher quality or fewer delays in treatment than the public system, or complementary where it covers services excluded from the public scheme.[9] From the introduction of Medicare, Australian health insurance filled a supplementary role. Certainly, it was originally envisaged as a luxury good, and population coverage could be left to decline until it reached some stable level, which was expected to be somewhere between 30% (because that was the experience in Queensland where public hospitals had provided universal free treatment since the post-war period) and 10% or less (based on the UK experience). However, it is important to note that private insurance was not proscribed as in Canada, even though Canadian Medicare provided the basic model for Australian Medicare. Private insurance was seen as providing something of a safety valve for pressures in the public system.

Medicare was established in the face of fierce political and medical opposition. At its most extreme, doctors withdrew their services from NSW public services.

Health policy had remained a significant difference between the two major political parties since the 1970s. Even after Medicare was established and popular, the Liberal (conservative) Party maintained a policy of repealing the Medicare legislation and returning to private health insurance for a period of over 20 years, but this changed following their election loss in 1993, which was partly attributed to their plans to dismantle Medicare. The Liberals won the 1996 election with a health policy of continuing Medicare and supporting private health insurance.

By the mid-1990s, the health system was portrayed as in crisis. On 7 February 1996, the *Sydney Morning Herald* proclaimed, 'It is no accident Medicare has come to resemble the people it serves – the only difference is our national health system is sicker than we are'. And the fundamental cause of the crisis was seen to be people eschewing private insurance and relying on the public hospital system: 'The decline of private health funds has been blamed for significantly increasing the pressure on public hospitals, with those leaving private funds joining public waiting lists' (*The Age*, 23 September 1998). In this way the 'health policy' problem was constructed as the need for more private health insurance to complement and take pressure off the public system, although this was not stated as an explicit objective of the policy changes. In fact, it was unlikely that higher insurance would reduce public hospital utilisation, as there were waiting lists, and individuals remained eligible for free treatment. Now, the policy objective, as quoted in the introduction to this chapter, is framed in terms of choice.

The impact of the insurance strategy

The timing of the policy changes and the private health insurance coverage of the population are presented in Figure 12.6. There was little change in the proportion of the population with private health insurance following the first step of the private insurance incentives. Pursuant to the second stage, the universal 30% subsidy to private health insurance, the decline in insurance coverage was arrested; and after the announcement of Lifetime Health Cover, insurance coverage increased dramatically from 32% to 45% of the population. In fact, as the deadline for purchasing insurance at the base premium approached, and encouraged by a comprehensive media campaign, the insurance funds were so swamped with applications that the deadline had to be extended to give sufficient time for processing. Just under 44% of the population now has insurance for private hospital treatment; the coverage for ancillary services is slightly lower at 41.5% (March 2003).

In 1995 the regulatory structure had been changed to allow private health insurers to contract with hospitals and individual doctors on price, with the aim of reducing patients' out-of-pocket health expenditure – a change opposed by the medical profession.[10] Further legislation enacted in 2000 as part of the private health insurance incentives allowed health funds to eliminate gaps without the need for doctors to enter into contracts. The level of no-gap services has been increasing since their introduction; by mid-2003, 81% of all in-hospital private medical services did not attract out-of-pocket payments.

The cost of the 30% rebate was $2.1 billion in 2000–1,[11] making health insurance one of Australia's most heavily subsidised industries.[12] Insurance

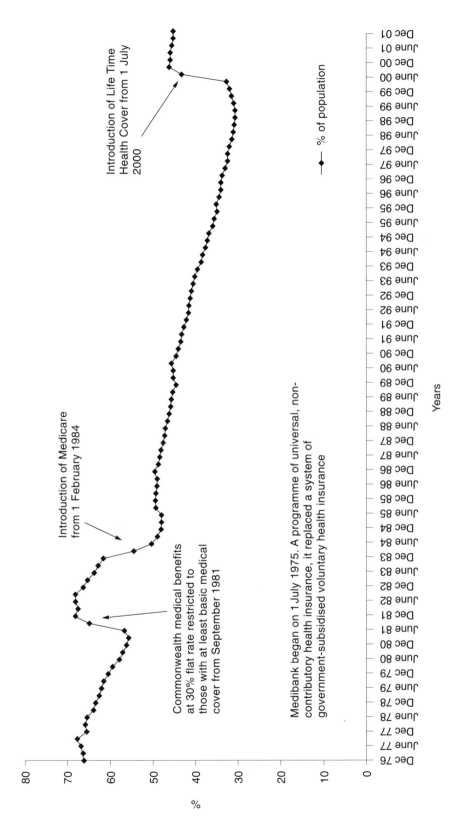

Figure 12.6 Total hospital insurance coverage of the population and the timing of the private health insurance incentives.

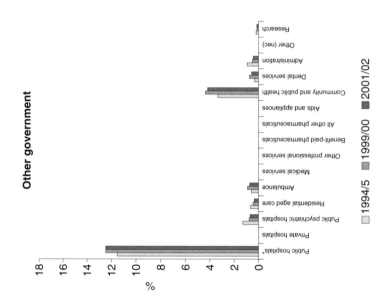

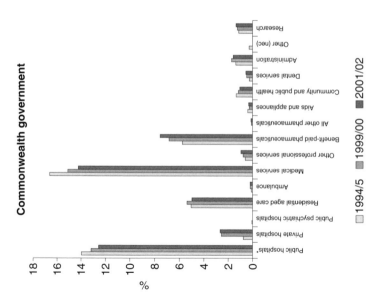

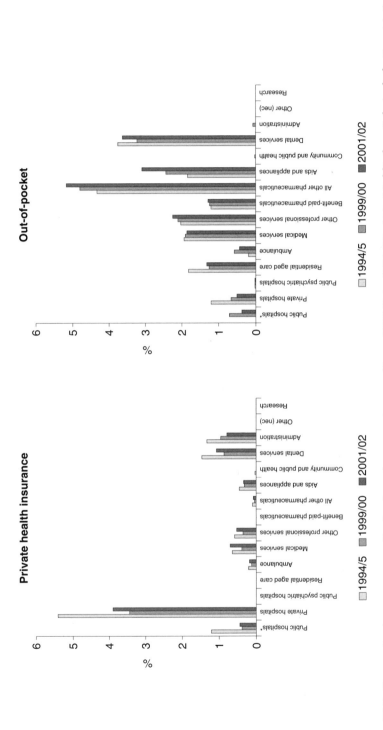

Figure 12.7 Change in the percentage distribution of recurrent expenditure 1994/5 to 2001/02. *Note* *Public hospitals include Repatriation hospitals in 1994/5. *Source:* Australian Institute of Health and Welfare (2003) *Health Expenditure Australia 2001–02*, Appendix Tables.

spokespersons like to point out that, although this seems expensive, for every 30 cents of government expenditure, another 70 cents is raised from private sources, implying that the system is 70 cents better off than if government had contributed the money directly. But for every 30 cents the government spends to attract one new member of an insurance fund (so generating the additional 70 cents of private expenditure), it must spend almost 60 cents on the rebate to existing members. The additional 70 cents from private sources actually costs government 90 cents. The net impact of the rebate has been to increase the Commonwealth share of recurrent healthcare expenditure, from 47.3% in 1994–5 to 48.5% in 2001–2 and reduce the private insurance contribution from 11.4% in 1994–5 to 8.1% in 2001–2. The Commonwealth contribution to private hospitals expenditure has increased. There is also an increase in the Commonwealth contribution to the costs of dental care, covered by private insurance; this comes after a substantial reduction in Commonwealth-funded public dental programmes.

The impact of this strategy on the allocation of health expenditure can be seen by comparing expenditure shares before its inception with the most recently available levels. Figure 12.7 shows trends in recurrent expenditure shares between 1994–5 and 2001–2. Overall, the shares financed by both the Commonwealth and state governments and by individuals grew, while the private health insurance share fell to about 40% of the out-of-pocket share of individuals. The breakdown of Commonwealth expenditure indicates reductions in the share for public hospitals and for medical services and increases for private hospital and pharmaceuticals. Because the Commonwealth has withdrawn funding from public dental services, the higher Commonwealth contribution to dental services arising from the apportioned private health insurance subsidy to ancillary services, benefits a very different client group.[5] The lower Commonwealth share on public hospital expenditure is mirrored by higher State government and out-of-pocket shares. The contributions from private health insurance have fallen for all categories of healthcare expenditure (except for medical services in 2001–2), reflected in the higher public share from the 30% subsidy to the cost of insurance.

Figure 12.8 shows the impact of the incentives on the age structure of the insured population over time. Lifetime Health Cover clearly had the largest impact on coverage. The largest percentage increase (of over 20%) was for those aged 45–49 years. There were also large impacts for those aged over 30 and the increase in under-18s is explained as the children of both these age groups. Perhaps surprisingly, there were increases in coverage even for age groups unaffected by Lifetime Health Cover, in particular those aged 20–30.

The resulting change in the age structure of the insured population meant that the proportion of insured individuals aged 65 or more with private cover fell from a high of 14.8% in the September quarter of 1998 to 10.5% in the September quarter of 2000 following the introduction of Lifetime Health Cover. There has since been a decline in the coverage of younger groups and an increase for most groups aged 55 or over. As a result, the proportion of the insured population aged 65 or more increased to 11.8% by June 2003. Hospital episodes per 100 insured persons fell from 6.5 in the final quarter of 1999 to 4.8 in the September quarter of 2000. The decline was partly caused by new entrants having to wait a 12-month period before being eligible to claim for many procedures, but the end of

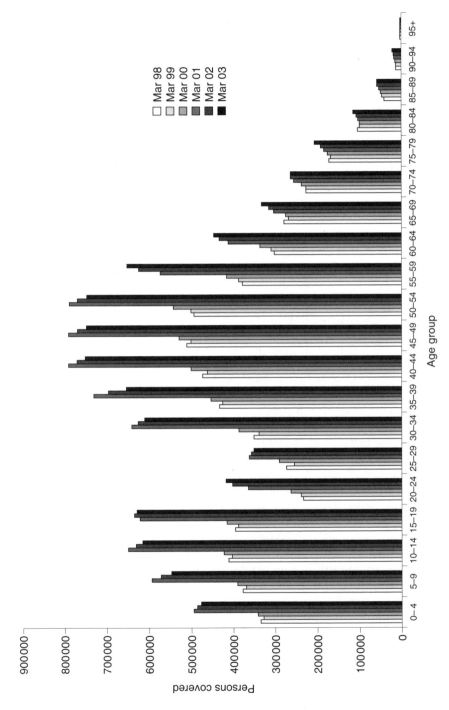

Figure 12.8 Number of persons insured by age, 1998–2003.

Table 12.4 Monthly benefit required from private insurance for lifetime health cover to be equivalent to delayed entry

		Current age		
		30	40	50
Age at entry	65	$106	$100	$92
	60	$104	$99	$92
	50	$97	$89	–
	40	$87	–	–

Notes: Basic rate premiums are assumed to increase with the CPI.
The real discount rate applied in the calculations is 6% per annum.

waiting periods and the higher age of entrants after 2000 have meant that the level has not been sustained.

It certainly seems that the regulatory (and cheap) change, rather than the subsidy, was the most effective in increasing coverage.[13] The introduction of Lifetime Health Cover was accompanied by an extensive and aggressive advertising campaign with the slogan 'Run for Cover', though why it should be so effective is unclear. Even without changes in the cost of the base premium, individuals would be more likely to benefit from saving the cost of insurance premiums until they expected to use private treatment, as can be illustrated by comparing the value of lifetime contributions to private insurance at different entry ages. Lifetime Health Cover presents consumers with two options: (a) insurance can be purchased over their lifetimes, with payment of the basic rate premiums; (b) entry may be delayed, avoiding the cost of insurance over the period that they are not privately insured, but when they choose to join, they pay the basic rate premium plus a loading (the size of which varies with age at entry). To investigate these alternatives, Table 12.4 presents calculations of the monthly benefit a family would need to derive from private insurance (over and above public hospital treatment as a Medicare patient) to make the value of the two options equal in current dollars. The calculations are for a typical hospital insurance package with no excess, and life expectancy is fixed at 85 for both partners.

For example, a family with both partners aged 30 can purchase insurance now or delay their purchase until a later age. Compared to delaying their entry until 65, this family would need to derive $106 worth of benefits from insurance for each month of the extra 35 years they are insured to make the two options equal in value. For a couple currently aged 50, the monthly benefits would need to be $92. These calculations indicate that the benefits of insurance would need to be large and sustained to make insurance cover over the lifetime an attractive option. However, for many higher earners, the rebate combined with the Medicare Levy surcharge results in a negative price as private insurance can be purchased for less than the additional tax.

The growth in private health insurance benefits paid for private hospital treatment between 1998 and 2003 is shown in Figure 12.9. There is a dramatic growth across most age bands following the introduction of Lifetime Health

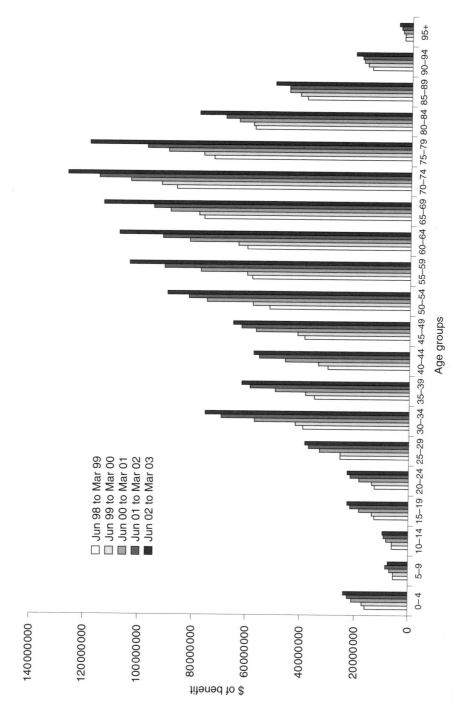

Figure 12.9 Annual hospital benefits by age, 1998–2003.

Cover, despite new entrants facing waiting periods for claims related to existing conditions. The trend to increased benefits has continued, with dramatic growth for those aged over 50. Increases were driven, not by increased episodes or increased length of stay for the insured population, but primarily by large growth in benefits paid per day. This is shown in Figure 12.10.

The cost of hospital care is the other, and more important, factor affecting benefit payouts and as a consequence, insurance premiums. Policies guaranteeing no out-of-pocket costs, no gap cover, are a component of that increase. Development and promotion of no gap cover continues to be government policy.[14] At best, this involves a redistribution of out-of-pocket expenses to private insurers, with an upward effect on payouts and premiums, but if providers respond to the moral hazard of insurance by increasing their fees, this inflationary pressure will be exacerbated. The impact of higher private insurance cover on length of hospital stay and other health service utilisation is a further important issue. While there is a large body of research on the factors influencing the insurance choice, there is not yet any analysis comparing new entrants and those insured prior to the incentives. Information on linking insurance status and utilisation is also limited. Administrative data indicate that, prior to the recent changes, the average length of stay for nine out of ten of the most common diagnosis-related groups was longer in private than in public hospitals. Furthermore, evidence would suggest that individuals with private health cover undergo higher rates of procedure than those without.[15]

The Australian Bureau of Statistics National Health Survey of 1989–90 is the only available dataset linking insurance status to hospital length of stay for private hospital patients. Analysis of these data indicates that when the individuals are matched according to their predicted probability of insurance (controlling for chronic conditions, incomes, sex of head of family, age, family structure, country of birth, alcohol and smoker status, employment status, education and region) the effect of insurance on length of hospital stay can be substantial. The ratio of duration of insured to uninsured is illustrated in Figure 12.11 for individuals from five family types. Significantly longer private hospital stays are found for privately insured patients from some family types: couples with dependants (about 50% longer), couples with head aged over 50 (about 90% longer) and single persons aged over 50 (about 60% longer). Similar results are obtained from hospital duration regressions, taking into account the endogeneity of the insurance decision.[16] If this behaviour persists in the current population of insured patients, the effect of increased coverage on total health expenditure and breakdown by funding source could be substantial.

Private health insurance, and therefore the 30% rebate, applies to ancillary services, which include dentistry, optometry, physiotherapy, and lifestyle and fitness, as well as to hospital stays. The levels of insurance benefits paid for the largest ancillary services are shown in Figure 12.12. Dental treatment involves the largest expenses claimed on insurance, followed by chiropractic, physiotherapy and optical services. The large expansion in insurance coverage with Lifetime Health Cover was followed by a major growth in payouts for ancillary services. Most expenditure is about 50% higher than in 1999, with natural therapies and acupuncture benefits more than doubling. The growth of benefits paid for fitness and lifestyle courses and equipment was over 900% of the 1999 level. The policy of allowing the 30% rebate to cover ancillary services has been widely criticised;

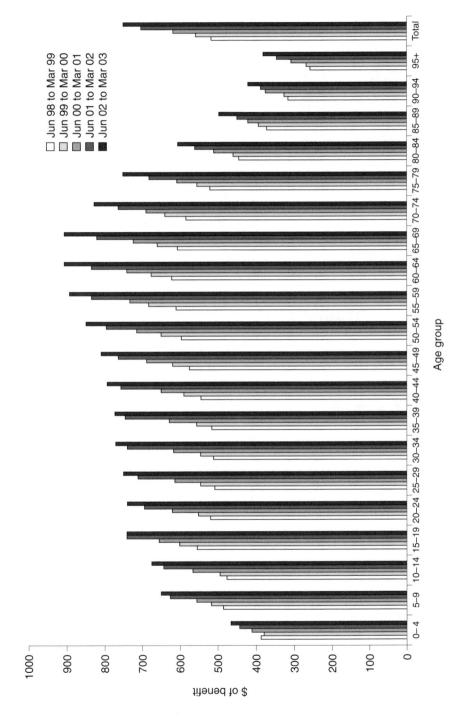

Figure 12.10 Hospital benefits per day by age, 1998–2003.

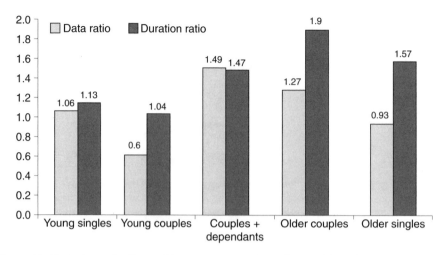

Figure 12.11 Estimated effects of insurance on private hospital length of stay by family type. *Source*: Savage (2002).[16]

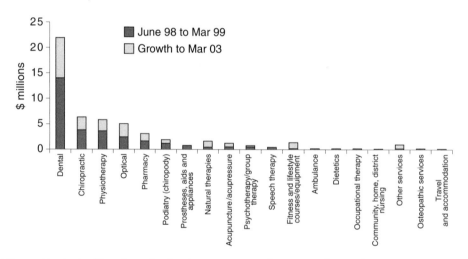

Figure 12.12 Ancillary benefits for the year to March 1999 and growth to March 2003 for major ancillary services. *Note*: Benefits less than $40 000 in 1999 are excluded.

the Australian government and the insurance industry has agreed to phase out insurance coverage for 'sport, recreation or entertainment'.[14]

The inclusion of cover for ancillary services may be an important factor in attracting and keeping the younger and healthier groups paying their insurance premiums. The attractiveness of ancillary cover is not so much as an insurance, but a partial reimbursement of expenses that would be incurred in any event (e.g. preventive dentistry, optometry). Although these low-risk groups are necessary to keep the cost of premiums down, the means to do this will entail increasing benefit payouts and consequently increase premium costs.

The Pharmaceutical Benefits Scheme

The Pharmaceutical Benefits Scheme (PBS) is a universal programme covering around 600 prescription drugs outside public hospitals; public hospitals negotiate separately with the industry. Under the PBS, the patient pays a fixed co-payment, currently $22.40 per script; pensioners and holders of other entitlement cards pay a concessional rate of $3.60. At present, 85% of PBS prescriptions are concessional.[17] Safety-net provisions reduce the standard co-payment to the concessional rate once out-of-pocket expenditure for a person or family reaches $686.40 in a calendar year; the concessional rate is reduced to zero once expenditure reaches $187.20 (52 prescriptions).

In the 1960s, the Pharmaceutical Benefits Pricing Tribunal was established to negotiate prices on behalf of the Commonwealth government, in response to concerns that Australia was being charged higher than world average prices. Subsequently, the use of this purchasing power has led to substantially lower drug prices in Australia than in the US, Canada and Sweden. Australia's public expenditure on pharmaceuticals is relatively low: 0.5% of GDP in 1999 compared with an average of 0.7% for other OECD countries. Industry concerns about the effect of low prices led to the Tribunal being transformed into an independent authority, which is required to consider the manufacturing company's Australian activity in negotiating price. The prices paid for recent innovative drugs are much closer to world prices.[18]

In spite of the industry concern about low prices, the PBS is the fastest growing area of public health expenditure. The total government cost of PBS drug subsidies was $4.2 billion in 2000–1, an 18.8% growth over the previous year[11] (Table 14, p. 20). Between 1991 and 2001 the volume of prescribed drugs grew by 50% and the level of the patient co-payment by 120% (*Australian Financial Review*, 18 March 2002). Eligibility for the higher concessional subsidy has also been extended to those of pensionable age with incomes less than $50 000 per annum.

The listing of new drugs on the PBS is controlled by the Pharmaceutical Benefits Advisory Committee (PBAC). In 1993, Australia became the first country to require an economic evaluation for drugs applying for listing on the PBS, though it is not clear that this was intended as a cost-control mechanism. It can also be seen as a means to determine appropriate prices through comparison with drugs with a similar level of effectiveness. However, the PBAC does not negotiate prices and indeed the cost-effectiveness analysis may use a price which is far from the final negotiated price.

Published guidelines on how to conduct and present the economic evaluation, and an economics subcommittee which scrutinises the submission, ensures some uniformity in the analyses. The Minister is bound by legislation not to accept a drug for PBS listing after a negative recommendation; they can, however, reject a positive PBAC recommendation for listing.

Developments in the PBS

Not only has the PBS been experiencing growth in excess of other programmes, but the growth has been substantially in excess of forecasts. The September 1999 growth forecast was 8.4% for 1999–2000, compared with actual growth of 14.1%. In 2000–1, the rate of growth increased to 18.8%. Most of this is due to new products being approved for use, as new, more complex and expensive drugs replace less costly established agents, and new classes of drugs are developed and approved. For example, the anti-smoking drug, Zyban, cost $80 million in PBS subsidies in 2001, 1.8% of total PBS expenditure; the arthritis drug Celebrex cost more than $160 million; and the cholesterol-lowering drug Simvastatin cost $270 million (statins were the highest cost class of medication comprising more than 10% of PBS expenditure). And newer, even more expensive agents are on the horizon.

The guidelines for PBS economic evaluations require a comparison with the best available alternative drug therapy. In the case of Zyban, there were no comparisons of cost-effectiveness compared to other approaches, such as behavioural therapy. Furthermore, the process was initiated and the analysis prepared by the manufacturer, and the manufacturer specified the indications/conditions for which PBS listing was being sought. However, once listing has been approved, there are no limitations on prescribing the drug. Although direct marketing to the public is prohibited, drug companies have well-established links with their clinical customers and, apart from direct marketing, they sponsor continuing medical education and research, both of which provide avenues to promote and establish their products. The PBS describes the wider prescribing of drugs found to be cost-effective for specific conditions as leakage, and this is a growing problem. Common examples are Celebrex, which was prescribed at about three times the forecast rate, and Losec, a proton-pump inhibitor, which was prescribed to over five times the number of people meeting the conditions indicated for access to the drug (*Australian Financial Review*, 18 March 2002).

The PBAC took a stand and rejected listing new drugs on the basis of their cost and likely usage, Viagra being the most prominent example. The manufacturer, Pfizer, then took the government to court, arguing that the overall budgetary impact of drug listing fell outside the PBAC legislation, although this argument was rejected in the judgement. A further Pfizer submission demonstrated that Viagra was more cost-effective than the listed treatment for impotence and the Minister's response was to de-list the existing treatment. But the government's response is not always to withstand the political pressure. For example, Herceptin, a new and expensive treatment for breast cancer, was rejected by PBAC on cost grounds. As noted above, the Minister cannot overturn a negative recommendation, but the then Minister could, and did, make the drug available through a special funding programme outside of the PBS.

Concern about industry influence and pressure on the operation of the PBS came to a head with the government's appointment of a former pharmaceutical industry consultant to PBAC. In the public controversy, which followed, the government dismissed all members of PBAC in December 2000 and instituted a new committee, including the former industry consultant.

There have been several strategies introduced to reduce expenditure growth, including enabling pharmacists to substitute cheaper equivalent drugs, higher patient co-payments for more expensive brands and, in response to leakage, some price-volume agreements with suppliers, to which the pharmaceutical companies are strongly opposed (*Australian Financial Review*, 22 March 2002). Members of the previous PBAC committee have proposed a tiered pricing system in which drug companies would be paid a lower price when health benefits are low (such as when anti-inflammatory drugs are prescribed for minor aches).

In the 2002 budget, the Government proposed a 30% increase in PBS co-payments. The legislation has since been rejected by the Upper House of the Commonwealth Parliament. The industry, in response to concerns about increasing drug expenditure, has agreed to a code of conduct that aims to end all 'non-essential hospitality' to doctors as part of a wider strategy to ease the pressures on the PBS budget (*Sydney Morning Herald*, 2 September 2002). Yet, at the same time, there are increasing advertisements aimed directly at consumers which, without nominating specific drugs, advise them to 'see their GP' to get help with a particular problem. The industry has also recommended higher co-payments for those who can afford them and, in the evaluation process for new drugs, that benefits be expanded to include future savings in healthcare expenditure flowing from drug treatment.

The Government's response to the continued growth of pharmaceutical expenditure has been to emphasise that drug costs are the major driver of increases in public health spending. The 2002 Budget papers included an Intergenerational Report forecasting growth in public expenditure, which predicted that PBS subsidies would increase from 0.6% of GDP in 2001–2 to 3.35% in 2041–2. In 2003 a new government campaign, advertising directly to consumers, aimed to reduce the number of prescription drugs. At the same time the industry, in concert with several disease advocacy groups such as Cancer Councils, has been raising consumer awareness of the problems of sustaining the current system of public finance and universal unlimited access.

Medical services – from surplus to shortage

For most of the period since Medicare was established, the challenge for medical workforce planning has been to deal with the perceived surplus of medical practitioners.[19] More sophisticated approaches to workforce planning have distinguished between specialist components of the medical workforce and GPs. While several specialty areas have been judged to be undersupplied, as recently as 2000 the Australian Medical Workforce Advisory Committee considered the GP workforce to be oversupplied.[20] This workforce increased by 43% from 1984 to 1998–9, or a 20% increase net of population growth.[21] The rise in GP numbers has slowed in more recent times, with only a 12% increase in ten years to 1998–9 or a 2% increase net of population growth over the same period[22] – yet by mid-2003 the perceived shortage of GPs had prompted a major proposal from the Government, and counter-proposal from the Opposition, to change the structure of general practice.

The distribution of the general practice workforce does not match the population, with GP to population ratios being much higher in the capital cities and metropolitan areas than in rural and remote areas. The apparent shortages in the latter have been highlighted by cases of country towns losing their single GP and finding it impossible to attract a replacement. There are various reasons why country practice is less appealing than work in city and metropolitan areas.

The maldistribution of the workforce is not new and was certainly in evidence prior to the introduction of Medicare, but as the supply of doctors has increased, the differences in cover between city and country have also increased. For example, in 1984–5 small rural centres had 94% of the number of GPs per capita as capital cities; in 1999–2000 this had fallen to 79%. The 1998–9 spatial distribution is shown in Table 12.5.

Differences in the availability of doctors are reflected in both consultation rates and bulk-billing rates, with both decreasing in areas of lower doctor supply. The average number of GP encounters was 6.7 per capita in the capital cities in 1998–9 compared to 5.9 in small rural centres. Bulk-billing rates ranged from 85% to just under 60% for the same areas.[20]

However, since 2000 the overall bulk-billing rate has dropped, with the March quarter data showing rates of 77% in 2001, 74% in 2002 and 68% in 2003. The cause of this decline in bulk-billing rates has been popularly construed as the shortage of GPs and the failure of the Australian government-determined bulk-billing fee to rise in line with price increases. The decline has also been interpreted as a threat to the viability of Medicare, with families unable to find bulk-billing general practices and so facing out-of-pocket expenses, or joining the queues at the already overstretched public hospital emergency departments. Bulk-billing rates reached their highest level, 80%, in 1998–9, having grown steadily since their starting point of 53% in 1984–5. It is clear that there was nothing in the original framing of Medicare that implied a desirable rate of bulk-billing; the scheme was considered a success at bulk-billing rates well below their recent levels.

The Australian Government's response is termed 'A Fairer Medicare'. It proposes to address the shortage of doctors by increasing medical school intakes, increasing GP training and increasing the use of practice nurses. The cost of these strategies is estimated at $295.8m over 4 years. The proposal to address the patient cost of GP visits includes:

- incentive payments for practices to bulk-bill concession card holders
- providing these concession card holders with a safety net to limit out-of-pocket costs, which will cover diagnostic and specialist services out of hospital, as well as GP visits
- allowing general practice to bulk-bill the Medicare rebate for all GP fees, thus reducing the patient's upfront costs
- allowing private health insurance to cover the remaining co-payments, all costing an estimated $893 million over four years.

The Opposition proposal is focused on increasing the rebates and offering financial incentives for the achievement of a practice bulk-billing rate that varies spatially (from 80% in metropolitan areas to 70% in remote areas).

'A Fairer Medicare' would alter the structure of the system in several ways. First, the rebate offered would differ for concession card holders and others, giving different population groups different entitlements, ostensibly under the same universal scheme. Second, the direct billing of the rebate component of the fee would reduce the charge the patient sees. Third, covering out-of-pocket costs with the safety net or private insurance may remove doctors' reluctance to increase their charges – though increases have happened already, as bulk-billing rates have fallen and average co-payments have risen even without these changes. Perhaps more importantly, the involvement of private insurance in out-of-hospital services presages a much greater role for this component of the

Table 12.5 Spatial distribution of full-time workload equivalent Medicare primary care providers, 1998–9

Location	FWEs per 100 000 pop	Population per FWE
Capital	95.7	1045
Other metropolitan	89.7	1115
Large rural	84.1	1190
Small rural	75.3	1328
Other rural	59.2	1690
Remote central	51.2	1952
Other remote	37.4	2674
All	86.8	1153

Source: Commonwealth Department of Health and Aged Care, 2000, Table 2.18, p. 62.

private sector. The future is uncertain at the time of writing. Doctors' groups have criticised the changes for not delivering enough additional funding and not tackling other perceived problems in the health system. A Ministerial reshuffle has instated a new Health Minister who has agreed to a review of the package, with a commitment to increased funding and with medical indemnity insurance to be rolled into the same set of issues.

Conclusions and international lessons

In the Australian health system private financing, both through some form of insurance and out-of-pocket payments, has been significant even under Medicare. The current arrangements owe more to the political responses to the 'strife of interests' than rational planning. Their complexity across levels of government, between public and private providers, and public and private payers has led to substantial opportunities and incentives for cost shifting and barriers to co-ordination across health services.[3]

The private hospital sector has changed considerably in recent years to become dominated by major national and even international for-profit corporations. These enterprises are becoming vertically integrated with the acquisition of pathology and diagnostic providers, and now general practices. It is too early to see what effect this will have on efficiency and equity of access, but clearly it changes the market structure so that governments and insurers are facing suppliers with more market power. The hospital corporations are, in turn, dealing with medical providers who, though less organised formally, are not used to being treated as employees – as some hospital groups have discovered.

The public sector has found it difficult and costly to contract directly with the private sector. Even if private sector prices could be reduced, there remain substantial problems in monitoring contracts, particularly around the quality of services provided. Given the expanding role of private insurance, it seems likely that the contracting and monitoring function will move to the insurers, and it is not clear that they are better equipped than government to handle it. The impact of private health insurance subsidies has been to make the private sector ever more dependent on public payments. At the same time, there is an increasing coalition of interests between insurers and private hospitals on the one hand, and insurers and government on the other.

Although private health insurance in Australia has always been high, relative to countries with similar health systems, its contribution to total expenditure (at around 10%) has been quite small. Yet it has been a major focus of political and policy attention. The level of government involvement in the industry, even prior to the subsidy, has meant that government is seen to have responsibility for adverse trends in insurance such as premium increases.

There is no doubt that the cumulative effect of private health insurance incentives has been to increase the number of people buying health insurance. Although much of the public dissatisfaction with private health insurance was focused on price, it was not the price reduction (the effect of the subsidy) that triggered the reversal in declining membership, it was Lifetime Health Cover. Why this should be the case is not clear, as even simple arithmetic shows that to be repaid the additional costs of buying health insurance over 20, 30 or 40 years, the consumer would need to making claims worth $1200 annually. There are two, not mutually exclusive, explanations for the increase in coverage. First, many people believed that Lifetime Health Cover at the base premium rate meant that their current premiums would not rise. The premium increases in 2002 were greeted with public outrage, with many media reports replaying the previous Minister for Health promising that premiums would not rise and may even fall. Second, people mistrusted the government's commitment to the universality of Medicare in the longer term. It is interesting to note that the big increases in coverage affected those in their forties and fifties, many of whom were old enough to remember previous dismantling of universal, tax-financed healthcare.

Whether increased coverage will be sustained is open to question. Some argue that the recent decreases in coverage of individuals aged less than 55 is the beginning of another downward spiral, as new purchasers gain experience with health insurance and find that they are not using it. However, since 2000, new entrants to private insurance are predominantly over 55. This is somewhat surprising, since such individuals were eligible to be 'grandfathered' in at the base premium merely 12 months previously and are now paying 50% above the base premium. These new purchasers have very different, and more expensive, claims than similar existing customers, suggesting that a change in their health status has initiated their move into insurance. The funds also hope these will be 'hit-and-stay' customers rather than the 'hit-and-run' phenomenon targeted by Lifetime Health Cover, though if their higher claims experience continues, the funds may prefer them to drop out.

In many ways, private health insurance funds face a dilemma. The success of the incentives has increased both the visibility of and government's contribution to insurance. Yet rather than attracting premium-paying, low-claiming cus- tomers, the insurers are facing increasing average payouts, with the inevitable effect on premiums. They will need to become proactive in managing care, through restricting choice of provider to those with whom they have negotiated favourable prices, and through denying benefits for what they deem unnecessary services, such as longer stays in hospital. Yet choice of provider and unrestricted access to services have been the most heavily marketed advantages of being privately insured. The way forward is unclear.

Among the government's objectives was a degree of reduction of pressure in the public system without increased public expenditure. Were this achieved, and the difference between public and private treatment made less stark, it would, paradoxically, further decrease the attractiveness of private insurance. There has not been a downturn in public hospital activity, but this would not be expected if there were unmet or queued demand. At the same time, there has been an increase in private hospital activity, but it is not possible to tell whether this represents activity displaced from the public system or whether it is insurance-induced demand. The private health insurance incentives have proved to be expensive, and indeed have increased the Commonwealth government's share of total healthcare expenditure. The impact has been regressive, with proportionately more of the benefits accruing to higher income groups.

The pharmaceutical industry provides another illustration of the entanglement of private interests and public subsidies. The PBS has ensured that all Australians have access to a wide range of prescription medicines, a factor valued by the Australian public as an essential component of Medicare. The Government wants to maintain the appeal of the scheme, in which all essential medicines are covered by the PBS, but if it is not prepared to meet an increasing pharmaceuticals bill, it will have to find new ways of restraining expenditure. The pharmaceutical industry has benefited from the higher sales volume assured by universal subsidies and has successfully argued its own importance to the Australian economy. However, the advent of extremely expensive new drugs, with potentially wide application, will challenge the current balance between co-payments and government expenditure. In 2002, an interdepartmental committee was set up to review all aspects of the PBS but as yet no findings have been made public.

General practice provides the next challenge for the interplay of public and private interests. The most pressing current policy issue is to simultaneously solve the perceived shortage of GPs, increase their remuneration and reverse the decline in bulk-billing. Increased GP incomes have to come either from tax revenues or consumer charges. The Government and Opposition have different policy solutions and this was set to be a major issue at the 2004 election.

The recent reform of the Australian healthcare system has been narrowly focused on the radical private funding experiment. The underlying problems in the public provision of primary and secondary care remain considerable, with public debate about the remuneration of GPs and cost sharing in primary care and timely access to high-quality hospital care. As the policy focus shifts to issues such as these, which consume over 90% of Australian healthcare expenditure, a remaining challenge is the systematic evaluation of the Howard reforms. Was this a high-profile, inefficient and inequitable diversion or a beneficial innovation that improved the public health of Australians?

References

1 Commonwealth Department of Health and Ageing (2003–4) *Portfolio Budget Statements – Budget Related Paper no. 1.11.* Canberra: Commonwealth Department of Health and Aged Care.

2 Crichton A (1990) *Slowly Taking Control?: Australian governments and healthcare provision, 1788–1988.* Sydney: Allen & Unwin.

3 Sax S (1984) *A Strife of Interests: politics and policies in Australian health services.* Sydney: Allen & Unwin.

4 Australian Institute of Health and Welfare (2003) *Australian Hospital Statistics 2001–02.* Canberra: AIHW cat. no. HSE 25.

5 Commonwealth Department of Health and Aged Care (2003) *General Practice in Australia.* Canberra: Commonwealth Department of Health and Aged Care.

6 Spencer A (2001) *What Options Do We Have for Organising, Providing and Funding Better Public Dental Care.* Sydney: The Australian Health Policy Institute and the Medical Foundation, University of Sydney.

7 Grbich C (2002) Moving away from the welfare state: the privatisation of the health system. In: Gardner M, Barraclough S (eds) *Health Policy in Australia.* Melbourne: Oxford University Press.

8 Duckett SJ, Jackson TJ (2002) The new health insurance rebate: an inefficient way of assisting public hospitals. *Medical Journal of Australia.* **172**: 439–42.

9 Davies P (2002) *When 'universal' is not enough: policies for voluntary health insurance.* Paper presented at the Commonwealth Fund International Symposium on Health Policy, Washington, DC, October.

10 Industry Commission (1997) *Private Health Insurance.* Belconnen, ACT: AGPS.

11 Private Health Insurance Administration Council (2003) *Health Insurance Statistics.* Belconnen, ACT: AGPS.

12 Hilless M, Healy J (2001) *Health Care Systems in Transition: Australia.* London: European Observatory on Health Care Systems.

13 Australian Institute of Health and Welfare (2002) *Health Expenditure Australia 2000–01.* Canberra: AIHW.

14 Butler JRG (2001) *Policy Change and Private Health Insurance: did the cheapest policy do the trick?* Canberra: National Centre for Epidemiology and Population Health.

15 Robertson IK, Richardson JRJ (2000) Coronary angiography and coronary artery revascularisation rates in public and private hospital patients after acute myocardial infarction. *Medical Journal of Australia.* **173**: 291–5.

16 Savage E (2002) *Does private health insurance lengthen hospital stays? Matching estimates for Australian private hospitals.* Paper presented to conference 'Regulating Private Health Insurance', ANU.

17 Pharmaceutical Benefits Pricing Authority (2001) *Annual Report for the year ended 30 June 2001.* Canberra: Australian Government Publishing Service.

18 Harvey K (2002) The Pharmaceutical Benefits Scheme under threat. *Health Issues Journal.* **71**.

19 Scotton R (1999) The doctor business. In: Mooney G, Scotton R (eds) *Economics and Australian Health Policy.* Sydney: Allen & Unwin, 72–92.

20 Australian Institute of Health and Welfare (1999) *Medical Labour Force 1997.* Canberra: Australian Institute of Health and Welfare.

21 Australian Medical Workforce Advisory Committee (2000) *The General Practice Workforce in Australia: supply and requirements 1999–2010.* Sydney: Australian Medical Workforce Advisory Committee.

22 O'Loughlin MA (2002) *Conflicting interests in private hospital care.* Paper presented to conference 'Regulating Private Health Insurance', ANU.

Chapter 13

Common challenges in healthcare markets

Alan Maynard

Introduction

The American political scientist Ted Marmor, of Yale University, opines that 'what is regular, is not stupid'. Healthcare markets throughout the world are never free of private and government regulation. The processes by which doctors and other healthcare workers are trained and employed are regulated by private professional bodies and public agencies to ensure 'fitness to practice'. Pharmaceutical markets are regulated by patents, safety controls in the production processes and the regulation of consumer access by restricted prescribing. Hospitals are regulated to ensure some, often limited, consumer protection, and funders, whether private insurers or governments, have their freedom constrained by rules to ensure probity and financial prudence. The ubiquitous nature of regulation in healthcare markets reflects rational responses to common problems.

The first part of this chapter examines how healthcare markets are regulated in an attempt to overcome market failures. It demonstrates that there is a continuing historical debate about regulation, but that it is inevitable and necessary to give consumer protection. In the second part of the chapter, the need to clarify policy objectives when reforming healthcare is discussed. It is in the interests of politicians to be obtuse about their policy goals, as this makes it more difficult for their opponents and the public to hold them to account. Most decision makers pursue, directly and indirectly, three policy objectives: macro economic expenditure control; efficiency or 'value for money' in the use of resources; and equity. The ranking or emphasis on each of these goals varies internationally and from sector to sector.

In the US, where the healthcare system consumes nearly 15% of GDP, the primary concern is cost containment. Improving the efficiency of the US system is seen as a potential means of controlling costs. For the liberal left, the inequity of the US system, with 42 million uninsured, is seen as a matter of concern.

In Europe, some healthcare systems can control total expenditure with fiscal policy but face criticism over access to care and waiting times (e.g. UK, Scandinavia and the Netherlands). Furthermore, parsimony can lead to deficits in quality (e.g. UK). Other Bismarckian systems, such as France and Germany, have weak expenditure control that fuel breaches of EU and national fiscal targets, creating pressures for radical reform which are politically very difficult to meet. Often equity concerns are muted by a cacophony about waiting times and expenditure control. The challenges of articulating and ranking these targets are great and often result in political 'muddling through' that preserves inefficiency and inequity.

Why is it necessary to regulate markets?

What is a market? Simply a network of buyers and sellers, who may be exchanging cabbages, beer, banking services or healthcare for money. Leading liberals have consistently recognised the need for market regulation. Ronald Coase of Chicago University took the epitome of the market – stock exchanges – and argued:

> It is not without significance that these exchanges, often used by economists as examples of a perfect market and perfect competition, are markets in which all transactions are highly regulated (and this quite apart from any Government regulation there may be). It suggests, I think correctly, that for anything approaching perfect competition to exist, an intricate system of rules and regulations would normally be needed.[1]

Regulation may be provided by private or public organisations. Its purpose is to influence the prices, volumes and qualities of the goods and services that are being produced and traded and ensure that the performance of markets is more consistent with social goals. But why is it that markets do not achieve these goals and why do we need to regulate their design and performance?

There are a number of causes of 'market failure' that provide a rationale for regulation either by private organisations, like the stock exchange, or by the state. In healthcare, they include the existence of monopoly or sole-seller power, the problem of asymmetric information, with doctors knowing more than patients about the benefits of care, the presence of moral hazard in funding arrangements and the problems created by the unequal distribution of income and wealth.

Market structures and monopoly power

Liberals regard the eighteenth-century Scottish political economist Adam Smith as the doyen of free-market advocacy. However, he and other founding fathers of the discipline of economics, such as John Stuart Mill, recognised that regulation of the market was essential for its efficient functioning.

Smith and Mill emphasised the need for clear ownership or property rights and basic legal structures to facilitate exchange between buyers and sellers. Without contracts and the ability to enforce them, market transactions become risky and expensive. However, capitalists can be the enemies of capitalism and the efficient working of markets. Smith noted:

> People of the same trade seldom meet together, even for merriment and diversion, but the conversation ends in a conspiracy against the public, or in some contrivance to raise prices.[2]

Smith went on to argue that whenever such trades set up registers of members and begin to tax themselves to help the disadvantaged, the resultant corporations will coerce their members and inhibit competition. It is this characteristic that dominates all healthcare markets. In countries such as the UK, Canada, New

Zealand and Australia, the Royal Colleges are bulwarks, which, in the name of 'quality control', can resist innovations in skill-mix and create bureaucratic restraints, inhibiting change while failing to demonstrate that they work in the public interest to enhance quality control and ensure consumer protection.

These structures are supported by trades unions, such as medical associations, that can sustain not only the management of activities which could be delegated cost effectively to other skill groups, but also ensure, through their controls on the number of practitioners in the market-place, that their members receive high levels of remuneration. Friedman argued that the 'American Medical Association is perhaps the strongest trade union in the United States'.[3]

Smith's discussion of the power of professions, and in particular the medical professions, exhibited some contradictions. For instance he argued that:

> We trust our health to the physician; our fortune and sometimes our life and reputation to the lawyer and the attorney. Such confidence could not be reposed in people of a very mean or low condition. Their reward must be such, therefore, as may give them that rank in society which so important a trust requires. The long time and the great expense which must be laid out for their education, when combined with this circumstance, necessarily enhance still further the price for their labour.[2]

Separately, in correspondence with Dr Cullen, he remarked:

> The title of Doctor, such as it is, you will say, gives some credit and authority to a man upon whom it is bestowed, it extends his practice and consequently his field for doing mischief. It is not improbable too that it may increase his presumption and consequently his disposition to do mischief.[4]

More recently, Friedman recognised the inhibiting effects of corporations or occupational licensure on the practice and cost of medicine.[3] He emphasised the use of professional power to control numbers entering medical practice, and to increase the remuneration of practitioners. He explained that medical practitioners typically carry out tasks best delegated to other groups and that this reduces their ability to focus on and practice those skills for which they have the greatest expertise. This is exemplified by medical practitioners carrying out administrative tasks best delegated to secretaries and clerical assistants. Thus, restrictions on entry may reduce both the volume of care available and the average level of competence of the medical labour force. Friedman demonstrated that there are many alternative forms of regulation to the medical licensure seen at present, but such demonstrations have little effect on policy. Worldwide, physicians control, explicitly and implicitly, the ways in which medicine is practised and in doing so raise its cost (and their income) while failing to demonstrate efficient levels of consumer protection, in particular good patient outcomes, evidence-based practice and the management of practice variations.

So although libertarians such as Smith and Friedman point out the potential of freer markets for the provision of better patient care, this potential is rarely exploited because, as Stigler has emphasised, regulation favours the regulated:[5] the regulated exploit the political processes to protect their advantages. The reasonable desire to protect patients from 'quacks' and other deficient practitioners has led to the medical profession capturing control over the supply of doctors and the supply of healthcare.

The uncritical acceptance of this monopoly of power results in the profession controlling both the number of practitioners in the NHS and other healthcare systems and the ways in which they practise. This is costly, requiring high levels of remuneration, and is inefficient in that it inhibits the capacity of the NHS to 'act smarter' as demanded by Prime Minister Blair as part of the 'modernisation' of the NHS.

Asymmetric knowledge

The resilience of common deficits in the performance of the NHS and other healthcare markets is reinforced by the asymmetric nature of knowledge about healthcare. Medicine can be complex and technical with the consumer relatively uninformed about the costs and benefits of diagnostic, therapeutic and rehabilitative interventions. Patients, as a consequence, become dependent on the medical 'experts' and cede their rights as consumers to physicians and other professions who, in turn become the primary determinants of the demand for healthcare. While it is the patients who make the initial decision to demand healthcare, once they are in the healthcare system, it is the doctors who determine what care will be provided, how and when.

The consequence of the asymmetry of knowledge between patient and practitioner is that doctors act as the patients' agents and demand access to care on their behalf. A consequence of this relationship can be that doctors will make unnecessary increases in the demand for healthcare in order to enhance their incomes.

There is a substantial international literature on the effects of the agency relationship and considerable methodological and empirical controversy about the resultant research.[6] One plausible explanation of doctors offering high levels of service input is that they may in this way reduce their uncertainty about diagnosis and appropriate treatment. Their 'wasteful' investigations and their use of multiple interventions may be the product of efforts to reduce the risks of misdiagnosis and inappropriate treatment. Such risk management or patient experimentation is resource intensive and may enhance practitioners' incomes indirectly rather than directly through inappropriate practice.

The continuing absence of rigorous evaluations and the translation of evidence into practice, and the continuing relative ignorance of patients about the health attributes of their medical care ensures the survival of both the agency relationship and public tolerance of the beneficial and negative aspects of the monopoly power of doctors. These characteristics ensure that the healthcare market cannot be 'free' and unconstrained by regulation unless significant regulatory investments are made to protect patient interests.

Moral hazard

Healthcare markets, whether public or private, reduce the price barriers to consumption. The purchase of private health insurance entitles the consumer to a prescribed benefit package, which, subject to co-payment rules, entitles the beneficiary to free care at the point of consumption, usually up to a financial ceiling. Public healthcare systems similarly, and subject to co-payment regulations, offer patients free care at the point of consumption. In both the public and private healthcare markets, the patient has no financial incentive to economise, as healthcare is 'free'.

Consumption choices by patients do, of course, have opportunity costs, though these costs fall largely on the funding agencies in the private and public sectors. The primary decision makers in these markets, patients and professionals, may bear none of the financial consequences of their behaviours, making the healthcare market unusual as the consequent lack of incentives to economise, or moral hazard, may lead to overconsumption.[7] Such propensities will be reinforced by the asymmetry of information, with the patients' professional agents not only being able to induce demand for their services but also shifting the cost of their decisions onto the funders, public and private.

Equity

A common assumption among the advocates of 'free' markets is that it is possible to turn a blind eye to the issue of the unequal distribution of purchasing power, in particular inequalities in income and wealth. The remarkable attribute of these distributions in the late 1970s was that, relative to the rest of Western Europe, the degree of income inequality in the UK was high and that it was rivalled only by the US. At that time, inequality in the UK wealth distribution was markedly high both in terms of its European neighbours and the US. The Conservative governments of Thatcher and Major made these inequalities even sharper and although the rhetoric of the Blair administration has been in favour of reducing them, its success has been limited, in large part because of its reluctance to increase progressive income taxation and fund its activities with 'stealth' and other taxes (e.g. national insurance contributions, which are proportional to income).

With citizens in all healthcare markets having unequal endowments of income and wealth, their capacity to 'vote' for more care by buying it is also unequal. The principal rationale for government provision of healthcare has been the equity argument, i.e. giving disadvantaged groups access to care. Instead of access to care being determined by ability and willingness to pay, the price barriers to care were removed so that the poor could consume.

Thus, the UK Coalition Government led by Churchill declared in its NHS White Paper in 1944 that:

> The Government . . . want to ensure that in the future every man and woman and child can rely on getting the best medical and other facilities available; that their getting them shall not depend on whether they can pay for them or on any other factor irrelevant to real need.[8]

Translation of such brave sentiments into practical policy has been difficult. The assumption for some decades after the creation of the NHS was that the removal of the price barrier to consumption would remedy the access problem, completely ignoring the existence of non-price barriers to use. The NHS inherited a bed and workforce stock that was very unevenly distributed. The large geographical inequalities in facilities were supported by large geographical inequalities in NHS funding.[9,10] Political recognition of the situation emerged in the late 1960s with Richard Crossman and was initially tackled by Keith Joseph in the Conservative Administration of 1970–4. The first thoroughly designed policy was not introduced until 1976 with publication of the Resource Allocation Working Party (RAWP) report.[11]

The RAWP formula and subsequent formulae in England and the other constituent parts of the UK began to mitigate inequalities in the financial capacity of health authorities within each of the four countries but did not reduce the inequalities which continue to exist between them.[12] Furthermore, reducing inequalities in financial capacity does little to resolve those in the utilisation of care. Dixon *et al.* (2003) argued that, although the evidence is complex and confusing:

> It seems reasonable to conclude that the NHS is indeed inequitable in key areas of healthcare provision. It seems likely that where the poor consume similar levels of care compared to the middle classes they present later in illness episodes and consequently utilisation may be less effective. These issues remain clouded by inadequate research.[13]

Policies to mitigate inequalities in geographical financial capacity to provide healthcare and social class inequalities in its use may or may not impact on the health status of individuals and local populations. The increased disparity in the distribution of income and wealth in the UK over the past 20 years has been correlated with increased disparity in health status. Outcome indicators such as infant mortality and expectations of length of life at birth and through the life cycle have improved; the gap between the rich and the poor peaked in the early 1990s and has declined since then, but it remains at a higher level than that of the early 1970s. In 1997–9 male life expectancy at birth for the unskilled manual class was 71.1 years compared to 78.5 years for professional classes. This male gap of 7.4 years was higher than the female life expectancy difference for these classes of 5.4 years.[14]

Male children born in affluent Rutland in 2000–02 were likely to live 8.5 years longer than children born of the poor in Manchester. For female children, the difference was 6.8 years. Furthermore, the children of the affluent, like their parents, are likely to live not only longer but also enjoy better quality of life.

There remains considerable debate and some uncertainty, in terms of a poor evidence base, as to whether such inequalities are best mitigated by investment in the NHS or whether it would be more cost-effective to invest in other social and economic policies that affect the life cycle income and health of individuals.[15–17] Politically it may be more convenient to focus on the role of the NHS, as conventional political wisdom appears to rule out the use of progressive direct taxes and redistributive income and social security policies.

The pronounced inequalities in the UK distributions of income and wealth are paralleled by high relative inequalities in healthcare and health. These have been successively charted nationally by the Black Report in 1979[18] and the Acheson Report in 1998.[19] Wanless highlighted similar problems.[14]

Systematic research work by Wagstaff, van Doorslaer and colleagues have used household expenditure surveys and other national material to explore internationally the financing and utilisation of healthcare, as well as related health issues. While UK funding, being tax-financed, scores relatively well in terms of redistributive effects, results on health were less impressive. For instance, they showed that health inequalities in the UK and US were particularly high, while in countries such as Finland and Sweden they are low. Across all the countries they analysed, there was a strong association between inequalities in health and inequalities in income.[20,21] Studies such as these promoted a considerable increase in knowledge of health and healthcare inequalities during the past 15 years. However, translation of this knowledge into more sophisticated research (e.g. improving health measures), let alone policy change, is quite modest.

Conclusions

The market and competition are powerful means by which change can be created in the delivery of healthcare, though it is difficult to create and sustain competition because of persistent market failures and inequity in income and wealth distribution. It is salutary to note that market-oriented reform plans in healthcare, be they those of the Thatcher Government in the UK[22] or the Jackson Hole Group in the USA,[23] have failed to produce the promise of their architects. Despite this evidence, renewed hope springs regularly on both sides of the Atlantic and throughout other healthcare systems in Australasia and continental Europe that competitive forces can be engineered to improve resource allocation.

Reforming healthcare: setting goals and incentivising change

Healthcare is a labour-intensive service and its decision makers are constantly changing their activity in response to often non-evidence-based advocacy of care by commercial (e.g. the pharmaceutical industry) and non-commercial organisations (e.g. the Medical Royal Colleges) and in response to non-evidence-based policy change. The marked propensity of policy makers worldwide to respond to often ill-defined 'crises' in their healthcare systems by 'redisorganising' the structures of healthcare provision and finance, while neglecting to evaluate such change, ensures a vicious circle of management activity which fails to focus on the fundamental problems of healthcare markets.

The waste inherent in such social experimentation without evaluation can be mitigated by clarity in the goals of managerial and policy change, and the better use of incentives to alter behaviour. Although the fundamental goals of healthcare policy are value for money, or efficiency and equity, all governments are concerned with the control of expenditure. Each of these goals will be briefly examined.

Expenditure control

It is common for healthcare reformers to focus on financial reform, be covert about their redistributive goals and imply, without evidence, that this will affect the efficiency of the delivery of healthcare.

All healthcare funding comes from householders. It is they who own the assets that produce income (rent, interest and profits from property, and wages from labour). To fund healthcare, householders can be obliged to give up their incomes either by taxation (where progressive income tax is the most effective way of redistributing income), by social insurance contributions (which are *de facto* taxes and usually levied in proportion to income), by private insurance contributions (which in a system like the US where the majority of the working population are covered by private insurance, can be regressive) and by co-payments or user charges (which are regressive).

The choice of funding source is essentially about the distributive goals that a society or its government wishes to achieve. Reformers on the right will seek to shift the burden of financing away from their supporters, the relatively affluent, towards poorer groups in society. This is epitomised both by the Howard Government in Australia (*see* Chapter 12) and UK advocates of user charges as the 'remedy' for NHS underfunding.[24] Those on the left used to advocate increased funding financed by income taxes. This was the response of the French Government (*see* Chapter 8), although in the UK this was seen as difficult, and a less redistributive financing source (national insurance contributions) was used by the Blair Government to fund its 'modernisation' of the NHS.

Generally, such choices are made with little reference to who should bear the burden of increased funding and are accompanied by assertions about how the funding will 'transform' healthcare delivery. This is simple nonsense, as increasing aggregate funding is unlikely to have any effect on the behaviour of the provider and is rarely accompanied by policies that address the fundamental failings of healthcare markets. Thus the British decision to increase NHS funding levels was accompanied by the setting of ambitious, largely uncosted and unprioritised access and quality targets, but did not address whether existing assets could be better incentivised to reduce practice variations and improve outcomes for patients from existing funding. The structural reforms implemented were largely non-evidence-based.

An important aspect of healthcare funding choice is whether the method used ensures expenditure control. In this era of emphasis on fiscal prudence, budget deficits are regarded as unwise (except in the US!), even if they are necessary in Keynesian terms for reflating economies such as those in France, Germany and Japan. Political adherence, or lip service at least, to the ideology of the 'small government' exerts considerable pressure on public funding of healthcare.

Household funding of healthcare creates the income of healthcare providers. Consequently, provider advocacy of increased funding is inevitable, as seen in the activities of professional organisations such as the British Medical Association and the Medical Royal Colleges, as well as commercial beneficiaries such as the pharmaceutical industry. Assessment of such provider advocacy has to examine the public interest as well as the providers' concern to increase their income and employment. This inflationary pressure, intensified by asymmetric information and other market failures, can be countered by market competition and government funding, which is cash limited.

Both methods of cost containment are imperfect. While market-oriented economists continue to advocate competition as the means to controlling aggregate expenditure, it is difficult to both create and sustain that competition. Thus Enthoven has repeatedly and logically set out the necessary design characteristics for a market in healthcare to work in principle, but managed care in the US failed because those conditions were ignored.[23] The performance of so-called healthcare markets like those in the US, Australia and Switzerland, epitomise the failure of private insurers to be effective in controlling activity levels and prices in healthcare. Such control is complicated by the fragmented nature of funding with a multiplicity of public and private agencies countervailing each other. In such countries, there are large public and private sectors and an attempt to limit expenditure in one sector can merely increase expenditure in another sector with no overall control of total funding. Competition as a means of controlling healthcare expenditure has not worked. Its advocates continue to assert, like the novelist GK Chesterton argued about Christianity: it has not failed; it just has not been tried properly!

Government control of public expenditure has been effective in many countries; indeed some might argue that prior to 1999 in the UK such controls were too successful in constraining NHS spending. The success of countries such as Sweden (when it cut expenditure to meet EU entry requirements) and New Zealand is evidence that if governments wish to control funding they can do so. Of course, such choices will be affected by the political climate and impending elections may lead to expenditures to buy votes in marginal constituencies. Thus government funding of healthcare may provide the necessary conditions for control, but not sufficient conditions, given the nature of the political marketplace. The evidence about the apparent beneficial attributes of national health insurance in terms of its control over expenditure, lower administrative costs and universal access continues to fuel advocacy of such funding methods in the US and elsewhere.[25]

The efficiency goal

Whatever the level of funding available in a healthcare system, the challenge is to ensure that that budget is used to create the highest level of increase in population health that is possible. Efficiency is a concept that links inputs to outputs or the value of what a society gives up – the opportunity cost – and what it gains – the value it places on improvements in health. Whether the country is Malawi, one of the ten poorest countries in the world, or Britain, one of the most affluent, the policy challenge in public healthcare systems is to use available resources to produce health gain at least cost. Decision makers in private healthcare systems are rewarded for providing what people are willing to pay for and if market preferences are for health gain maximisation, then private healthcare systems also will strive after value for money or efficiency and seek to achieve the greatest health improvement for clients at least cost.

Whatever the level of expenditure and however efficient the delivery of healthcare, rationing is unavoidable. Rationing involves depriving patients of care from which they would benefit and which they would like to receive. Rationing is unavoidable because life is finite, the product of a terminal sexually transmitted disease, and demand can be infinite. In the face of the ubiquitous scarcity of resources, the problem is not whether to ration but how. This universal problem was discussed by Fuchs 30 years ago when he quoted the Book of Atonement (Yom Kippur) prayer book:

> *Who shall live and who shall die, who shall fulfil his days and who shall die before his time . . .*[26]

Rationing can be carried out in relation to patients' willingness and ability to pay or in relation to need. Most healthcare systems have elements of both the market and non-market mechanisms, although in Canada private healthcare insurance is not permitted. In the publicly funded systems, need can be defined as the ability of the patient to benefit from care. In such a system and if resources are to be used efficiently to maximise achievable population health gain, resources have to be targeted at those patients who can gain most from care. Where healthcare interventions are inefficient and of little benefit to patients, they may be left in pain and discomfort, and ultimately to die. This outcome is inevitable for us all eventually. When cure is impossible, it is important to ensure that the path to death is supported efficiently and in a humane manner. In the most expensive *public* healthcare system in the world (US), access is determined by the rules in Medicare, Medicaid and Veterans Administration systems. Consequently access to pharmaceutical benefits for the elderly under Medicare are poor, while in the UK NHS they are extensive with no co-payment.

In private healthcare systems, those without health insurance, for instance the 42 million Americans who have no insurance, may receive care, but it may bankrupt them. In some economies, like China, those able to pay can access highly sophisticated care, while the 800 million poor rural people get poor access, and when in need face penury and premature death. The benefits of private insurance packages are always finite and annual renewal can lead the ill to lose cover and face substantial bills.

Rationing is ubiquitous and the form it takes varies between healthcare systems, as well as within healthcare systems, as practitioners use often arbitrary rules to determine access to care. Recently the English Government has ruled that interferon beta should be given to those multiple sclerosis patients who, at particular stages of their disease, can benefit from it. Prior to this, local decision makers had different rules about availability of this drug, which is low in cost-effectiveness. In the Lothian region around Edinburgh, the drug was not available. In North Yorkshire it was available subject to strict local criteria. This postcode rationing was the product of different conclusions about cost-effectiveness arrived at by local experts. Now that the drug is supposed to be available within limiting criteria in England, take-up remains uneven because of local priorities and the availability of resources to implement change.

The pursuit of efficiency requires the continuous development and updating of the evidence base and its appropriate application. Unfortunately, the investment in improving the knowledge base of medical practice remains inadequate and medical practice can be slow to change outside the pharmaceutical practices, where change can be induced both quickly and inefficiently.[27–29]

Equity

The original rationale of increased government activity in healthcare markets worldwide was the failure of private markets to deliver care to the poor. This failure is unsurprising, as private insurance is designed to support those with the resources to purchase cover. Typically, governments have supported private initiative (e.g. the Friendly Societies which provided some cover in the nineteenth century), then provided cover for the labour force for reasons such as heading off workers' discontent (Bismarck's reforms in Germany in the late nineteenth century) and improving population health (e.g. when many army recruits for the Boer War were found to be in poor health), and then finally, usually in a piecemeal fashion except in countries such as the UK and New Zealand which developed national health services (1938 and 1948 respectively), full cover for the whole population has been developed.

However, it is evident from research that this has failed to deal with significant inequalities in access, funding and health. Initially, 'free' at the point of consumption care was assumed to have dealt with the equity in utilisation issue, but the research literature denied this.[19,30] By the late 1960s in Britain, there was acceptance of geographical inequalities in NHS funding and the emergence of formulae in the constituent parts of the UK to mitigate them.

Discussion of health inequalities was stymied during the period of the Conservative Government (1979–97) and, for ideological reasons, income and wealth inequalities, usually highly correlated with health inequalities, were allowed to increase. The Blair Administration declared itself intent on reducing disadvantage in the public sector, but progress in the health sector has been limited. The primary cause of this is the unusual adherence of the Government to one of its election pledges: not to raise income tax. So while the tax burden has increased considerably since 1997, and there has been some progress in reducing child poverty, significant reductions in income and wealth inequalities remain elusive, as do reductions in health inequalities.

The Government has Wanless investigating these issues, with an English remit and its initial focus is rather narrow, i.e. addressing inequalities in the length of life, rather than quality-adjusted length of life. Even if income redistribution were politically possible, Wildman has shown that policies designed to maximise health and reduce health inequalities as proposed by the Labour Government[31] can be incompatible. Furthermore it has been shown that health promotion policies can increase income inequalities because, for instance, the poor's feelings of hopelessness may lead to lower take-up rates of health-improving behaviours. The consequence of this is that, with the middle class adopting health promotion messages more rapidly, health inequalities may widen.[15,32]

Another approach to the inequality issue is the use of equity weights in prioritising healthcare investments. At present, technology appraisals, such as those carried out by the National Institute for Clinical Excellence (NICE), focus on the clinical and cost-effectiveness of new technologies, with guidance being determined largely by economic considerations. A NICE policy issue is whether measures of cost-effectiveness should be weighted by equity, i.e. any technology that improved the health status of the poor more than the middle classes might be given some greater preference.

The leading proponent of this is Williams, who has proposed the 'fair innings' approach.[33] His preferred measure of the success of a technology is the quality-adjusted life-year or QALY.[34] He argues that society prefers to direct resources to those who have not had a fair innings, at the expense of the elderly. This alleged preference needs careful empirical measurement to determine how much resource should be shifted from the relatively efficient treatment of the elderly to the inefficient treatment of chronically ill younger patients. Even if Williams' fair innings approach is not accepted, some form of equity weighting of treatments for the disadvantaged, however determined, may be socially acceptable. If so, such redistribution through the healthcare system may reduce inequalities in health, particularly if the focus of measurement is not mere length of life but also its quality, or QALYs.

Overview

What are the goals of healthcare policy? It is difficult to achieve expenditure control, efficiency and equity together, and as a consequence choices have to be made about the ranking of these goals and the acceptable trade-offs. The simplistic interpretation of the mandate of public healthcare systems is that they should maximise improvement in population health, i.e. they should pursue efficiency.

However, these systems were created because of equity concerns. If we assume that the goal of healthcare is to improve health, this equity goal has to be defined as reducing inequalities in both the duration and quality of life of poor and middle-class citizens. It seems likely that society cannot pursue effective reduction in health inequalities before it first addresses inequalities in income.[15] Without this, interventions in the NHS are likely not only to be difficult to implement but also to have limited effects on the considerable inequalities in health that continue in healthcare systems such as those in the UK.

Creating change

Inefficiency such as variations in clinical practice and the failure to measure success with appropriate measures of health outcome, together with persistent inequalities in health, are sustained by well-chronicled failures in public and private markets. These market failures and the inefficiency and inequalities they sustain are perpetuated by the unwillingness of governments to define clearly their goals and their failure to incentivise change with better evaluation and reward systems. Instead, governments prefer to reform healthcare structures and processes continually and blindly, reluctant to learn from their continual social experiments and refusing to accept that their success is dependent on the evidence base about practice and policy.

A nice example of this blind approach to the policy process is general practice fundholding. The Conservatives adopted this from academic debates.[35] This reform or social experiment merited careful evaluation but the Government denied this and asserted that it was obviously going to be successful!

Both this arrogant belief and that of the Opposition, which rejected the policy as 'divisive and inefficient', was based on opinion rather than evidence. When Labour came into power they pledged to abolish GP fundholding and this they did in 1999. In 2003, a study showed nicely that GP fundholding had reduced hospital admissions.[36] If general practice is to be incentivised, some form of fundholding will have to be reintroduced.

Campbell argued over 35 years ago that all reforms are social experiments.[37] He emphasised the need to evaluate these experiments so that future change could be evidence based. His pleas remain largely unheard and politicians continue to experiment in ways that potentially damage patients' welfare. Reform that is not informed by the evidence base uses resources that could be used to treat patients. Denying patients care by well-meant but ill-considered changes in organisational and incentive structures is clearly inefficient and unethical. But as Marmor has remarked, 'what is regular, is not stupid'. The inefficient pursuit of healthcare reforms may bring few benefits to taxpayers and patients, but enhances the fortunes of their political architects and the provider interests they champion.

References

1 Coase R (1988) *The Firm, the Market, and the Law.* Chicago: University of Chicago Press.
2 Smith A (1776 and 1976) *An Inquiry into the Nature and Causes of the Wealth of Nations.* Campbell RH, Skinner AS (eds). Clarendon Press: Oxford.
3 Friedman M (1962) *Capitalism and Freedom.* Chicago: University of Chicago Press.
4 Rae J (1895) *Life of Adam Smith.* London: McMillan & Co.
5 Stigler GJ (1974) Free riders and collective action: an appendix to theories of economic regulation. *The Bell Journal of Economics and Management Science.* **5**(2): 359–65.
6 McGuire TG (2000) Physician agency. In: Culyer AJ, Newhouse JP (eds) *Handbook of Health Economics*, vol. 1A. Amsterdam: Elsevier.
7 Zweifel P, Manning WG (2000) Moral hazard and consumer incentives in health care. In: Culyer AJ, Newhouse JP (eds) *Handbook of Health Economics*, vol. 1A. Amsterdam: Elsevier, pp. 409–59.
8 Ministry of Health (1944) *A National Health Service.* London: HMSO.
9 Cooper M, Culyer AJ (1970) *An economic assessment of some aspects of the operation of the National Health Service.* In: *Health Services Financing*, Appendix A. London: British Medical Association.
10 Cooper M, Culyer AJ (1971) An economic survey of nature and intent of the British National Health Service. *Social Science and Medicine.* **5**: 1–13.
11 Department of Health and Social Services (1976) *Sharing Resources for Health in England: Report of the Resource Allocation Working Party.* London: DHSS.
12 Maynard A, Ludbrook A (1980) Applying resource allocation formulae to constituent parts of the UK. *Lancet.* **i**: 85–7.
13 Dixon A, Le Grand J, Henderson J, Murray R, Poteliakhoff E (2003) *Is the NHS equitable? A review of the evidence.* London School of Economics Health and Social Care Discussion Series: DP11.
14 Wanless D (2003) *Securing Good Health for the Whole Population: population health trends.* London: HM Treasury.
15 Wildman J (2003) Income related inequalities in mental health in Great Britain: analysing the causes of health inequality over time. *Journal of Health Economics.* **22**: 295–312.
16 Atkinson AB (1999) Income inequality in the UK. *Health Economics.* **8**: 283–8.
17 Grossman M (1972) On the concept of health capital and the demand for health. *Journal of Political Economy.* **80**(2): 223–55.
18 Black Report (1980) *Inequalities in Health: report of a research working group.* London: DHSS.
19 Acheson D (1998) *Report of the Independent Inquiry into Inequalities in Health.* London: Stationery Office.
20 van Doorslaer EV, Wagstaff A, Bleichrodt H, Calonge S, Gerdtham U, Gerfin M *et al.* (1997) Income-related inequalities in health: some international comparisons. *Journal of Health Economics.* **16**: 93–112.
21 Wagstaff A, van Doorslaer E (2000) Equity and the distribution of healthcare and healthcare finance. In: Culyer AJ, Newhouse JP (eds) *Handbook of Health Economics.* Amsterdam: Elsevier.

22 Department of Health (1989) *Working for Patients.* Cmnd 555. London: HMSO.

23 Ellwood PM, Enthoven AC, Etheredge L (1992) The Jackson Hole initiatives for a twenty-first century American health care system. *Health Economics.* 1(3): 149–68.

24 Healthcare 2000 (1995) *UK Health and Healthcare Services: challenges and policy options.* London: Healthcare 2000.

25 Woolhandler S, Campbell T, Himmelstein DU (2003) Costs of health care administration in the United States and Canada. *New England Journal of Medicine.* 349(8): 768–75.

26 Fuchs VF (1924) *Who Shall Live? Health economics and social choice.* New York: Basic Books Inc.

27 Bloor K, Maynard M (2005) International pharmaceutical policy – health creation or wealth creation? In: Freemantle N, Hill S (eds) *Evaluating Pharmaceuticals for Health Policy and Reimbursement* (in preparation).

28 Maynard A, Chalmers I (eds) *Non Random Reflections on Health Services Research: the 25th anniversary of AL Cochrane's effectiveness and efficiency.* London: British Medical Journal Publishing.

29 Chalmers I (2003) Trying to do more good than harm in policy and practice: the role of rigorous, transparent, up-to-date evaluations. *Annals of the American Academy of Political and Social Science.* 589: 22–40.

30 Townsend P, Davidson N, Whitehead M (eds) *Inequalities in Health: the Black Report and the health divide.* New York: Penguin.

31 Department of Health (1998) *Our Healthier Nation: a contract for health.* (Rep. No. 1998h). London: The Stationery Office.

32 Contoyannis P, Forster M (1999) Our healthier nation? *Health Economics.* 8: 289–96.

33 Williams A (1997) Intergenerational equity: an exploration of the 'fair innings' argument. *Health Economics.* 6(2): 117–32.

34 Williams A (1985) The economics of coronary artery bypass grafting. *British Medical Journal.* 291: 326–9.

35 Maynard A, Marinker M, Gray DP (1986) The doctor, the patient and their contract III. Alternative contracts: are they viable? *British Medical Journal.* 292: 1438–40.

36 Dusheiko M, Gravelle H, Jacobs R, Smith P (2003) *The Effects of Budgets on Doctors Behaviour: Evidence from a Natural Experiment.* CMPO Working Paper Series No. 03/064.

37 Campbell DT (1969) Reforms as experiments. *American Psychologist.* 24(4): 409–29.

Chapter 14

Enduring problems in healthcare delivery

Alan Maynard

Introduction

Since the publication of the first Nuffield volume on *The Public–Private Mix for Health* over 20 years ago,[1] healthcare systems have experienced significant increases in funding and many well-intentioned reforms, both structural and financial. Despite these activities, much is unchanged in European, North American and Antipodean healthcare. Acrimonious debates continue as to the level and distribution between income groups of the funding of healthcare. While vague agreement exists about the need to improve the efficiency of healthcare provision with better performance management and market-like incentive structures, there is a lack of clarity concerning the goals of such innovations and a failure to evaluate outcomes systematically in all the countries that have experimented in this way. These omissions are, in part, a product of ideological debate and in part of the public and private reformers' unwillingness to address fundamental inefficiencies that reflect international medical practice.

Fundamental inefficiencies in the delivery of healthcare

Analysis of healthcare markets, whether in Canada, the US, Australia, Scandinavia, Germany, New Zealand, France or elsewhere, is characterised by common, well-researched and durable manifestations of inefficiency. Regardless of the public–private mix for healthcare, medical practice internationally exhibits substantial unmanaged variations in clinical practice and a reluctance to measure the success of healthcare systems by their success in improving the health of populations.

Variations in clinical practice

For over three decades, researchers at the Dartmouth Medical School in the US have been exploring variations in clinical practice in the US. An early, dramatic example of this work compared beneficiaries of the US Medicare programme in Boston and New Haven, places which are not only the homes of the famous universities Harvard and Yale, but also have similar demographic characteristics. The federal Medicare programme provides healthcare benefits for the elderly. Wennberg and his colleagues found that for beneficiaries in these two similar East

Coast cities, the adjusted rates of discharge from hospital, readmission rates, hospital length of stay and reimbursement varied by 47, 29, 15 and 70% respectively. Furthermore, even though expenditure in Boston was nearly double that of New Haven, the mortality rates in the two areas were identical. An obvious question arose from this work: what was the extra spending in Boston buying and could its expenditure be reduced to New Haven levels without affecting its mortality rate?[2,3]

These variations may be caused by demand or supply-side factors. In most studies, the impact of the former is controlled by selecting similar populations for comparison and adjusting the data for remaining differences. Variations appear principally to be caused by supply-side behaviours. Thus Wennberg and Gittelsohn concluded:

> *The amount and cost of hospital treatment in a community has more to do with the number of its physicians, their medical specialties and the procedures they prefer, than the health of their residents.*[4]

The work of the Dartmouth group has stimulated studies of variations throughout the world. For instance, McPherson has found similar variations in the UK and has charted differences in these variations between the US and Western Europe.[5,6] This established body of knowledge has had surprisingly little effect on the design and execution of healthcare reforms.

Wennberg developed the US work into an atlas of variations in medical practice in the US.[7] In recent publications, his associates have re-emphasised the importance of these variations in the US. Fisher and colleagues have noted that US Medicare expenditure per capita in 2000 varied from $10 550 per enrollee in Manhattan to $4823 in Portland, Oregon. These differences were a result of volume effects rather than differences in illness rates, socioeconomic status or the price of services:[8–12]

> *Residents in high spending regions received 60% more care but did not have lower mortality rates, better functional status or higher satisfaction.*[8]

Separately, Fisher noted that there were potential savings for Medicare of 30% of the budget with no adverse effects on patient health if high spending areas reduced expenditure and provided the safe practices of conservative, low-spending areas.[13]

As well as the slight impact this literature has had on healthcare policy and the practice of doctors, related knowledge is equally slow in its effect on practice and policy. Controversy is rife over efforts that have been made to explore the appropriateness of healthcare. Robert Brook's pioneering work in the US was criticised because the definition of what was appropriate for a patient in particular circumstances was inevitably a combination of objective evidence and subjective judgements (in particular, expert opinion and consensus statements made to compensate for incomplete knowledge).[14]

However, while bearing such reservations in mind, the results of this type of research are striking and merit careful evaluation when considering whether resources are allocated efficiently or wastefully in contemporary healthcare systems. For example, American and British clinicians collaborated in a study of the appropriateness of coronary artery bypass surgery (CABG) and coronary angiograph interventions in the Trent region of the English NHS. They used two separate expert panels to determine appropriateness, one American and the other English, concluding that:

> *Inappropriate care even in the face of waiting lists, is a significant problem in Trent. In particular, by the standards of the UK panel, one half of the coronary angiographs were performed for equivocal or inappropriate reasons, and two fifths of the CABGs were performed for similar reasons. Even by the more liberal US criteria, the ratings were 29% equivocal or inappropriate for coronary angiograph and 33% equivocal or inappropriate for CABGs.*[15]

Absence of practice guidelines, based on the best available evidence of cost-effectiveness, and lack of incentives and performance management methods to enforce such guidelines, ensures the maintenance of practice variations and inappropriate care. The waste this imposes on all healthcare systems is considerable and begs the question: is increased investment in healthcare merited when remedying existing inefficiencies would free up considerable resources to improve access and outcomes for patients?

A good example of this inefficiency is brought to light in work in England that has used hospital episode statistics (HES). Yates has published extensively and worked with the Department of Health to identify the causes of lengthy waiting times, and his research on process management has unblocked capacity and lowered waiting lists by reducing variations in activity caused by organisational failures.[16,17]

More recently, research funded by the Department of Health and undertaken by Bloor and her colleagues at York University, has demonstrated the considerable variations in the activity rates of NHS surgical consultants in England. In Figure 14.1, this distribution shows activity by consultant in ascending order from the right, with vertical lines illustrating the activity rates for individual consultants in a particular and anonymous hospital.

The challenge for local managers, clinical and non-clinical, is to explain these variations in consultant activity. The first cause of variation is invalid data. While hospitals are required to collect data on activity (finished consultant episodes, FCEs), the incentives to perform this task accurately are small, as its accuracy affects neither personal nor institutional income. So although HES has cost millions of pounds to collect each year since 1987, its routine use in the NHS has been minimal.

Other causes of variation in activity are public sector bottlenecks, private sector work, the work/leisure choices of practitioners and the quality of some doctors. Yates has demonstrated nicely that activity may be low in the NHS because of local shortages of nurses and beds (often due to delayed discharging of the elderly who should be in social care), and lack of theatre capacity (sometimes occurring when theatre capacity is under-utilised). These problems can be resolved by often quite inexpensive local solutions.[18]

Another possible cause of variation in NHS clinical activity is private work. This may take the form of time given to trade union activities (i.e. the British Medical Association), work for professional organisations (e.g. the Royal Colleges) and private clinical practice. The usual argument about private practice is that practitioners who do this type of work neglect NHS patients. However, Bloor and colleagues[18] have shown that NHS consultants in surgery with maximum

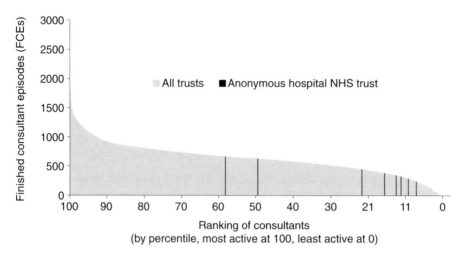

Figure 14.1 Ranked activity per consultant surgeon, FCEs, trauma and orthopaedics.

part-time contracts (who can undertake private practice) do more work for the NHS than full-time consultants in surgery.

Yet another possible cause of variation in clinical activity is the quality of practice. Small numbers of consultants may be incompetent to practice or restricted by their local employers to low levels of activity in simple cases. The extent to which this creates difficulty is unknown, as such problems are regulated imperfectly, with most practitioners having job tenure for life.

Another aspect of the inefficiency inherent in medical practice variation is the failure of healthcare systems to deliver what is appropriate for patients. From the evidence base it is clear that there is a package of interventions which is demonstrably cost-effective, cheap and often not delivered to patients. Identification and management in primary care of conditions such as hypertension, diabetes, asthma and high cholesterol can avoid emergency admissions to hospital and enhance the length and quality of patients' lives. A US study[19] has shown that Americans receive only about half the care they need. In the UK, the Government has recognised similar deficits in the delivery of appropriate primary care and has incentivised a quality framework with fees for service.[20]

The evidence of medical practice variation is extensive, long-standing and depressing. While variation is human, the observable extent of unmanaged variation demonstrates that the available endowments of primary and secondary care, if deployed more efficiently, could produce more population health. Such inefficiency is unethical, depriving patients of care from which they could benefit.

Measuring success: why is outcome measurement absent?

Advocacy of outcome measurement is an ancient practice. In the Babylonian Laws of Hammurabi, there is a clear attempt to measure success and link it to rewards.

> If a surgeon has made a deep incision in the body of a man with a lancet of
> bronze and saves the man's life, or has opened an abscess in the eye of a man

and has saved his eye, he shall take 10 shekels of silver. If the surgeon has made a deep incision in the body of a man with his lancet of bronze and so destroys the man's eye, they shall cut off his hand. (BC 1792)

Florence Nightingale took the success measures of Lunacy Act legislation, which required hospitals to measure whether a patient was dead, relieved or unrelieved, and advocated its more general use. Psychiatric hospitals such as Bootham in York and acute facilities such as St Thomas' in London used this classification until the creation of the NHS. Nightingale argued for this form of measurement in sharp, Thatcherite, value-for-money terms:

> *I am fain to sum up with an urgent appeal for adopting this or some uniform system of publishing the statistical records of hospitals. There is a growing conviction that in all hospitals, even in those which are best conducted, there is a great and unnecessary waste of life. . . . In attempting to arrive at the truth, I have applied everywhere for information, but in scarcely an instance have I been able to obtain hospital records fit for any purpose of comparison. If they could be obtained, they would enable us to decide many other questions besides the ones alluded to. They would show subscribers how their money was being spent, what amount of good was really being done with it, or whether the money was doing mischief rather than good.* (F Nightingale, *Some Notes on Hospitals* (3e), 1863)

The high mortality rates in nineteenth-century hospitals affected not only Nightingale but also other leading policy advocates. Semmelweis identified the effects of poor hand hygiene in a study of maternal mortality in Vienna in the 1840s.[21] But such work had all too little consistent and long-term effect on the practice of medicine. A literature review on hospital-acquired infections 15 years ago noted problems similar to those 100 years earlier – and with the additional problem of antibiotic resistance![22]

More recently, there has been an increased interest in medical errors following the publication of a US Institute of Medicine report.[23] Extrapolating data from local studies to create a national estimate of the mortality effects, it was concluded that medical errors kill between 44 000 and 98 000 Americans each year, i.e. more than motor vehicle accidents (43 458), more than HIV/AIDS (16 516) and more than breast cancer (42 297). Medication errors alone kill three times as many Americans annually as died in the New York Twin Towers on 11 September 2001. Mistakes, surgical errors and poor hand hygiene are all well-known risks, which are badly managed worldwide.

Australian studies have revealed error rates of 16%, i.e. 16 in 100 hospital admissions are subject to errors. When the Australian data are mapped onto the more conservative American methodology, their error rate falls to 10%.[24] This is the error rate claimed to exist in the UK NHS, although the only empirical study is a small-scale retrospective analysis of one London hospital.[25]

Another manifestation of medical errors in England has been a series of cases demonstrating that practitioners have killed or significantly impaired the functional health of a large number of patients. Wishart, a practitioner in Bristol killed 29 children and damaged others with defective paediatric surgical interventions that were evident to local and national management for many years. Two gynaecological surgeons, Neale and Ledward, damaged dozens of women in

North Yorkshire and Kent. Shipman, a general practitioner, may have killed over 200 of his patients with lethal morphine injections. These tragic episodes demonstrate that retrospective analysis of routine NHS data (HES) showed the damage done by Ledward and in Bristol. Unfortunately, their management systems failed to use these data and act on them.

These examples of failure, together with academic publications,[26] have focused greater attention on outcome measurement in the NHS, although this focus has been very limited and often restricted to mortality rates. Dr Foster, a private organisation, has employed Jarman's approach, producing an annual report on hospital staffing and the standardised mortality rates of each institution. While this work offers a useful focus on outcomes for patients, it is quite limited, as the numbers are small and the source, Hospital Episode Statistics (HES), requires careful validation.

Most patients entering the healthcare system, whether in primary or secondary care, survive. The relevant measure of success is, therefore, the effect of interventions on the health-related quality of life (HRQoL) of patients. Validated generic HRQoL figures exist and have been used in hundreds of clinical trials and to measure population health (www.sf36.org and www.euroqol.org). An example is the application of SF36 to privately treated patients in the hospitals of the British United Provident Association (BUPA). Their use of an HRQoL was brought about by the damage Ledward inflicted on their private patients. To enhance 'consumer protection' they now ask their patients to complete SF36 at entry to hospital and three months after discharge. The data they collect indicate restoration of physical, social and psychological functioning, and BUPA concentrates its management efforts on practitioners three standard deviations from the average. The SF36 data informs those interactions and facilitates greater understanding of failures.[27]

While such measures are used by groups of practitioners in healthcare systems, not all countries have implemented system-wide use of such measures. There is a strong case for careful piloting of the use of HRQoL on populations, as without it policy and practice will focus on performance measures of process (e.g. activity rates and waiting times) and mortality outcomes that are of limited use. With such measures particularly, if they are linked across primary and hospital care, it will be possible to measure the success of interventions over time for episodes of ill health as well as to provide long-term population measures to inform epidemiology and prevention policies.

Overview

The long-standing and relatively well-researched nature of variations in clinical practice is remarkable. These characteristics are paralleled with the associated problem of the poor evidence base of medical practice. Cochrane remarked 30 years ago that only about 10% of medical practice was supported by evidence that it did more harm than good.[28] The evidence base has since improved, but many interventions are of uncertain benefit to patients. This improvement is the product of, among other things, the Cochrane Collaboration – an integrated network of researchers working to common techniques of systematic review and evaluation.[29] Practitioners and policy makers still have to be reminded to be modest in their claims of being able to heal the sick:

Because professionals sometimes do more harm than good when they intervene in the lives of other people, their policies and practices should be informed by rigorous, transparent and up to date evaluations.[30]

This chronic, well-evidenced propensity to deliver healthcare of uncertain clinical and cost-effectiveness to patients is coupled with the evident reluctance of practitioners and policy makers to translate evidence into practice. Why does this market continue to fail the patient, in the face of well-researched evidence about medical practice variations, of evidence of what works and what is unproven by the Cochrane Collaboration, and of an obvious need to measure success in terms of the effects of healthcare providers on population health?

Obstacles to change

Separating ideological from empirical issues

In health policy, there are some areas where the competing public and private parties can agree to an agenda for collaborative work, and others where values will always differ and the parties should recognise this. The latter are illustrated in Tables 14.1–14.3.[31]

The Libertarian–Conservative–Republican camp believes freedom to be the supreme goal for society. Government is seen as a threat to freedom, which can only be protected and furthered by private markets and competition.

The Egalitarian–Socialist–Democrat perspective focuses principally on creating and sustaining equality of opportunity. Government is not seen as a threat, but the means by which private markets are corrected so that individuals achieve greater real freedom.

The two groups, Libertarian and Egalitarian, argue about health policy from their own perspectives of an ideal healthcare system (Table 14.2). They have very different views about the demand and supply characteristics of their systems and disagree about adjustment mechanisms and the criteria by which they judge their systems to be successful. In the Libertarian system, success is judged by consumers in relation to getting what they want, how and when they want it. In the Egalitarian system, the electorate would ideally judge success in relation to the extent to which population health is improved and from the available budget.

These ideals can be compared with the actual performance of the private and public systems. Both systems may fail as shown, in terms of demand and supply, adjustment mechanisms and success criteria. In the private system, consumers will judge success in relation to their accessing care without being bankrupted or experiencing sharp increases in their premium rates. In the public system, success measurement will focus on mortality, and the success of the system in terms of improving the patients' health-related quality of life is ignored.

These three tables summarise the essence of the ideological debate about healthcare. That debate often creates little agreement and enlightenment and consumes large volumes of scarce resources, in particular, political and research capacity. It is imperative to agree a research agenda which bridges the ideological divide and which facilitates the creation of a better knowledge base about what works in health policy.

Table 14.1 Attitudes typically associated with viewpoints A and B

	Viewpoint A (Libertarian)	*Viewpoint B (Egalitarian)*
Personal responsibility	Personal responsibility for achievement is very important, and this is weakened if people are offered unearned rewards. Moreover, such unearned rewards weaken the motive force that assures economic well-being and in so doing they also undermine moral well-being, because of the intimate connection between moral well-being and the personal effort to achieve	Personal incentives to achieve are desirable, but economic failure is not equated with moral depravity or social worthlessness
Social concern	Social Darwinism dictates a seemingly cruel indifference to the fate of those who cannot make the grade. A less extreme position is that charity, expressed and effected preferably under private auspices, is the proper vehicle, but it needs to be exercised under carefully prescribed conditions, for example, such that the potential recipient must first mobilise all his own resources and, when helped, must not be in as favourable a position as those who are self-supporting (the principle of 'lesser eligibility')	Private charitable action is not rejected but is seen as potentially dangerous morally (because it is often demeaning to the recipient and corrupting to the donor) and usually inequitable. It seems preferable to establish social mechanisms that create and sustain self-sufficiency and that are accessible according to precise rules concerning entitlement that are applied equitably and explicitly sanctioned by society at large
Freedom	Freedom is to be sought as a supreme good in itself. Compulsion attenuates both personal responsibility and individualistic and voluntary expressions of social concern. Centralised health planning and a large governmental role in healthcare financing are seen as an unwarranted abridgement of the freedom of clients as well as of health professionals and private medicine is thereby viewed as a bulwark against totalitarianism	Freedom is seen as the presence of real opportunities of choice; although economic constraints are less openly coercive than political constraints, they are nonetheless real and often the effective limits on choice. Freedom is not indivisible but may be sacrificed in one respect in order to obtain greater freedom in some other. Government is not an external threat to individuals in the society but is the means by which individuals achieve greater scope for action (that is, greater real freedom)
Equality	Equality before the law is the key concept, with clear precedence being given to freedom over equality wherever the two conflict	Since the only moral justification for using personal achievement as the basis for distributing rewards is that everyone has equal opportunities for such achievement, then the main emphasis is on equality of opportunity; where this cannot be assured, the moral worth of achievement is thereby undermined. Equality is seen as an extension to the many, of the freedom actually enjoyed by only the few

Table 14.2 Idealised healthcare systems

	Private	Public
Demand	• Individuals are the best judges of their own welfare • Priorities determined by own willingness and ability to pay • Erratic and potentially catastrophic nature of demand mediated by private insurance • Matters of equity to be dealt with elsewhere (e.g. in the tax and social security systems)	• When ill, individuals are frequently imperfect judges of their own welfare • Priorities determined by social judgements about need • Erratic and potentially catastrophic nature of demand made irrelevant by provision of free services • Since the distribution of income and wealth is unlikely to be equitable in relation to the need for healthcare, the system must be insulated from its influence
Supply	• Profit is the proper and effective way to motivate suppliers to respond to the needs of demanders • Priorities determined by people's willingness and ability to pay and by the costs of meeting their wishes at the margin • Suppliers have strong incentive to adopt least-cost methods of provision	• Professional ethics and dedication to public service are the appropriate motivation, focusing on success in curing or caring • Priorities determined by where the greatest improvements in caring or curing can be effected at the margin • Predetermined limit on available resources generates a strong incentive for suppliers to adopt least cost methods of provision
Adjustment mechanism	• Many competing suppliers ensure that offer prices are kept low and reflect costs • Well-informed consumers are able to seek out the most cost-effective form of treatment for themselves • If, at the price that clears the market, medical practice is profitable, more people will go into medicine and hence supply will be demand responsive • If, conversely, medical practice is unremunerative, people will leave it, or stop entering it, until the system returns to equilibrium	• Central review of activities generates efficiency audit of service provision and management pressures keep the system cost-effective • Well-informed clinicians are able to prescribe the most cost-effective form of treatment for each patient • If there is resulting pressure on some facilities or specialties, resources will be directed towards extending them • Facilities or specialties on which pressure is slack will be slimmed down to release resources for other uses
Success criteria	• Consumers will judge the system by their ability to get someone to do what they demand, when, where and how they want it • Producers will judge the system by how good a living they can make out of it	• Electorate judges the system by the extent to which it improves the health status of the population at large in relation to the resources allocated to it • Producers judge the system by its ability to enable them to provide the treatments they believe to be cost-effective

Table 14.3 Actual healthcare systems

	Private	Public
Demand	• Doctors act as agents, medicating demand on behalf of consumers • Priorities determined by the reimbursement rules of insurance funds • Because private insurance coverage is itself a profit-seeking activity, some risk-rating is inevitable; hence, coverage is incomplete and uneven, distorting personal willingness and ability to pay • Attempts to change the distribution of income and wealth independently are resisted as destroying incentives (one of which is the ability to buy better or more medical care if you are rich)	• Doctors act as agents, identifying need on behalf of patients • Priorities determined by the doctor's own professional situation, by his assessment of the patient's condition and the expected trouble-making proclivities of the patient • Freedom from direct financial contributions at the point of service and absence of risk-rating enables patients to seek treatment for trivial or inappropriate conditions • Attempts to correct inequities in the social and economic system by differential compensatory access to health services leads to recourse to healthcare in circumstances where it is unlikely to be a cost-effective solution to the problem
Supply	• What is most profitable to suppliers may not be what is most in the interests of consumers and since neither consumers nor suppliers may be very clear about what is in the former's interests, this gives suppliers a range of discretion • Priorities determined by the extent to which consumers can be induced to part with their money and by the costs of satisfying the pattern of 'demand' • Profit motive generates a strong incentive towards market segmentation and price discrimination and tie-in agreements with other professionals	• Personal professional dedication and public-spirited motivation likely to be corroded and degenerate into cynicism if others, who do not share those feelings, are seen to be doing very well for themselves through blatantly self-seeking behaviour • Priorities determined by what gives the greatest professional satisfaction • Since cost-effectiveness is not accepted as a proper medical responsibility, such pressures merely generate tension between the 'professionals' and the 'managers'

Adjustment mechanism	• Professional, ethical rules are used to make overt competition difficult • Consumers denied information about quality and competence and, since insured, may collude with doctors (against the insurance carriers) in inflating costs • Entry into the profession made difficult and numbers restricted to maintain profitability • If demand for services falls, doctors extend range of activities and push out neighbouring disciplines	• Because it does not need elaborate cost data for billing purposes, it does not routinely generate much useful information on costs • Clinicians know little about costs and have no direct incentive to act on such information as they have – and sometimes quite perverse incentives (i.e. cutting costs may make life more difficult or less rewarding for them) • Very little is known about the relative cost-effectiveness of different treatments and even where it is, doctors are wary of acting on such information until a general professional consensus emerges • The phasing out of facilities that have become redundant is difficult because it often threatens the livelihood of some concentrated specialised group and has identifiable people dependent on it, whereas the beneficiaries are dispersed and can only be identified as statistics
Success criteria	• Consumers will judge the system by their ability to get someone to do what they need done without making them 'medically indigent' and/or changing their risk-rating too adversely • Producers will judge the system by how good a living they can make out of it	• Since the easiest aspect of health status to measure is life expectancy, the discussion is dominated by mortality data and mortality risks to the detriment of treatments concerned with non-life-threatening situations • In the absence of accurate data on cost-effectiveness, producers judge the system by the extent to which it enables them to carry out the treatments that they find the most exciting and satisfying

Seven areas for research

In evaluating practice and policy and improving the evidence base, answers to the following research questions continue to be of importance, but the gathering of evidence to answer them remains elusive.

1 What are the objectives of the healthcare system, regardless of the public–private mix? What ordering or weight do these objectives get and how are these changing over time? Equity in terms of distribution and access is important and covers most systems; also, what weight is being given to the priorities which have emerged as a result of 55 years of experience of the NHS? How are they likely to be affected by change in the public–private mix? An analysis of public statements could identify the clarity or contradictions in objective setting and make possible the determination of consistent sets of possible objectives for the healthcare system, public and private.

2 Who is really responsible for control of the system(s): and who controls resource use at the 'margins' or boundaries of care, e.g. the boundaries between hospital and primary and social care; the boundary between capital and current revenue allocation; the boundary between capital and labour; and the boundaries between the public and private sectors? Who controls any movements in these boundaries? What criteria are used to determine policy making at these boundaries? Why is it that insurance principles and practice, seem to gravitate only towards institutional care and particularly for acute (mainly surgical) cases, and not for general practice, prevention, the care of the elderly and other services for the chronically ill?

3 What incentives (monetary and non-monetary) are there (or lack of them) to achieve efficiency for individual clinical and non-clinical managers and for institutions in the public and private sectors? Why do decision makers at the boundaries behave as they do? What incentives motivate public and private action, and the interaction between the public and private sectors? Is inefficient behaviour in labour, capital and service provision markets an inevitable product of poor incentives? For example, is the long-term survival of clinical variations a product of rational behaviour? Is it likely that research in this area could identify how behaviour in the public and private sectors could be altered with new incentives to make it more consistent with policy objectives? (as in 1 above).

4 Who rations what and how? What criteria are used by what decision makers in the public and private sectors to allocate scarce healthcare resources which have effects at the micro (operational) level? Is the allocation that results consistent with the avowed rationing criteria of the sector and the policy objectives of that sector or system?

5 How is success determined at the level of the patient, the practitioner and institutions such as GP practices and hospitals? Is measurement and management of activity, access, waiting times and failures due to medical errors as measured by mortality data an adequate proxy for 'success'? How is health to be described? How are alternative states of health to be valued relative to each other? Whose values for different health states should be elicited and how should they be aggregated? How are views about 'equity' to be incorporated

into the measurement process? What are the obstacles to the use of health-related quality-of-life measures in routine medical practice?

6 Who in effect decides, and what are the investment criteria used in the public and private healthcare sectors? Are the techniques of investment appraisal used? If so, how? If not, what criteria decides who will get a new hospital or a new piece of medical equipment, and are they consistent with policy objectives and the optimum use of resources?

7 What are the major unresolved problems in the healthcare system? This question takes us back to question 1. Are outcomes, in terms of efficiency (e.g. improving patient health at least cost) and distributional equity, however defined, consistent with policy objectives or does the system (and its public and private sectors) fail to meet its objectives?

The purpose of acquiring answers to this research agenda is to clarify the goals of public and private healthcare systems, understand how decisions are made and better appreciate how performance can be improved. Appreciation of these processes is an essential element in the design of any reform of a healthcare system.

The roles of decision makers

The organisation and funding of this research agenda and the translation of evidence into practice by cautious and gradual reform requires changed behaviour from decision makers at all levels of healthcare systems such as the NHS.

Central government

Were health policy reform to be based on evidence and properly evaluated, its pace would be much slower and achievements more substantial. An observer of the New Zealand health policy argued that much of the 'change' created by reforms was, in fact, illusory and best described as 'jumping on the spot'.[32] As can be seen from the material in the preceding chapters, this conclusion is also valid for many healthcare reform efforts elsewhere and in recent decades. The failure to define the problem, or problems, appraise options for change in relation to the not inconsiderable evidence base that is available and evaluate reform to improve that evidence base wastes enormous amounts of managerial effort.

For central government to become more rational, given the many exigencies of the political system in which it works, it needs more analytical capacity, better information systems and a more fruitful system of collaboration with the research community. Researchers are often accused of failing to communicate their knowledge to the 'practical' men and women who work in government. There are such failures in academia, but one of the principal causes of such imperfect communication is the inability of policy makers, civil servants and health service managers to understand the rudiments of economics, statistics, epidemiology, clinical trial design and medical sociology.

There will always be tension between researchers and policy makers. This was neatly summarised by Nobel Laureate, George Stigler:

> *A scholar ought to be tolerably open minded, unemotional and rational. A*
> *reformer must promise paradise if his reform is adopted. Reform and research*
> *seldom march arm in arm.*

Despite these conflicting priorities, greater effort by both groups is essential if reforms are to be better designed and implemented. An essential element of this is the professionalisation in terms of analytical skills of civil servants, managers and other policy makers. It is unfortunate that downsizing in 2003–4 in the English Department of Health seems likely to have the opposite effect.

Professional organisations

The governance of the healthcare professions is often poor but rarely subject to public debate. The Royal Colleges in Britain grew out of the professionalisation of 'barber-surgeons' and 'apothecaries' centuries ago, and recently have proliferated into 18 institutions. These bodies control entry into medical practice with the General Medical Council (GMC). It is they who control the undergraduate curriculum and the acquisition of postgraduate qualifications and College membership, which in turn determines entrance into specialist status. Similar politically powerful mechanisms exist in other countries.

If there is gross malpractice, the GMC may strike practitioners off their register. However, its work and that of the Colleges is not informed by the systematic management of data about activity, failure (e.g. mortality) and success (improved health-related quality of life). Recent scandals (e.g. in Bristol) have led to GMC reforms but these appear to be weak and there is a risk that reaccreditation processes may remain focused on qualitative rather than quantitative data.

This amateur approach does not create the protection against 'quacks' and malpractice promised in the ancient charters of the Royal Colleges. Furthermore, their activities are subsidised by government with direct allocations of funding and tax subsidies.

It is timely for the regulators, the Royal Colleges and parallel organisations elsewhere, to be better regulated. They should lead change so that practitioners translate evidence into practice and validate their performance data and use it with non-clinical colleagues to better manage the use of taxpayers' money. There is some evidence of such change (e.g. www.rcplondon.ac.uk/healthinformatics) but some Colleges seem locked into ancient practices of little merit in the twenty-first century.[33]

Nursing and other professions in the NHS have been subjected to considerable regulatory change. The challenge is to recognise that for both medical practitioners and nurses, the delivery of care is a team activity and outcomes, good and bad, are their joint responsibility. Illuminating these processes requires sophisticated data as, for instance, an adverse outcome after surgery may be caused by neither the surgeon nor the nurse, but by the anaesthetist. The fragmentation of both regulation and data collection and management makes effective analysis of the patient pathways complex and difficult.

The NHS

Media and political rhetoric tends to depict expenditure on healthcare management and administration as wasteful and unnecessary. In fact, without better management taxpayers' resources will be wasted. The NHS problem is not too much management but too little. Some NHS managers are extraordinarily skilled but even they tend to focus on tactics (e.g. surviving the demands of government access and financial targets) rather than strategy. Most NHS managers do not have the skills and time to concentrate on evidence-based, data-driven decision making. Few of them know what their consultants do in terms of activity and outcomes. The superficiality of management in the NHS, and all other healthcare systems, is astonishing, with both public and private systems held together by independent and isolated medical practitioners who churn patients often very successfully in a largely data-free environment.

The development of the World Wide Web, with access to over 300 000 websites (of very variable quality) on healthcare means that consumers and their carers are now better informed. There is some recognition that NHS management also needs to be better informed, although it is debatable whether spending £4 billion on new information systems is the best policy!

Such a debate has to focus on the incentives needed to get such an IT system designed and used efficiently. The crucial element in this process is the doctors. If they are not involved in the design of the systems, trained in their use and given strong incentives, they will not use them. Hopefully, this lesson has been learned in previous wasteful IT ventures in the NHS. What is needed is careful and clear definition of the necessary core data set and how it will facilitate the identification and erosion of inefficient practices.

Conclusions

The market for healthcare, whether it is private or public, will always be an area of contention and with a high public profile. The competing political parties will continue to manufacture attacks and defences, reforms and counter reforms, which have multiple purposes. Politicians in power have to react to the pressure of their rivals and the media. However, when they use the evidence base, the outcomes can be beneficial as epitomised by the robust defence of the MMR vaccine and the challenge of poor science.[34]

The media and political rivals can create 'crisis' frenzies and it is in their interest to do so. There is an inclination for the public to regard death as a failure rather than an inevitability, a view which is supported by a media that offers uncritical reporting of new and often very expensive technologies that give patients a few more months of sometimes poor-quality life, e.g. the use of the drug taxane for the treatment of certain cancers. Healthcare can repair some of the ravages of living, but peoples' life expectancy and the quality of their lives is more likely to be influenced by their genetic make-up and behaviour over their lifetimes.

As societies spend increasing proportions of their rising GDP on healthcare, more realism about its productivity in terms of improving the health of the population is needed. But this is not in the interest of the media, politicians and commerce. Promising miracles increases their income and power!

The role of academics is to counter the turbulence of the political market-place with the creation and dissemination of the best available evidence. Convincing those in receipt of their messages that there is no quick fix is not easy. Nevertheless, that is the message. We must not be cynical about the healthcare industry, but forever sceptical about its evidence base and its capacity to improve the length and quality of patients' lives.

The healthcare industry of 2005 is remarkably similar to its predecessor of 20 years ago. It is now more expensive, with some significant interventions of proven cost-effectiveness capable of transforming human life. However, large and unexplained variations in clinical practice continue and the measurement of success in terms of improved health is absent. Too much remains, both in the therapeutic area and in the reform of the healthcare system, which has no evidence base. The challenge is to make both health policy and medical practice more evidence-based and accountable. Hopefully, over the next 20 years we will be even more successful in managing the enduring problems in healthcare delivery than we have been in the last two decades!

References

1 McLachlan G, Maynard A (eds) (1982) *The Public–Private Mix for Health*. London: The Nuffield Provincial Hospitals Trust.
2 Wennberg JE, Freeman JL, Culp WJ (1987) Are hospital services rationed in New Haven or over-utilised in Boston. *Lancet*. 23 May: 1185–8.
3 Wennberg JE, Freeman JL, Shelton RM, Bubolz TA (1989) Hospital use and mortality among Medicare beneficiaries in Boston and New Haven. *New England Journal of Medicine*. **321**: 1168–73.
4 Wennberg JE, Gittelsohn A (1982) Variations in medical care among small areas. *Scientific American*. **264**(4): 120–34.
5 McPherson K (1990) Why do variations occur? In: Anderson TF, Mooney G (eds) *The Challenges of Medical Practice Variations*. Basingstoke: Macmillan Press, pp. 16–35.
6 McPherson K, Wennberg JE, Hovind OB, Clifford P (1982) Small-area variations in the use of common surgical procedures: an international comparison of New England, England, and Norway. *New England Journal of Medicine*. **307**(21): 1310–14.
7 The Dartmouth Atlas of Health Care Project. Center for the Evaluative Clinical Sciences at Dartmouth Medical School, Hanover, New Hampshire. [Online] [accessed February 2004] Available from URL www.dartmouthatlas.org/99USlinks/chap_3_SCV.php
8 Fisher ES, Wennberg DE, Stukel TA, Gottlieb DJ, Lucas FL, Pinder EL (2003) The implications of regional variations in Medicare spending. Part 2: health outcomes and satisfaction with care. *Annals of Internal Medicine*. **138**: 288–98.
9 Fisher ES, Wennberg DE, Stukel TA, Gottlieb DJ, Lucas FL, Pinder EL (2003) The implications of regional variations in Medicare spending. Part 1: the content, quality, and accessibility of care. *Annals of Internal Medicine*. **138**: 273–87.
10 Phelps CE (2003) What's enough, what's too much. *Annals of Internal Medicine*. **138**: 348–9.
11 Shine KI (2003) Geographical variations in Medicare Spending. *Annals of Internal Medicine*. **138**: 347–8.
12 Wilensky GR (2003) The implications of regional variations in Medicare – what does it mean for Medicare? *Annals of Internal Medicine*. **138**: 350–1.
13 Fisher ES, Wennberg JE, Stukel TA, Sharp S (1994) Hospital readmission rates for cohorts of Medicare beneficiaries in Boston and New Haven. *New England Journal of Medicine*. **331**: 989–95.

14 Brook RH, Kamberg CJ, Mayer-Oakes A, Beers MH, Raube K, Steiner A (1990) Appropriateness of acute medical care for the elderly: an analysis of the literature. *Health Policy.* **14**: 225–42.

15 Bernstein SJ, Kosecoff J, Gray D, Hampton JR, Brook RH (1993) Appropriateness of the use of cardiovascular procedures: British vs US perspectives. *Int J Technol Assess Health Care.* **9**: 3–10.

16 Yates J (1995) *Private Eye, Heart and Hip.* London: Churchill Livingstone.

17 Yates J (1987) *Why Are We Waiting?* Oxford: Oxford University Press.

18 Bloor KE, Maynard A, Freemantle N (2004) Variation in activity rates of consultant surgeons, and the influence of reward structures in the English NHS: descriptive analysis and a multilevel model. *Journal of Health Services Research and Policy.* **9**(2): 76–84.

19 Rand Corporation. The First National Report Card on Quality of Health Care in America. [Online] [accessed May 2004] Available from URL www.rand.org/publications

20 Maynard A, Bloor K. Do those who pay the piper call the tune? *Health Policy Matters.* **8**. Department of Health Sciences, University of York. [Online] [accessed May 2004] Available from URL www.york.ac.uk/healthsciences/pubs/hpmindex.htm

21 Pittet D, Boyce JM (2001) Hand hygiene and patient care: pursuing the Semmelweis legacy. *Lancet.* **April**: 9–20.

22 Currie E, Maynard A (1989) *Economic Aspects of Hospital Acquired Infection.* University of York: Centre for Health Economics.

23 Kohn LT, Corrigan JM, Donaldson MS (1999) *To Err is Human: building a safer health system.* Washington, DC: National Academy Press.

24 Wilson RM, Runciman WB, Gibberd RW *et al.* (1995) The Quality in Australian Health Care Study. *Australian Medical Journal.* **163**: 458–71.

25 Vincent C, Neale G, Woloshynowych M (2001) Adverse events in British hospitals: preliminary retrospective record review. *British Medical Journal.* **322**: 517–19.

26 Jarman B, Gault S, Alves B, Hider A, Dolan S, Cook A *et al.* (1999) Explaining differences in English hospital death rates using routinely collected data. *British Medical Journal.* **318**: 1515–20.

27 Vallance-Owen A, Cubbin S (2002) Monitoring national clinical outcomes: a challenging programme. *British Journal of Health Care Management.* **8**: 412–17.

28 Cochrane AL (1972) *Effectiveness and Efficiency: random reflections on health services.* London: Nuffield Provincial Hospitals Trust. (Reprinted in 1989 in association with the *BMJ*.)

29 Maynard A, Chalmers I (eds) (1997) *Non-random Reflections on Health Services Research: on the 25th anniversary of Archie Cochrane's 'Effectiveness and Efficiency'.* London: BMJ Publishing Group.

30 Chalmers I (2003) Trying to do more good than harm in policy and practice: the role of rigorous, transparent, up-to-date evaluations. *Annals of the American Academy of Political and Social Science.* **589**: 22–40.

31 Maynard A, Williams A (1984) Privatisation and the National Health Service. In: Le Grand J, Robinson R (eds) *Privatisation and the Welfare State.* London: George Allen & Unwin.

32 Cooper MH (1984) Jumping on the spot – health reform New Zealand style. *Health Economics.* **3**: 69–72.

33 Maynard A (2004) *Can the Royal Colleges improve their performance?* Mimeograph, University of York.

34 Taylor B, Miller E, Farrington CP, Cetropoulos MP, Favour-Mayaud JL, Waight P (1999) Autism and measles, mumps and rubella vaccine: no epidemiological evidence for a causal association. *Lancet.* **353**: 2016–29.

Also from The Nuffield Trust

The Public–Private Mix for Health: the relevance and effects of change
Edited by Gordon McLachlan and Alan Maynard
ISBN 0 90057 438 0
Published 1982

This earlier collection of essays gives the views of a number of distinguished analyses in the UK and in seven foreign countries on policy issues of the time, concerned with the public–private mix for healthcare with particular reference to the financial systems. It can be read as a companion to this volume and gives a perspective on healthcare policy and financing which is particularly useful in today's climate.

Index

Page numbers in *italics* refer to figures or tables.

Aaron, Henry 84
access to healthcare
  and GP fundholding 27
  ideological considerations 9–10, 11–12
  and prescription charges 50–1
  private insurance systems 57
  Australia 273–5
  New Zealand *230*
  US healthcare 30, 33, 86–7, 108–9
  see also equity; health inequalities; risk
    selection
Accident Compensation Corporation
  (ACC) 220
Acheson report (1998) 75
activity levels 72, 78
  consultants 295–6, *296*
  New Zealand *229*, 232
  see also capacity constraints
administration costs
  GP fundholding 27
  international comparisons 105
  performance data 72
  prescription charges 50–1
  private insurance systems 100, 105,
    132–3
  US healthcare 100, 105, 132–3
adverse events *see* medical errors
Agenda for Change (DoH; NHS
    Modernisation Agency) 75
alternative therapies *see* complementary
    therapies
ambulatory care
  France 151–2, *152*, 157
  Germany 211–12
  see also primary care
amenity beds 45
Association of Accredited Service Providers
    194, 195
audit arrangements 68
  see also activity levels; inspection and
    regulation; performance management
Audit Commission 68
Australian healthcare system 247–77
  background and structure 247–51, *249*
  dental services 251
  expenditure 248–51, *250*

funding arrangements 248–51, *250*
hospitals 251–5, 275–6
insurance rebate schemes 259, 260–4,
  268
international comparisons 275–7
Life Time Health Cover 259, 260–70,
  276
out-of-pocket payments 255–8, *257*, *263*
Pharmaceutical Benefits Scheme (PBS)
  271–3
private health insurance 251, 255–60
reforms and incentives 258–70
viability of Medicare 274–5, 276–7
workforce planning 273–5

Barnett formula 64
benchmarking 192
Beveridge System 162–3, *163*
Bismarck System 162–3, *163*, 191–3
Blair Government reforms 50, 58, 67–9,
  289, 290–1
block-funding 23, 25
Blue Cross/Shield schemes 34
Book of Atonement (Yom Kippur) 287–8
Bristol Children's Hospital 297
British Household Panel Survey 27
British Medical Association (BMA), on
    insurance-based healthcare 48–9
budget allocations *see* healthcare
    expenditure; NHS funding
budgetary caps, France 148–9, 150–1,
  153–5
bulk-billing 248, 274
BUPA 78, 298
Bush, George HW 85

California State Medicaid programme 30,
  33
Canadian Health and Social Transfer
  (CHST) 127–9
Canadian healthcare system 117–37
  economic growth patterns 119–22
  federal government transfers 127–9, *128*
  healthcare expenditure over GDP 121–2,
    121
  inflationary pressures 122, 132–3, 134–6

Canadian healthcare system (*cont.*)
  provincial government expenditure
    122–3, 125–6, *127*
  regressive income distribution policies
    130–5
  tax revenue cuts 129–32, *130*
capacity constraints 69, 70–1
  Australia 273
capital investments 52, 71
  see also PFIs (Private Finance Initiatives)
capping *see* budgetary caps; drug
    regulation
Castle, Barbara 46
catering services 52, 70
Celebrex 272
change costs
  GP fundholding 27
  vs. potential benefits 49
change creation 290–1
  areas for research 304–5
  ideology as obstacle 299–303
  role of Government 305–6
  role of professions 306
CHEs (Crown Health Enterprises) 227–8
cleaning services 52, 70–1
clinical governance 68
clinical need 239–40
  see also rationing
clinical practice variations 293–9
  evaluation 296–8
  and private work 295–6
cliniques privées 148–9, 150
Clinton, Bill 108
CMU *see Couveture Maladie Universelle*
co-payments
  Australia 271
  France 142–3, 145–6
  Germany 194, 199–201, *200*
  Scandinavian healthcare 164, 168–9,
    169
  US 90–2, *91*
  see also prescription charges; user
    charges
Coase, Ronald 280
Cochrane Collaboration 298–9
Commission for Health Improvement
    (CHI) 56, 68
Commission for Healthcare Audit and
    Inspection (CHAI) 68
Commonwealth funding 248, *249*, 252,
    254
competition 201, 203, 286–7
complaints management 56

complementary therapies 53, 58, 251, 268,
    270
consultants
  activity levels 295–6, *296*
  fees 45, 54, 56
  new contract arrangements 55–6, 73
  private practice incomes 54
  working practices 45–7, 54–5
  see also specialists
consumer-driven healthcare systems 35–6,
    301–2
contracting-out services 52, 55, 70–1
  Scandinavian countries 175–6
Contribution au Remboursement de la Dette
    Sociale (CRDS) 144–5
Contribution Sociale Généralisée (CSG) 144
'corporisation' of hospitals 176–7
  see also Foundation Hospitals
cosmetic surgery 54, 57–8, 227
cost and volume contracts 25
cost-containment programmes 285–7
  Australia 271–3
  France 152–6
  Germany 203–6, *205*
  New Zealand 238–9
  see also rationing
Couveture Maladie Universelle (CMU) 143,
    145–6
'cream skimming' *see* risk selection
'crowding-out/in' 109, 125–6, 129

'Dekker' reforms 24, 210
Denmark *see* Scandinavian healthcare
    systems
dental charges 50
  Australia 251
  Germany 212, 214
  Scandinavian countries *166*
diagnosis related groups *see* DRGs
    (diagnosis related groups) use
disability support
  New Zealand 223
  see also elderly care provisions; long-
    term healthcare
discharge rates *see* hospital discharge rates
DRGs (diagnosis related groups) use
  France 145
  Germany 213
  Scandinavian countries 177–8, *179*
  UK 76–7
  US 85
  see also Health Resource Groups

drug costs 68–9, 122, 132–3, 135, 272
  patent vs. off-patent 135
  and price discrimination 105–6
  see also drug regulation
drug funding
  Canada 122
  France 142–3, 145–7, 152, 154–6
  Germany 213, 214
  Scandinavian countries 168–9, *169*
  UK 26, 50–1, 58
  US 90–2, *91*
  see also co-payments; drug regulation;
    prescription charges
drug regulation
  Australia 271–3
  France 155–6
  New Zealand 238–9
Dutch healthcare systems 24

efficiency evaluation 22–3
  and ideology 7–10, 287–8
  privately-financed systems 30–4
  publicly-funded systems 24–8
  see also activity levels; evidence-based
    evaluation
egalitarian ideology 10–11
  see also equity
elderly care provisions
  Australia 264, 266–8, *267, 269*
  Canada 134
  Germany 193
  New Zealand 223, 224
  UK 51, 52, 59
  US 89–93
  see also long-term healthcare
elective surgery 54, 57–8, 71
electronic patient records 72
  US IT systems 107–8
emergency care, and fundholding 26–7
Employee Retirement Income Security Act
  (1974) 98
equality 10–13, *10*
equity 57–8, 75–6, 283–4, 288–300
  and fundholding 27
  and price discrimination 105–6
  Canadian experiences 130–7
  New Zealand *230*
  Scandinavian countries 180–1
  see also access to healthcare
equity stakes 71
error rates *see* medical errors
ethical considerations, healthcare
  distribution 12–13, 136–7

European Union
  on competition 201, 203, 287
  on public deficit reductions 157
evaluation schemes *see* evidence-based
  evaluation; quality indicators
evidence-based evaluation 17–18
  and clinical variability 294–8
  and NHS organisational changes 76–7
  New Zealand 24–5, 228–32, *229–30*
  Scandinavian countries 180–1
  see also efficiency evaluation
expenditure control 285–7
  efficiency goals 287–8
  see also cost-containment programmes;
    rationing

'fair innings' approach (Williams) 289–90
Family Doctor Act (1994) 171
federal veterans programme 91–2
fee for service (FFS) schemes 29–33, 66,
  72–3, 74
  France 145–7, 152
Feldstein, Martin 108–9
FFS *see* fee for service (FFS) schemes
Finland *see* Scandinavian healthcare
  systems
fiscal policies 285–6
  taxation v. social insurance 49, 129–33
  France 141–4, 156–8
  Scandinavian countries 169
  UK 47–8
  US 86–9, *87, 88, 89*
fiscal transfers (US) 96
'Flexible Spending Accounts' (FSA) 98–9
'for-profit' healthcare providers 53–4
  see also private healthcare (UK)
Foundation Hospitals 28, 59, 76–7, 242
French healthcare systems 141–58
  ambulatory care 151–2, *152*, 157
  co-payment systems 142, 145, 146
  coverage issues 144–5
  expenditure patterns 141–4
  fee for service (FFS) schemes 145–7, 152
  financing arrangements 142–4, *143*
  future challenges 156–8
  global capping arrangements 148–9,
    153–5
  hospital care provisions 147–8
  refunding 142, 146–7
  regional discrepancies 150–1
  user charges 145–7
front-end deductible insurance (FED)
  schemes 255

General Medical Council (GMC) 306
geographical health inequalities
  clinical practice variability 293–4
  funding 64, 284, 294
German healthcare systems 191–216
  Bismarck's social health insurance (SHI)
    model 191–7, *193, 197*
  co-payments 199–201, *200*
  dental care 212, 214
  effects of competition 208–9
  expenditure patterns 197–9, *198, 199*
  financing arrangements 196–7, *197,*
    206–8, *207*
  future considerations 208–11
  hospital care provisions 194, 212–13
  private sector 199–203, *200, 202*
  reforms 203–6, *205*
  sickness funds 195–6
'goodwill' purchase/sale 74
GP contract 73–4
GP fundholding 23–4, 35, 300
  administration costs 27
  evaluation 26–7, 75

health inequalities 284–5
  see also access to healthcare; equity
health insurance funds *see* national health
    insurance programmes; private
    insurance schemes
Health Insurance Portability and
    Accountability Act (1996) 107–8
health maintenance organisations (HMOs)
    21, 29–34, 110
health outcomes
  New Zealand 231
  see also quality indicators
Health Resource Groups 241
health status
  US systems 85–6, *86*
  see also risk selection
healthcare distribution 130–4
  ethical objectives 12–13
  geographical variations 64, 284, 293–4
  ideological considerations 11–12
  statistical analysis 14–16, *15*
  theoretical models 22–3
  see also equity; NHS funding
healthcare expenditure 64–5
  background history 44–51
  current fiscal policies 52–9, 64–5
  future targets 65
  as percentage of GDP 43, 48, 64, *65*
  public–private funding streams *44*, 52

sustainability issues 117–19, 134–7
  Australia 248–51, *250*
  Canada 121–4, *121*, 124–7, *127*
  France 141–4, *143*
  Germany 197–9, *198, 199*
  New Zealand *220, 225, 234, 235, 236*
  Scandinavian countries 164, *165*, 183
  US 84–9, *87, 88, 89*
HMOs (health maintenance organisations)
    21, 29–34, 110
hospital closures 25–6
hospital 'corporisation' 176–7
  see also Foundation Hospitals
hospital discharge rates 69
Hospital Episode Statistics (HES) 72, 298
hospital expenditure patterns
  New Zealand 226–7
  UK 1991–4 25–6
  US healthcare 30–1, 33–4
hospital pay beds 45–6
  see also private hospitals
HRQoL (health-related quality of life)
    indices 298
HSAs (Health Savings Accounts) 99

ideology 299–303
  defined 16
  and empirical issues 299, *300–3*
  and evidence-based evaluation 17–18,
    290–1
  health objectives 11–12
  rival positions 10–11
  trade-offs 12–13, 17
  value-compatibility 16–17
  and *World Health Report 2000* 14–16
incentive schemes 304
  Australia 252, 274
  Scandinavian countries 177–8
  UK 70
Independent Treatment Centres (ITCs)
    71
individual health status *see* risk selection
inflationary pressures
  administration costs 100, 105, 132
  consumer-driven demand 35–6, *301–2*
  pharmaceutical costs 68–9, 122, 132–3,
    135, 272, 288
  profession-led 280–2
information technology
  electronic patient records 72
  international comparisons 107
  US healthcare systems 106–9

inspection and regulation 56, 68
   Germany 213, 215
   see also performance management
insurance schemes *see* national health
      insurance programmes; private
      insurance schemes
interferon beta 288
internal market 23–4
   background history 48–9
   ideology 7–8, 17
   New Zealand comparisons 240–2
   see also purchasing entities; quasi-market
      reforms
IPAs (independent practice associations)
      32–3

Jackson Hole Group 285
junior doctors 70
Juppé health reforms 144–5, 150–2, 157

legislation, cost-containment measures
      203–6, *205*, 273
libertarian ideology 10–11
Life Time Health Cover 259, 260–70, 276
litigation 56
local level fund systems 192–3
London hospital closures 25–6
long-term healthcare 51, 52, 59
Losec 272

managed care systems (US) 29–30, 35–6
   evaluation 30–4
MBS (Medical Benefits Scheme) 248–52
measures of central tendency 8–9
Medicaid programme 87, 94–7
medical errors
   and clinical governance 68
   as evaluation tool 34, 297–8
Medicare programmes 87, 89–90, 109–11,
      137
   Australia 248–52, 259–60, 273–5, *275*
   Canadian experiences 122
   eligibility 89–90
Medicare + Choice/Advantage
      programmes 92–3, 110–11
*Medicare Prescription Drug, Improvement and
      Modernization Act* (2003) 90, 92, 99,
      109, 111
mental health targets 74
mergers and acquisitions 34
mortality rates 297
mutual aid funds 143

National Audit Office 68
National Clinical Assessment Authority
      (NCAA) 68
national health insurance programmes
   arguments for/against 123–4, 287
   see also local level fund systems; NHI
      (National Health Insurance) funds;
      sickness funds
National Institute for Clinical Excellence
      (NICE) 59, 68–9, 289
national insurance (UK)
   NHS contributions 47
   vs. taxation 49
National Patient Safety Agency 68
National Service Frameworks (NSFs) 28,
      69
national tariff systems 76–7
New Zealand healthcare system 23–4,
      219–43
   key information *219*
   disability support 223
   evaluation 24–5, 228–32, *229–30*
   expenditure *220, 225, 234, 235, 236*
   financing arrangements 220–1, 221–6,
      221
   hospitals 226–7
   out-of-pocket payments 224–6
   patient prioritisation initiatives 239–40
   primary care 221–3, 227, 232
   private health insurance 224–6, *225*
   public–private finance changes 233–8,
      234–6
   quasi-market reforms 227–33
   user charges and subsidies 221–3, 241
NHI (National Health Insurance) funds
      142–3, *143*
   refunding arrangements 142, 146–7
NHS funding 63–5
   background history *44*, 47–51
   and expenditure control 285–9
   geographical variations 64, 284
   revenue sources 47, 49, 63–4
The NHS Plan (DoH 2000) 55, 65, 70
NHS reforms
   background history 43–51
   and change directions 307
   comparisons with New Zealand 240–2
   policy approaches 290–1
   post-1991 funding 52–9, 63–4
   see also Foundation Hospitals; GP
      fundholding; internal market; Primary
      Care Trusts
Nightingale, Florence 297

Nixon, Richard 85
Northern Ireland healthcare funding 64, 76
Norway *see* Scandinavian healthcare systems
nursing practice changes 74

OECD Economic Surveys (2004) 69
ONDAM (*Objectif National des Dépenses d'Assurance-Maladie*) 150–1, 153–5
optician charges 50
OQN (*Objectif Quantifié National*) 149–50
out-of-hours payments 73–4
out-of-pocket payments
  Australia 255–8, *257*
  France 145–7
  New Zealand 224–6
outcome evaluation 284, 289–90, 296–8
  New Zealand 231
  see also quality indicators

Pareto analysis 9
partnership ideology 55
'patient choice' 12–13, 15, 55, 286–7
  pitfalls 35–6, 283
  New Zealand *230*
  Scandinavian countries 178
  US healthcare 103–4
patient health risk *see* health status; risk selection
patient prioritisation initiatives
  New Zealand 239–40
  see also rationing
patient rights 179
pay beds 45–6
PBMs (pharmaceutical benefit management companies) 91–2
PCOs (preferred provider organisations) 29–30
peer review 154
performance data 72
  see also activity levels
performance management 70, 295–6
  France 150–1, 156
  Germany 203–6
  see also activity levels
performance targets, hospital star ratings 71
PFIs (Private Finance Initiatives) 52, 71
  Australia 254–5
PHARMAC 223, 238–9
pharmaceutical benefit management companies (PBMs) 91–2

Pharmaceutical Benefits Scheme (PBS) 271–3
pharmaceutical industry
  marketing vs. research and development 135, 156
  Australia 271–3, 277
  Canada 122
  France 152–3, 154, 155–6
  Germany 192, 213, 214
  New Zealand 238–9
  Scandinavian countries 177–8, 179
  UK 26, 50–1, 58, 68–9
  US 90–2, *91*, 105–6
  see also cost-containment programmes
Pharmaceutical Pricing Authority (PPA) 72
political influences *see* ideology
postcode prescribing 70, 289
prescription charges
  exemptions 50–1, 58
  and fundholding 26
  see also co-payments; pharmaceutical industry; user charges
price discrimination 105–6
primary care 64
  background 45
  budget limiting 76
  Australia 248–51, *250*, 277
  New Zealand 221–3, 227, 232
  Scandinavian countries *165*, *166*, 170–2
  UK 27–8, 66, 73–4
  see also ambulatory care
primary care trusts (PCTs) 27–8, 67–8
  primary care expenditure 74–5
prioritisation initiatives, New Zealand 239–40
private healthcare (UK)
  background history 44–51
  current situation 52–8, 64–5, 71, 242
  comparative studies 43–4, *44*, 48, 58
  complementary therapies 53, 58
  employee insurance schemes 47, 53, 58, 64
  'for-profit' providers 53–4
  ideological considerations 12
  public purchasing 29–34, 52–3, 55–6, 59, 71
  self-financed and non-insured 53–4, 57–8, 64, 288
  see also prescription charges; user charges
private hospitals
  Australia 251–5, *253*, 275
  France 147–8

New Zealand 226–7
  Scandinavian countries 172–3
  UK 53
private insurance schemes
  administration costs 100, 105, 132
  premium charges 53–4, 266–70, 276
  rebate schemes 259, 260–4, 268, 273
  self-financed 53–4, 57–8, 64
  Australia 251, 255–60, 276
  Germany 192–3, 201, *202*, *207*, 210
  New Zealand 224–6, *225*
  Scandinavian countries 164–8
  UK 47, 53, 64
  US *87*, *88*, 97–9, 132
private non-insured healthcare 288
professional organisations
  and change creation 306
  and inflation 280–2
Programme Budgeting Marginal Analysis
  (PBMA) 238
purchasing entities
  key systems 21
  current challenges 36
  privately-financed schemes 29–34
  publicly-funded systems 23–8
  Scandinavian countries 177

quality indicators 27–8, 289–90
  HRQoL (health-related quality of life)
    indices 298
  France 148, 151
  New Zealand 231
  quality of life measures 78
  staffing levels/mortality rates 34
quasi-market reforms 227–33
  financial impact 233–8, *234–6*
  UK comparisons 240–2
  see also internal market

RAND Health Insurance Experiment (HIE)
  31–2
rationing 68–9, 242, 287–8, 304
  New Zealand 238–40
RAWP (Resource Allocation Working
  Party) 284
reaccredidation 72
Reagan, Ronald 85
rebate schemes, income-tested 259, 260–4,
  268, 273
recruitment and retention 70, 72
  overseas sources 70
Reid, John 75
Reinhardt, UE 136–7

research funding 24
  US healthcare systems 102
resource consumption 282–3
  and scarcity 117–19, *119*
  UK internal market reforms 26–7
  US healthcare systems 33–4
  see also rationing
resource distribution 10–13, 57–8
risk selection
  internal market systems 27
  Germany 208–9
  New Zealand 224–5
  privately-financed healthcare 29, 32,
    158
risk status *see* risk selection
risk-related premiums
  age-banding 224–5
  in public insurance funds 206
  see also private insurance schemes; risk
    selection
Royal Colleges 281, 286, 306

satisfaction surveys
  Scandinavian countries *182*
  US healthcare 103
Scandinavian healthcare systems 161–84
  co-payment arrangements 168–9, *169*
  current policies/changes 174–81
  dental care *166*
  evaluation 180–1, 183–4
  financing arrangements 163–4, *163*, *165*,
    166
  future trends 169–70, 182–4
  general practice *165*, *166*, 170–2
  hospitals *165*, *166*, 172–3, 176–7
  pharmacies *166*, 173
  private health insurance 164–8
Scotland healthcare funding 64, 75
selective contracting 30, 33
SHI (social health insurance) system
  191–6, 209–11
  financing 196–7, *197*
  see also German healthcare systems
Shipman, Harold 298
sickness funds 24, *193*, 195–6
significance levels 8
skill-mix changes 74
Smith, Adam 280–1
social insurance funds *see* national health
  insurance programmes
social welfare, ideological objectives 8–17
Southern Cross 224

specialists
  Australia 252
  France 153
  New Zealand 226–7
  see also consultants
star ratings 71
State Children's Health Insurance
    Programme (S-CHIP) 94, 109
statins 272
statistical analysis, and ideology 8–10,
    14–16
Stigler, George 305–6
subsidies, New Zealand 221–3, 225, 239
sustainability issues 117–19, 134–7
Swedish healthcare systems 23–4
  evaluation 25
  see also Scandinavian healthcare systems

tariff systems 76–7
taxation policies
  Canadian health funding 130–3
  New Zealand 224–5
  Scandinavian countries 169
  UK health funding 47
technological innovations
  Germany 192
  US healthcare 101–2
Thatcher reforms 48–9, 66–7, 283–4
  see also GP fundholding; internal market
Tomlinson report 26
trade union influence 280–2
training
  funding 24
  intake levels 70
Treaty of Amsterdam (1999) 201
Treaty of Maastricht (1992) 201
'two-tier' healthcare
  background 45–6, 56
  Germany 210

United States healthcare systems 29–34,
    83–111
  administration costs 105
  advantages and strengths 99–104
  coverage 108–9
  disadvantages and weaknesses 104–9
  federal funding 88–9, *89*, 91–2, 95–7
  funding patterns 86–9, *87, 88, 89*
  future trends 109–11
  information needs 106–9

  international comparisons 85, 100–1
  Medicaid programme 87, 94–7, 109–11
  Medicare programme 87, 89–90, 109–11
  Medicare + Choice/Advantage
    programmes 92–3
  private insurance schemes 86, *87, 88,*
    97–9
  regulatory mechanisms 84–5
  spending trends 104
  tax-financed expenditure levels 84,
    87–8, *88, 89*
  'veterans' health system 91–2
user charges
  France 29, 58, 145–7
  New Zealand 221–3, 241
  see also co-payments; prescription
    charges
utilisation rates *see* resource consumption

values
  and efficiency analysis 7–10
  and ethical discourse 12–13, 16–18
Viagra 272
Volume Performance Standard (VPS) 85
Vote Health 240, 241
vouchers, for private health insurance
  (US) 88

waiting lists 69
  causes 45–6, 54–5
  as evaluation tool 28
  Scandinavian initiatives 178–9
  targets 69
Wanless report (2002) 69, 241, 289
weighted measures 14–16, *15*
well-being measures 10–11
  see also quality indicators
Williams, A 289
working hours
  consultant's contract 73
  GP's contract 73–4
  junior doctors 70
Working for Patients (Secretaries of State
  1989) 23
World Health Report 2000 (WHO) 14–16, *15,*
  102–3
World Wide Web 307

Zyban 272